"Mark Kinet can plausibly defend the unique perspective of psychoanalysis because, unlike many of his colleagues, he embraces its theoretical and clinical diversity, and he remains abreast of developments in neighbouring fields: psychiatry, psychotherapy and neuroscience."

Mark Solms *is a neuropsychologist, psychoanalyst, and professor at the Neuroscience Institute of The University of Cape Town, Cape Town, South Africa*

"This is a timely and urgent book. It gives a clear insight from different perspectives and aptly outlines their interrelationship. The book demonstrates great knowledge and is enthusiastically written. It shows psychoanalysis as a rich world of thought, a unity in diversity, without nitpicking. It frees it from its excessive self-involvement and self-chosen limitation to 'pure psychoanalysis'. And it can help psychiatry – which has itself lost its way in a self-created maze of mental disorders and treatment modules – regain substance and get in touch with life lived."

Antoine Mooij *is a psychiatrist, philosopher, psychoanalyst and emeritus professor at Utrecht, Netherlands*

"This is one of the best attempts to bring Freudian psychoanalysis to the 21st century. Kinet takes you on a personal journey through the psychoanalytic landscape, reviewing and integrating Freudian and Lacanian approaches with object relations theory, neuropsychoanalysis and attachment approaches. There is always something new to discover for the reader. Recommended for both adventurers and the more cautious within the psychoanalytic tradition."

Patrick Luyten, *professor KULeuven (B) and University College London, United Kingdom*

"*Psychoanalytic Principles in Psychiatric Practice* is an excellent book. Mark Kinet, in his gracious and inimitable style, navigates the divergences and convergences of psychiatry and psychoanalysis. He weaves a rich tapestry of psychoanalysis' history, showing where it intersects with (and departs from) medicine, philosophy, and literature. Through its breadth and scope, it is a great introduction to psychoanalysis."

Arthur Eaton, *PhD, is a psychologist, philosopher, historian, journalist, and author in the Netherlands*

Psychoanalytic Principles in Psychiatric Practice

In this approachable book, Mark Kinet offers a unique methodology for integrating psychoanalytic work in the psychiatric setting.

Acknowledging the systemic rupture between psychoanalysis and psychiatric treatment, Kinet seeks to bridge the gap and offer a pathway for integrating the disciplines to provide integrative therapy for patients experiencing issues like personality problems, depression, anxiety and trauma. Integrating Freudian, Kleinian, Bionian, Winnicottian, Bowlbyan and Lacanian thought, Kinet provides an overview of psychoanalytic thinking and its benefits in a psychiatric setting. Kinet turns to philosophy, science, art and ethics to encourage a symbiotic relationship between the two disciplines.

Written in Kinet's trademark accessible and personable manner, *Psychoanalytic Principles in Psychiatric Practice* will inspire the training psychiatrist and psychotherapist, as well as the more experienced practitioner, to consider a more panoptic approach to working with patients.

Mark Kinet is a psychiatrist, psychotherapist and psychoanalyst. He has authored or (co-) edited some thirty books on psychiatry and psychotherapy, psychoanalysis and cultural issues. His most recent book is *The Spirit of the Drive in Neuropsychoanalysis*, Routledge (2024).

Psychoanalytic Principles in Psychiatric Practice

A Remedy by Truth

Mark Kinet

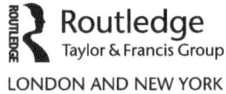

Routledge
Taylor & Francis Group
LONDON AND NEW YORK

Designed cover image: © Getty

First published 2025
by Routledge
4 Park Square, Milton Park, Abingdon, Oxon OX14 4RN

and by Routledge
605 Third Avenue, New York, NY 10158

Routledge is an imprint of the Taylor & Francis Group, an informa business

British Library Cataloguing in Publication Data
A catalogue record for this book is available from the British Library

Library of Congress Cataloging-in-Publication Data
A catalog record has been requested for this book

ISBN: 9781032698038 (hbk)
ISBN: 9781032686202 (pbk)
ISBN: 9781032698052 (ebk)

DOI: 10.4324/9781032698052

Typeset in Times New Roman
by Taylor & Francis Books

Contents

x Contents

Chapter 1

Prologue

A Psychodynamic Psychiatry

Michel Thys, former editor-in-chief of the Dutch-language *Tijdschrift voor Psychoanalyse*, used this title in a noted contribution: *Getting Better by Truth*.[1] Simplicity is the hallmark of the truth, and brevity is the soul of wit.[2] This statement, therefore, struck me as if by lightning. Psychic help is often offered in a chemical or magical way, but indeed, does psychoanalysis for remedy not primarily promote telling the truth? With thanks for his explicit permission, I am therefore happy to use Thys's formulation as the subtitle of this book. It is a thoroughly revised, substantially expanded, but above all brought up-to-date elaboration of my *Freud & Co in Psychiatry*, published as the third in the *Current Psychoanalytics* series in 2006.[3] We are now so many years and over thirty books further, and – fortunately – neither psychoanalysis nor I have stood still since then.

Meanwhile, we can compare well, for example, with two modern classics. Glen O. Gabbard's *Psychodynamic Psychiatry in Clinical Practice* is already in its fifth edition.[4] I agree with his reasoning, but my book is markedly different in outline and inspiration. First, mine is neither a textbook nor a course text. It contains no recipes, no concrete instructions or tools. Since I consistently think person-centred, not disorder-centred, I do not propose psychodynamic approaches to DSM-V disorders. While Gabbard is guided exclusively by the *International Psychoanalytical Association* and, in particular, the Anglo-Saxon tradition, like South Americans and South Europeans I am inspired by a broader culture. The ideas of the French and the Lacanian *World Association of Psychoanalysis*, for example, are strongly represented in my book. As a result, the psychoanalytic principles underlying my psychiatric practice are explained in a much broader and more detailed way. After all, before you can help people, you must understand how they or their minds work. Another modern classic is the *Handbook of Psychodynamic Approaches to Psychopathology*, edited by my compatriot Patrick Luyten et al. It won the Canadian Goethe Prize for psychoanalytic scholarship and contains a thorough inventory of the current scientific and empirical state of psychodynamic issues.[5] In it, the editors distinguish between two cultural currents within psychoanalysis.[6] The first is hermeneutic or interpretive: it attributes much importance to meaning, honours qualitative

DOI: 10.4324/9781032698052-1

research and prefers the individual case study. The second is empirical and neo-positivist, investigates causes and their effects, loves quantification and uses probabilistic data analysis in (preferably as large as possible) groups. While my book tries to draw from both traditions, it mainly aligns (certainly in terms of style) with the former direction.

Over the past three decades, I have worked exclusively in clinical practice, mainly in (semi-) residential psychiatric settings.[7] In terms of psychopathology, this primarily concerned anxiety, mood, post-traumatic stress and personality disorders in patients who did not request psychotherapy (and even less psychoanalysis) of their own accord. They were often initially treated within clinical psychotherapeutic, (re-)constructive, insight-giving and/or mentalisation-enhancing milieu therapy. The approach there is trans-diagnostic and intervenes in the psychodynamics and psychogenesis underlying many manifestations and surface phenomena. Psychotic and perverse or paraphilic disorders are rare and, therefore, receive little attention in this book. For me, psychoanalysis was and is, first and foremost, a practice aimed at people (called 'patients') who suffer psychologically.[8] As such, it has been in dire straits in recent decades. After all, mental health care is dominated by biological psychiatry with its high-tech research and pharmacotherapeutic treatment and by likewise primarily symptom-focused (mostly behavioural) therapy. For a long time, both could present better scientific credentials than psychoanalytic therapies. Luyten et al. argue and document why this lag has almost wholly caught up today. Nevertheless, psychoanalytic approaches do not convince the medical world and political and health authorities of their scientific and clinical value and relevance. Nevertheless, psychoanalytic thought remains quite virulent.

This is abundantly clear from the fact that many scientists or intellectuals spare neither time nor effort to challenge their principles nor fight with their representatives and their ideas. It remains surprising (and at the same time not) that the critical arrows are always pointed at psychoanalytic and not at other psychotherapeutic help or 'counselling'. Psychoanalysis is also wrongly identified by many, even within mental health care, with the psychoanalytic cure several times a week on the couch and with the analyst behind and outside the patient's field of vision. Just as physics did not end with Newton, psychoanalysis did not end with (much less with the person of) Sigmund Freud. Today, psychoanalytic therapists work in newborn and elderly care wards. They try to assist in the first contact between baby and parents, do play therapy with toddlers and primary school children, help adolescents find their way in terms of independence and sexuality, and work within medical-psychiatric and even forensic psychiatric facilities with the most diverse and severe psychopathology in adults. They do this in individual face-to-face talk therapy, in the playroom, in groups or couples and families, and with out-patient and (semi-) residentially hospitalised patients. However, these field workers, often absorbed full-time in psychiatric and/or psychotherapeutic care, very seldom contribute to publishing these psychoanalytic applications from their practice-oriented perspective.

The book contains reflections and data from psychiatric, psychotherapeutic and psychoanalytic practice. It comprises interrelated contributions that can also be read separately if desired. The words are then like paint thrown at an invisible man to at least make his outline visible. The process is also similar to what happens in the psychoanalytic process. Specific topics recur in variations on the theme. Repeating, repeating and repeating are always necessary to learn or unlearn. I have tried to address the broadest possible audience: beginners and insiders. Given the complexity of the subject matter, footnotes are frequently used. I hope they put you on track: they serve only for references or to clarify or specify specific details without disrupting the presentation flow. I have started from my experience in clinical psychotherapy, group psychotherapy, psychoanalytic psychotherapy and classical psychoanalysis. Because I want to make this book interesting and enjoyable, I expressed my thoughts personally and essayistically. In doing so, I deliberately used both poetic and schematic language.[9] The former predominates in much psychoanalytic theory, its imagery bubbling up in the therapeutic encounter, and is particularly valuable for the felt and lived understanding it seeks. The second aims to describe problems sparingly to enable more empirical description and research. Readers interested in clinical case material might wish to consult two forthcoming books in my 'trilogy'. In *Psychoanalytic Psychotherapy in Psychiatric Practice: Clinical Portraits*, I sketch patients' portraits and their issues, combining biography with radiography.[10] In the other, *Patient Testimonies of Psychodynamic Psychotherapy Processes*, patients testify uniquely about their psychotherapeutic evolution. The psychoanalytic principles set out in the present book are thus illustrated both vividly and realistically in psychiatric practice.

Notes

1 Michel Thys (2006). 'The psychoanalytic content of a treatment increases as truth-finding is accompanied by psychic change that alleviates the patient's suffering or as such psychic change is accompanied by an experience of truth concerning oneself' (p 140).
2 William Shakespeare. *Hamlet*. Excerpt from Polonius, in Act 2, scene 2.
3 Mark Kinet (2006).
4 Glen Gabbard (2014).
5 Luyten (2015) and Luyten et al. (2015).
6 Patrick Luyten (2006).
7 Throughout this book, I always speak of (semi-) residential versus ambulatory as two poles of a continuum qua degree of holding of the setting.
8 Consistently, I refuse to talk about clients or customers. Humans are not just consumers. Etymologically, the term 'patient' refers to both suffering and patience.
9 Shahar (2010).
10 Both forthcoming at Routledge.

Chapter 2

Psychiatry, Psychotherapy and Psychoanalysis
The Difference

1 Common Sense

Most people will not confidently give their opinion on the theory of relativity, pre-Colombian civilisations or the antics of the Colorado beetle. We gladly leave these matters to experts. It becomes very different when it comes to the issues of the heart. In these, many emerge as experts on a regular basis. Anyone who considers themself the happy possessor of common sense has valuable insights to contribute on emotional and relational problems. Sometimes unhindered by any knowledge, people start judging, looking for and often finding connections – if all psychological woes are not summarily reduced to downright simulation, that is.

People with genuine familiarity with psychoanalysis are somewhat less abundant. They are sometimes found in certain intellectual or artistic circles. Dropping Freudian- or Lacanian-inspired *bon mots* may create a semblance of profundity, but it often amounts to nothing more than a Homeric epithet. In the media, psychiatry is invariably bathed in a sensationalist atmosphere of scandal. Every television programme contains the inevitable close-up of a barred window or lingers over the relatively sparse furniture of an isolation cell. Feature films like *One Flew Over the Cuckoo Nest* [1] defined the image of the mental institution for decades, and thanks to the oeuvre of Woody Allen, analysts are no more than a running gag, at least when they are not portrayed as sexually frustrated shrinks who fool around with already traumatised patients.

Meanwhile, people who suffer psychologically try to hide rather than take care. They are ashamed, feel guilty and do not want to know (or to have known by others) that something is wrong with them. The world of psychiatry, psychotherapy and psychoanalysis is perceived by them as the unsafe playground of gurus or quacks, both sometimes even more daft than their patients. To them, it is all the same.

DOI: 10.4324/9781032698052-2

2 Shakespeare's Truth[2]

Before immersing ourselves in this pot to clarify this murky water, we start with a brief illustration from Shakespeare's *Macbeth*. Believed to have been written in 1606, the play is widely regarded as the one in which the author delves most deeply into 'the anatomy of evil'.[3] In this tragedy features one of the most famous psychiatric patients in world literature: Lady Macbeth. In a nutshell, the state of affairs. Macbeth murders King Duncan of Scotland partly at the instigation of the three witches and partly at that of his wife to take his seat on the throne. From then on, what French playwright Jean Cocteau[4] would call the 'infernal machine' kicks in. The blood keeps flowing, and Lady Macbeth goes mad. She is tormented by droves of intrusive thoughts that no longer allow her to sleep. She becomes confused, feels haunted by the projected phantoms of her conscience, becomes afraid in the dark and compulsively tries to wash her hands to clean away imagined crimes. Macbeth does what one would do even now. He calls in a doctor. Then comes the question:

> Canst thou not minister to a mind diseased,
> Pluck from the memory a rooted sorrow,
> Raze out the written troubles of the brain,
> And with some sweet oblivious antidote
> Cleanse the stuffed bosom of that perilous stuff
> Which weighs upon the heart?

To which the doctor replies: 'Therein the patient/Must minister to himself.' Not surprisingly, this attitude finds little favour with Macbeth: 'Throw physic/To the dogs; I'll none of it.'[5]

Already in this ancient fragment, we meet the patient who wants to be cured by a doctor's prescription and, at the same time, does not want to know about confronting himself. We will see later that Jacques Lacan and Wilfred Bion, two leading post-Freudians, give this not-wanting-to-know the status of a passion: Lacan's passion of ignorance (*la passion de l' ignorance*)[6] or Bion's *minus Knowledge* (-K).[7] For Lacan, not knowledge (*connaissance*) but mis-knowledge (*méconnaissance)* [8] constitutes the essence of our awareness. Indeed, according to him, this so-called consciousness is characterised by visual deception rather than vision. The core of the Ego and thus the core of the Cartesian *cogito*, according to him, is the blind spot. Therefore, 'We never knew'[9] frees us from all guilt because the best thing for a good conscience is a bad memory. We can also adopt Kaiser Wilhelm II's words about World War I: 'I never wanted that'.[10]

> This is the excellent foppery of the world, that, when we are sick in fortune, often the surfeit of our own behaviour, we make guilty of our

disasters the sun, the moon, and the stars; as if we were villains on necessity, fools by heavenly compulsion, knaves, thieves and treachers by spherical predominance, drunkards, liars and adulterers by an enforced obedience of planetary influence.

Shakespeare again, this time in *King Lear.* [11]

Now, what are answers that can be given by the 'doctor' to the question of psychological suffering? The options vary widely; the difference is tremendous. Although the distinction is not always clearly discernible from the various manifestations of mental health care, they turn out to be underlying and structural. I describe them first in their pure (à la Max Weber) 'ideal-typical' form.[12] In practice, of course, they always form an alloy between them.

3 Psychiatry's Answer

Psychiatry is a sub-specialty of medicine. Psychiatrist means 'soul physician'. In Dutch, this becomes 'nerve doctor': the soul has disappeared from it. Moreover, it is a recent sub-specialty of medicine. In its most basic form, it originated in the early nineteenth century. Until then, the insane stayed in dungeons, were tied to chains, and were locked in cages; in other words, they did not receive humane treatment. We are reminded of the opening images of the Oscar-winning feature film *Amadeus* [13] by Milos Forman.

In 1792, Philippe Pinel,[14] chief physician at Bicêtre, stripped the insane in the Hospice de la Salpêtrière of their chains. This counts as a historic moment. Psychiatry was born; that is, it liberated itself from prison. In my own country, in the early 1800s Ghent psychiatrist Jozef Guislain transferred the insane from the dungeons of the *Gerard de Duivelsteen* prison to the institution he designed and then pioneered, which still bears his name today. In the first phase, psychiatry was situated in and only in the asylum. The society of normals was protected by isolation of the insane, the psycho- and sociopaths. A pre-scientific *'traitement moral'*[15] was applied, based on ethical-religious principles, i.e. caring devotion on the one hand, responding to a sense of sin and guilt on the other, handling penance and punishment and improving virtues. Only in the second phase did psychiatry shift to the university and become more akin to medicine. Medicine had by then evolved into an applied natural science. It wanted to apply its experimentally acquired knowledge of nature to relieve people's distress, alleviate suffering, and cure diseases. In doing so, it looks for objectively ascertainable facts because the success of treatment rests on a correct assessment of these. This natural scientific model has been very successful. Everyone knows the explosion of medical science, and who does not applaud its often highly technological triumphs?

From medicine, psychiatry inherits not only a scientific orientation but also a modus operandi. The pattern is familiar. The doctor makes a diagnosis, suggests an aetiological (causal) hypothesis, pronounces the prognosis and institutes therapy. This has the status of a prescription. The patient must take that medicine and behave in such and such a way 'for his health'. To this end, the doctor derives authority and power from his or her experience and science. All this is very valuable, but it also carries a risk. The doctor may view the patient as a (suffering) object to be *treated*. Through their 'uninhibited' observation, they turn a subject into an object that carries complaints and symptoms (signs of disease) and develop a knowledge that counts as objective. Moreover, the source of evil is usually situated in the outside world and outside the patient's responsibility.[16] Suffering is the doctor's territory. Beneath the symptom, they expose the true cause. Sensory and equilibrium disturbances are the surface symptoms of multiple sclerosis; debilitation, various pains and weight loss signs of a cancerous tumour proliferating in silence; imperative auditory hallucinations, syncretistic thoughts and a 'weird' contact are indications of schizophrenic disorder. By definition, in all this, the doctor is not so much attentive to the particular in the patient as to what in that patient refers to a generality:[17] a syndrome, a disease, a disorder that has a place in the taxonomy ('nosology') in force at the time. 'Two ulcers and an intestinal colic have come in' or, for psychiatry: 'A suicide attempt, a compulsive neurosis and a vital depression'. The caricatured extreme of this method is the patient who does not speak, who lends themself to examination as a mere body, who does not ask questions and who is of goodwill in treatment, that is, conforms or folds to the doctor's knowledge of them.

Finally, there is also deontology or, if you like, the ethics that psychiatry inherits from medicine. For the demand, the complaint, the suffering, and the danger to life, the doctor has only one duty. To take care of the patient responsibly, that is, to provide obligatory and immediate assistance with expert knowledge. The imperative of deontology is a material act. Not words, but actions and without delay. The symptom must go away: the culprit caught, the flaw located, the rotten spot cut away. In short, the signs of disease must be eliminated, preferably *cito, tuto et iucunde*, i.e., quickly, reliably, and with minimal inconvenience to the patient.[18] Following Freud, it may be said that medicine is fundamentally unaccustomed to the psychic and the mental, and uncomfortable with words. And whatever forces it to watch helplessly or, in other words, fucks its illusion of omnipotence is pushed away, expelled. We think of the words: 'It's nothing; it's the nerves. It's psychological. There's nothing to be *done* about it'. Psychiatry may have been released from prison and adopted by medicine. Yet she is viewed with displeasure and suspicion by her adoptive mother and treated stepmotherly. Not only outside but also within the medical profession, psychiatrists and their patients are often met with a lot of disbelief.

4 The Answer of Psychoanalysis

If the birth of psychiatry falls around 1800, psychoanalysis can be roughly situated around 1900. Under the motto 'If I cannot appease the Gods, I will stir the underworld', Freud published *The Interpretation of Dreams*, his first *magnum opus*.[19] Freud had his reservations about the psychiatry of his time.[20] He noted that psychiatry could explain few psychopathological phenomena substantively. It could perhaps explain why a person develops jealousy delusions. However, it could not explain why exactly they were *jealous* delusions. According to him, psychiatry did not take into account the significance of psychopathological symptoms. By referring only to constitutional factors, it did not consider the life history or personality of the patient. He, therefore, compared psychiatry to a trickster who gives the patient more than they possess. He developed psychoanalysis (complementary to psychiatry) in the hole of its structural deficit. Still, in his introductory lectures, he went on to note that scientifically deepened psychiatry would no longer be possible without sufficient knowledge of unconscious processes.[21]

He laid the foundation of his science of the unconscious through some founding acts, which differ substantially from medical acts. To begin with, he gradually refrained from answering his patients' demands. He abstained from any prescription, encouragement, counsel or advice. For the establishment of his psychoanalytic technique, we see how he abandons first magnetism, later hypnosis,[22] the laying on of hands and suggestion. An almost complete therapeutic *reduction* takes place, suspending any material act. He does not answer the demand because he is honest enough to acknowledge that he (or that psychiatry) *has* no answer. This failure to answer the question (frustration) allows the lack to exist. It keeps the engine of speech running and the desire alive. Indeed, Freud's renunciation of immediate gratification is a driving force for the unconscious speaking or the speaking unconscious that gets to speak, thanks to the basic rule of free association. The manifest demand (e.g., 'deliver me from the anxiety that often overwhelms me in social situations') can thus meanderingly shift, and an unconscious motive unfolds (e.g. in a neurotic context: 'I want to show off my ability, but I'm afraid my rival won't tolerate it'.).

Furthermore, Freud suspended any material act and any pre-existing knowledge. Instead of looking at an object to be treated, he proceeded to *listen* as uninhibitedly as possible to the speech of the subject, the psychically suffering human being.[23] He cleverly kept a low profile and, in other words, employed a kind of Socratic ignorance, a *docta ignorantia* or learned ignorance.[24] He installed himself in the place of the object small a (Fr: *objet petit a*),[25] as Jacques Lacan would later call it. In the place of the letterbox in which, according to a typical Lacanian *plaything,* the patient can deposit not his letters ('*lettres*') but his rubbish ('*litter*'). Or, in other terms, at the place of Bion's big O:[26] where the analyst listens with free-floating attention, in reverie, so that a resonance arises between the subjectivity of both 'partners' and conversations at the frontier of dreaming can unfold.[27]

By suspending (not abolishing!) all knowledge, psychoanalysis can become a creative act for the patient. It creates a space where their private truth can come to the fore, a truth that guides the repetitive patterns of their life (e.g. repeated problems with the law, difficulties with divorce, a wrong choice of partner) and limits their existence. Moreover, they can also arrive at more conscious decisions within this space. In this way, Freud derived his authority to speak or interpret not so much from science but mainly from listening carefully to what the patient had unknowingly said. Freud renounced the therapeutic and educational pride in not identifying with the patient's transference, making the physician a supposedly all-knowing subject. He rejected the temptation to be the God of whom it is said, 'And He created man in His likeness.' Indeed, through this renunciation, the suffering but supposedly desiring subject can become itself. It can reach the position of what Lacan would later call *absolute difference* by arriving at more personal choices regarding love, work, relationships and so on.[28]

5 Right versus True

For psychiatry and medicine, the register of knowledge, right versus wrong, was at play. We think of school, of the master and his pupils. Of cartoonist Kamagurka's drawing of an eager little boy saying with a heated face from the back bench: 'Now I am still stupid, but at the end of the year, I will be smart'. This register of knowledge fits natural science and its progress. It has several characteristics that I borrow from Paul Verhaeghe.[29] It accumulates and increases. We now know more about chemistry, for example, than we used to. You can generalise. Every salt behaves similarly. You can teach it. We write it ready and clear on the board. It makes claims of completeness. What we don't know now, we may know tomorrow. Chemistry can become alchemy. It makes predictions based on its knowledge: please don't act like that; it explodes! Psychoanalysis, on the other hand, plays the register of truth. Our private truth. The register of true versus false. There are questions to which we know no better or more accurate answer now than we used to, and some of them have no better answer to be found. Mother, why are we alive? Why is it that there is war? Or like the title of that beautiful collection of short stories by Raymond Carver: 'What do we talk about when we talk about love?'[30] Truth cannot be generalised, cannot be taught, and does not allow for predictions (how can I raise my children to be happy people?). However, the same is true of both knowledge and truth: completeness is structurally impossible. There remain things that are unsayable and unthinkable. There remains a Kantian gap between *noumenon* and *phenomenon*.

Once again, I refer to Lacan and Bion. For Lacan, the symbol is the murder of the Thing.[31] Through language, the immediacy of being is lost.

Lacan also talks about the *mi-dire* of truth,[32] which can only be said halfway. At the core of our being, there is a gap or a lack that paradoxically drives us to want to eliminate it in all possible and impossible ways. This enterprise is inevitably doomed to (more or less glorious) failure. Feelings expressed in words turn, according to Haruki Murakami, into lies.[33] This aligns with what Wilfred Bion says: 'All thoughts are lies'. However, we must be careful with statements contrasting truth with lies. After all, to lie at all, don't you have to know the truth first? We might also paraphrase Winston Churchill: the truth is so precious that it must remain hidden in a fortress of lies!

Freud's original approach, abandoning traditional medical deontology and a sustained attitude toward scientific research,[34] led him to fundamentally new insights that are sufficiently well known. The principle of psychic (as opposed to physical or constitutional) causation. The symptom as an expression of an unconscious and intrapsychic conflict between different agencies.[35] The decisive effect of the unconscious on psychopathological, general psychological (the dream, the joke, the slip and so on) and cultural (religion, art) phenomena. The omnipotence of (early childhood) sexuality in its broader Freudian sense: the household of pleasure and enjoyment. The neurosis as a discontent in civilisation,[36] an essence of the human condition and so on.

6 The Symptom

There are numerous differences between (ideal-typical) psychiatry and psychoanalysis. I mention only a few of them, which will be discussed further. Psychiatry works with signs, and psychoanalysis with signifiers. Psychiatry works mainly with general/natural causes and psychoanalysis, particularly with private/cultural reasons. Psychiatry relies on statistics, psychoanalysis on uniqueness. Psychiatry cloaks itself in knowledge, psychoanalysis in ignorance. Psychiatry is characterised by intervention and psychoanalysis by presence. Psychiatric assistance is through irregular therapeutic consultation and psychoanalytic through a systematic therapeutic relationship.

However, I will mainly dwell on the symptom to further illustrate the difference between psychiatry and psychoanalysis. In psychoanalysis the symptom is entirely different from a disease sign that must be removed (preferably as quickly as possible). It is an involuntary phenomenon that repeats itself, whose meaning the patient does not understand, that implies a hidden demand on the other, and that gives rise both to suffering (e.g. at the level of the Ego) and to a strange kind of pleasure (e.g. at the level of the Superego that 'likes' to blame and punish). The symptom is a meaningful and creative attempt to deal with unbearable psychic contents or stimuli. In this sense, it is born as an attempt at self-help. The psychiatrist viewed the symptom as a sign of illness. Freud listened to it primarily as a meaningful, recurrent signifier[37] or story element. It is one of the pre-eminent formations of the unconscious alongside the dream, the slip, the transference, enactment or acting-out. The analyst lies in wait to enter the patient's history and inner world through one of these 'interstices'. For these chinks, as it were, psychoanalysts are on the hunt.[38]

A simple example. A patient complains of despondency and feels down and guilty without understanding why. The doctor inquires about sleep and appetite. Are there forgetfulness or concentration problems? In other words, are there enough signs of illness to speak of major depression according to his current diagnostic manual? This is important because if so, he has at his disposal a remedy whose effectiveness has been scientifically proven: anti-depressant medication or (in case of uncontrollable suicidal urges) electro-convulsive therapy. Psychoanalysis, on the other hand, according to the principle that 'the patient is always right'[39], assumes that there is an unconscious reason for the feelings of guilt. It will try, through patient listening, to seek whether they have been repressed because of forbidden unconscious (e.g. sexual or aggressive) tendencies. It follows that, according to psychoanalysis, the symptom should not be fought but understood. If one fights the symptom, the symptom will shift (e.g. the phobia disappears, but compulsive thoughts appear) so that the therapist eventually comes to the helpless conclusion that the patient does not *want to* heal, which – though misunderstood by both parties – is true!

7 The Answer of Psychotherapy

Just as psychiatry was adopted by medicine, psychoanalysis was adopted by psychiatry and –as will be seen – adapted. Indeed, psychoanalysis triggered a *boom* of psychological insights, some more popular than others. Nowadays, several principles are generally accepted: psychic causality in itself, the connection that may exist between psychopathology and (early) child development, psychopathology as an expression of discordant psychodynamic forces, the notion that psychotherapy is possible *at all* and that changes can be brought about merely by using psychological means. The result is the exponential development of various psychotherapeutic techniques and methods.[40] Psychotherapy, then, is the set of psychological treatments developed after psychoanalysis. Several of them have historically grown out of psychoanalysis, but three other main streams can be distinguished: behavioural therapy, experiential ('client-centred') therapy and systemic therapy. All are assisted to a greater or lesser extent by psychology as the wing-adjutant of psychiatry. We understand by this psychology a generalised knowledge, for example, about psychosexual development, about grief, about learning processes, about the stages of bereavement counselling and so on.

Psychotherapy consists of understanding a sick person and acting on them or their environment with words or behavioural prescriptions. It involves specific ways of personal influence to combat symptoms and/or correct behavioural disorders. In other words, it is always at the service of an (ideal) image of so-called normality, whether explicit or not, be it of autonomy, 'mature' love, authenticity or common sense. More technically, these are structured and methodically designed forms of help that can be distinguished from ordinary social contacts and start from a voluntarily-entered agreement or contract. They consist of a relational interaction of an expert therapist with one or more patients. They are based on a well-defined theoretical vision of psychosocial functioning and lead or aim to lead to a change in psychosocial functioning.[41]

This sounds clear, uncluttered, *clean* and scientific: adapted by psychiatry. One would say: come, let's get started, for happiness and health, blessed by Sacred Science and reimbursed by Social Security.[42] However, some problems arise. For instance, what do happiness and health exactly mean? And shouldn't illness and abnormality be distinguished from each other? The former implies a dimension of suffering, while normality (as the word indicates) refers only to a statistical norm.[43] Also, what does psychotherapeutic expertise mean? In my part of the world the title of psychotherapist is not even legally protected. Anybody can declare themselves a psychotherapist. Moreover, by no means all psychiatrists and psychologists have undergone full psychotherapeutic training.

Finally, for a principal problem, I sketch a short parable. A frog and a scorpion are standing on the bank of the river. The scorpion asks the frog: will you carry me across? The frog refuses. Are you mad? And if you sting me on the way? Of course, I won't sting you, replies the scorpion. Then we'd drown together! The frog agrees, and in the middle of the river, he is stung by the scorpion anyway. What are you doing? asks the frog dismayed. Ah, I couldn't resist, the scorpion admits.[44] Behold the shipwreck of psychotherapy as a 'voluntary commitment or contract'. Because all understanding notwithstanding, psychotherapy is not safe. Because it is forgotten that the unconscious is at play, and the drives applicable there are not clear, orderly and reasonable but take us beyond the limits of the impossible and the forbidden. Because perhaps our desire drives us instead to fly and drown, not to keep us afloat. It touches on those other elements of psychoanalysis that are more sensitive than the principle of psychic causation per se. Elements that also provoke a lot more resistance[45] and that make one seek detours and shortcuts that risk ending up in dead ends. For instance, the primordial influence of sexuality proved unpalatable even to some of Freud's closest collaborators[46] (such as Adler and Jung). For example, the demonic[47] of the unconscious, through which we keep repeating (even highly destructive) patterns. There is a possibility that the patient seems unconsciously not to *want to* heal. The irrational, inconsistent, inappropriate desire that curses with the myth of (wanting a) healthy life. Also, the fact that one cannot cure a man of his humanity, which is to say that one cannot cure him of his dividedness.

There is his conscious 'common sense' and good intentions on the one hand and unconscious irrationality and impulses on the other. By the way, the latter also applies to the therapist who sometimes dares to imagine himself as objective, endowed with common sense and 'normality'.

For behold, one of the fundamental assumptions of psychoanalysis is that there is no strict division between the observer and the observed, between us, the normals and them, the abnormals. From this, it follows that, as a therapist, you must know well what you want, learn as much as possible about your own (even unconscious) desire and question your position vis-à-vis your truth and your lack. Many lessons can be learned from the patient's resistance, but as Freud[48] says, no therapist goes further than his resistance and complexes allow him to.[49] Therefore, a sufficiently thorough personal analysis is the *sine qua non* of psychoanalytic work. Only this way the therapist will be able to locate their feelings and sensitivities enough to use them to understand what is going on in the patient and their mutual relationship.

8 Psychoanalytic Psychotherapy

Apart from the resistance (also within psychiatry) to psychoanalysis, another problem of applicability presents itself. Let us not forget that the insights of psychoanalysis came about in Sigmund Freud's private practice, i.e. the classical cure (on the couch, free association, abstinence and neutrality, high frequency of sessions) in well-developed and wealthy, primarily neurotic patients. Needless to say (although this is sometimes forgotten), psychoanalysis has not stood still over the past century. Several great authors (e.g. Sandor Ferenczi, Melanie Klein, Donald Winnicott, Jacques Lacan, Wilfred Bion, Heinz Kohut, Peter Fonagy, etc.) and their followers contributed not only to further theoretical development but also to a broader clinical practice, in which almost the full range of possible psychopathology can be approached employing an adapted psychoanalytic method and technique.

Today, psychoanalytic psychotherapists work clinically with the most diverse psychopathology and in the most varied settings. They are often experience-near rather than experience-distant in their theoretical insights.[50] They allow themselves not to be divided but inspired by the various theoretical and cultural developments that characterise the psychoanalytic movement. Freud's dream of a uniform psychoanalytic movement has long since been replaced by pluralism. Since the gentlemen's agreement within the British psychoanalytic association between the (Anna) Freudians and the Kleinians, there has been room within the international psychoanalytic movement for Bion and his modifications of Kleinism, for the object-relationalists (Fairbairn, Winnicott, Balint), for the hermeneuts (Ricoeur, Habermas). Even among North Americans, Kohut's Self Psychology did not offend Ego-psychological hegemony, nor did the developmental psychological perspective of Mahler, the relational turn and two-person-psychology, among others. Sporadically, even the silence between the *International Psychoanalytical Association* (IPA) and the (Lacanian) *Association Mondiale de Psychanalyse* (AMP) also gets broken.[51]

Meanwhile, amid this theoretical diversity, technically, quite a few converging trends are occurring where psychoanalytic psychotherapy is gradually emerging as *common ground* and preferred treatment for the vast majority of psychopathology, including neurosis.[52] Some distinguish within psychoanalytic therapies a spectrum going from 'pure' psychoanalysis[53] over psychoanalytic therapy to supportive psychotherapy.[54] In theory, this distinction would have to do with differences in technique and finality. With specific problems, it is clear from the outset which 'objective' is paramount: sometimes purely the restoration of psychological equilibrium, sometimes a more profound growth or psychological restructuring. In the first case, the work is mainly therapeutic and goal-oriented; in the second, free association (in its purposelessness) is primarily facilitated or encouraged. However, the difference can often only be established in retrospect and both supportive and exploratory episodes occur within the psychoanalytic process.[55]

For Freud, only those who took the facts of transference and resistance as their starting point were allowed to call themselves psychoanalysts.[56] The unconscious, repression, infantile sexuality and Oedipus complex are foundational concepts mentioned again and again throughout his theorising. According to John Rickman, in Freudian psychoanalysis, transference, resistance, and infantile sexuality are fundamental.[57] According to him, it is up to each analyst to develop his thinking and actions within these broad boundaries and take responsibility for them. Otto Kernberg[58] defines interpretation, analysis of transference and technical neutrality[59] as three essential features of the psychoanalytic method. Horacio Etchegoyen[60] describes it briefly as a method that recognises the past in the present and distinguishes them through interpretation. Finally, Jacques Lacan[61] considers the unconscious, repetition, transference, and drive the four fundamental concepts of psychoanalysis.[62] Indeed, for him, psychoanalysis is characterised not least by its ethics and epistemology focused on the subject and their private truth.[63]

9 The Demise of the Subject?

For it is this subject that today is once again in danger of being neglected by psychiatry. It is the flip side of the success of so-called biological psychiatry. Since 1938, with electroconvulsive therapy, lithium as a mood stabiliser in 1949, the first antipsychotics and antidepressants in the 1950s and the first benzodiazepine as a tranquilliser in 1960, biological treatment has gained a firm and indispensable place in psychiatric practice. More specifically, for the so-called major psychiatric disorders, such as schizophrenia, major depression and manic-depressive psychosis, aka bipolar disorder, these drugs represented a real breakthrough. Judicious use of psychopharmaceuticals according to evidence-based medicine[64] has, therefore, become a *must* for any right-minded psychiatrist. But in psychodynamic psychiatry, pills act more as a framework than a *passe-partout.* They create the enabling condition for the actual work.[65]

Psychiatry seeks to develop knowledge about the whole human being as a physical, psychological, social, and existential being. It applies this knowledge to dampen pain, ward off fear, alleviate suffering, or cure disease. But psychoanalysis, as a science of the unconscious, teaches that humans may seek health from their nature but, therefore, not from their culture.[66] 'I have a project: to go mad', says seventeen-year-old Fyodor Dostoevsky to his brother.[67] Charles Baudelaire speaks of *'la joie de descendre'* (a joyful descent), and Anatole France of *'la volupté de se perdre'* (losing oneself lustily).[68] It is not healthy, and it is not good, but it is true. And yes, we can unquestionably relate this descent/self-loss to the anatomy of evil from the prologue.

Within various therapeutic practices, there can be something psychoanalytically active. It revolves mainly around an ethical project. The patient is thereby considered, regardless of their capacity, vulnerability or psychopathology, as a subject in the making with their private truth that needs to be heard, however unbeneficial this truth may (initially) seem.[69] On the other hand, methods and techniques for working psychoanalytically will differ depending on whether the subject is a child or an adult, a psychotic or a neurotic.

According to Shakespeare, the world is a stage, and the fact that we who walk around on it are no more than actors reflects his belief that we do not easily escape the roles written for us. Each of us is involved in an unfolding drama whose plot keeps uncannily repeating itself. 'Character is destiny' is a statement attributed to the pre-socratic Heraclitus. In a modern psychoanalytic guise, the unconscious contains the knowledge of his repetition. Anna O., one of Freud's first patients, spoke of her private theatre.[70] Choosing the drama as a metaphor for psychic reality, Joyce McDougall tries to abandon standard psychiatric labels.[71] These labels can be stuck on symptoms but not on people. For that, everyone's personality is too complex, too subtle and, above all, too unique. Indeed, such labels are no more or no less than pseudo-mastering 'cover-signifiers'.[72] They put a point that prevents the patient from truly telling his story. Moreover, they promote the illusion that something pertinent would have been said about someone and imply that the diagnostician would be free of the psychodramas lying behind the symptoms. However, we all have our neurotic conflicts, our islands of hidden madness. We can all react psychosomatically under stress, and we are all capable of both perverse fantasies and impossible dreams. What distinguishes the sick from the healthy is their conflicts and how they try to resolve them in conscious and unconscious ways.

According to Freud, the difference between normal and abnormal ceases in our sleep when we all dream indiscriminately.[73] We are all troubled by forbidden sexual or aggressive tendencies: the theatre of the forbidden, of incest and parricide. And we are all bothered by the theatre of the impossible: we can never again be one with the all-powerful and all-good mother or father. We cannot control other people's thoughts, feelings and actions, and we cannot possess the power and sexual attributes of both parents at once. Neurosis is, in a sense, the default mode of the human condition. How each of us tries to settle or 'come' (to terms) with universal/existential themes. That's the question.

Notes

1 Milos Forman (1975).
2 Freud read Shakespeare from age ten and quoted him constantly in his letters and works (Gay, 1989; Bloom, 1998). Harold Bloom (1994) puts Shakespeare and Freud in positions 1 and 18 of his Canon.
3 Hunter (1968). Andre Green (1988 p 421–423) calls Macbeth Shakespeare's darkest 'démon du mal'.
4 Jean Cocteau (1934).
5 William Shakespeare. *Macbeth*. Act 5, Scene 1.
6 Jacques Lacan (1975a).
7 Bion (1962) promotes Knowledge to a fundamental passion alongside Love and Hate. Minus Knowledge (-K) represents its *counterpart*: knowing the truth but falsifying it, not wanting to see it.
8 Jacques Lacan (1950) in (1966 p 165).
9 'Wir haben es nicht gewusst' as Germany's initial reaction to the horror of the Holocaust.
10 'Ich habe es nie gewollt' in Peter Conrad (1999 p 48).
11 William Shakespeare. *King Lear*. Act 1, Scene 2.
12 The ideal type is an analytical comparison measure and methodological tool for describing social situations. It is a subjective abstraction in which the most essential characteristics are named. In reality, this ideal type never occurs purely.
13 Milos Forman (1984).
14 See 'Le mythe Pinel' (Postel, 1981).
15 Paul Verhaeghe (2002a p 85–86).
16 See Jacques Lacan's 'la belle âme' (1966a) in (1966 p 72), who denies any share of his own responsibility.
17 Ibidem p 15.
18 Sigmund Freud (1905b).
19 'Flectere si nequeo superos, Acheronta movebo'.
20 Sigmund Freud (1916–1917).
21 Sigmund Freud (1916–1917).
22 Freud inferred psychic causality from hypnosis. There is within us a knowledge we cannot know. The analyst analyses hypnotic transference. The patient is freed from the 'tyranny of suggestion'.
23 Medicine is the clinic of the gaze, psychoanalysis of the ear. For medicine, only the visible is *real*.
24 Socrates was the son of a midwife and used the maïeutic/midwifery method. In Plato's Meno, all knowledge is memory. It only needs to be 'liberated' from it.... *Docta ignorantia* is a concept of Nicholas of Cusa.

25 Given that this is a first mention, a brief explanation. This *objet petit a* is one of Lacan's most famous concepts. For him, it is psychoanalysis's (lack of) object (1956 p 12). It is a phantasmatic object that exists only in the relationship between man and language.

26 Wilfred Bion (1970 p 31).

27 Alluding to 'conversations at the frontier of dreaming' by Thomas Ogden (2002): '…just above sleep' (Bion 2013 p 56) 'to participate in dreaming the patient's undreamt dream' (Ogden 2004 p 1360).

28 The specificity of psychoanalytic ethics is expressed in the *choice process* rather than its *outcome*. See Jacques Lacan (1986) and Marc De Kesel (2002).

29 Paul Verhaeghe (1989).

30 Raymond Carver (1981).

31 '*Le symbole est le meurtre de la Chose*' in Jacques Lacan (1966a p 319) and the painting *La trahison des images/ceci n'est pas une pipe* by René Magritte see Kinet (2002 p 26).

32 Jacques Lacan (1991b).

33 Haruki Murakami (2008).

34 Extracted from what were considered meaningless waste products of the human mind.

35 Compromise between versus alloying different forces. Also, *within* psychic instances. See, for example, Donald Carveth (2023) within conscience.

36 By Freud's '*Kultur*' is meant 'the whole sum of achievements and the regulations which distinguish our lives from those of our animal ancestors and which serve two purposes - namely to protect men against nature and to adjust their mutual relations' (1930a p 89).

37 As a concept, the signifier does not appear in Freud's work. Signifiers are fundamental elements of language that differentiate among themselves. They do not express pre-existing meaning but produce meaning according to context. According to Lacan, the unconscious does not precede or underlie ('preverbal') language but, conversely, is instead its result. Only the speaking being has an unconscious.

38 Seneca: '*Errare humanum est; perseverare diabolicum*'. We can all make a mistake. Making the same mistake twice can raise eyebrows. A third time may involve something demonic/diabolic/of the unconscious. To be analysed! The devil/demonic lurks in the details. Short-story writer Donald Barthelme: 'Fragments are the only forms I trust'.

39 At least until he realises he is wrong.

40 Sigmund Freud (1933 p 16): 'The many psychiatrists and psychotherapists who cook soups on our fire'.

41 Pierloot & Thiel (1986 p 3–10).

42 Jean Florence (1985).

43 Illness is about the experience from a first-person perspective of 'not being able to'. Abnormality is more about the observation, from a third-person perspective, of a deviation from an average. This deviation acquired a moral connotation: 'abnormality' as the objectionable/a criterion for 'disease' (Kienstra, 2020). The WHO defines mental health as 'a state of mental well-being that enables people to cope with the stresses of life, realise their abilities, learn well and work well, and contribute to their community.'

44 Jean Florence (ibid. p 265).

45 Sigmund Freud (1925a): in addition to the narcissistic affront that man is not master of his own house (the unconscious in itself), the doctrine of repression (the not-wanting-to-know) and infantile, polymorphously perverse sexuality. He later adds a fourth: the hypothesis of the death or destructive drive, which he says meets with resistance even in analytic circles (1930b).

46 Sigmund Freud (1914a).
47 Resistance is like a demon that does not want to come into the light of day, knowing that this would mean its end (Verhaeghe (1996 p 18).
48 Sigmund Freud (1910).
49 Complex was a term coined by Carl Gustav Jung. In psychoanalysis, it is the set of affectively charged representations that strike interpersonal relationships and contain internal conflicts through which they cause defences (Laplanche & Pontalis, 1967).
50 Distinction by Robert Wallerstein (2002).
51 Horacio Etchegoyen and Jacques-Alain Miller (the then presidents) ensured this (fledgling) rapprochement (1996) thanks to personal meetings/sympathies.
52 Otto Kernberg (1999).
53 De Jonghe et al. speak of the 'utopian' analysis (1987, p 186). Freud contrasted the gold of psychoanalysis with the copper of suggestion (1919a, p 183). Psycho-analysis was long opposed to supportive components and denied their importance within its clinical applications.
54 See above or, e.g. E. Bibring, (1954), Rockland (1989), Derksen & Markx (1992).
55 Motto to be distilled from the *Menninger Foundation Psychotherapy Research Project:* 'Be as expressive as you can be, and as supportive as you have to be' (Wallerstein 1986 p 688).
56 Sigmund Freud (1914a).
57 Pearl King (2003) Bion was analysed with Klein and Rickman.
58 Otto Kernberg, (ibid. p 1079).
59 Technically characterised by equidistance: an equal (scientific) distance to Id, Ego and Superego.
60 Horacio Etchegoyen (1999 p 112).
61 Jacques Lacan (1973).
62 A high-speed comment on repetition and transference. Repetition stems from two forces: automatism on the side of the signifier and the always missing encounter with the object/Thing on the part of the drive. Lacan uses the term 'insistence' to name the repetition characteristic of the signifying chain in the unconscious. He defines the unconscious as a memory system. He elaborates (1994) on the para-doxical function of transference. In its symbolic aspect, the repetition helps the cure progress by revealing the signifiers of the subject's history. The imaginary (love and hate) aspect acts as a resistance.
63 There is something psychoanalytic like '*il y a du psychanalyste*' Jacques Lacan (2001 p 378–379). Psychoanalysis is not an (imaginary) identity but an activity: the analyst renounces the master position attributed to him by the patient see also Serge André (2003 p 10).
64 Guido Pieters (2000 p 124–134).
65 I mentioned psychodynamic pharmacotherapy in 2006. See Glen Gabbard (2014 p 149). 'Not whether but how the combination of psychotherapy and medication is beneficial' (ibid. p 157).
66 Philippe Van Haute (2000) or Paul Verhaeghe (2002a).
67 Jean Florence, ibid.
68 Bart Verschaffel (1989 p 19).
69 See Bion's '*truing*' (Grotstein,1983) or '*la vérité en état naissant*' (Lacan, 1978 p 22–35).
70 Sigmund Freud and Joseph Breuer (1895b).
71 Joyce McDougall (1982).
72 Hubert Van Hoorde (1992).
73 Sigmund Freud (1916–1917).

Part I

A Precise Position

Chapter 3

Psychoanalysis in Depth and Breadth

Size *Does* Matter

1 Curious

Until a stretch after World War II, psychoanalysis was all the rage. For instance, it was the primary treatment philosophy within psychiatry. In the words of Bruno Bettelheim: 'Just as the curing of physical illness was that of medicine'.[1] Later, in the sixties and seventies, there was the heyday of Wilhelm Reich and Herbert Marcuse's Freudomarxism. Portraits of Freud hung fraternally next to those of Che Guevara, Lenin or Mao. The atmosphere of sexual and other revolutions could be soaked up in many dormitories and student rooms. Apart from the social, psychoanalysis also left a significant mark on the scientific world. It was the leading explanatory model that affected the most diverse psychological and cultural phenomena with its 'universal acid'[2] just as happens today with neuro- and evolutionary biology. So, I was not the only youngster who started reading texts by and about Freud at the end of the last century. I found their reading a revelation both for the depth they penetrated and the breadth they covered. Size *does* matter.[3] Psychoanalysis knew a lot about the complexity of feelings. It breathed the perfume of the forbidden but also seemed to hold many keys to unlock one's and others' hidden rooms. It's a chicken and egg issue, but to this day, I owe partly to it a rather curious vocation. It ensures that I have never been bored for a second in my (though full-time) clinical work. So, the following quote by Dorothy Parker certainly fits the psychoanalytic bill. 'The cure for boredom is curiosity. For curiosity, there is no cure.'[4]

In brief, curiosity is one of the main foundations of the so-called desire of the analyst that Jacques Lacan talks about. According to his analysis, an analyst is neither 'clean' nor do they embody a stoic ideal. They can, in principle, cherish all human feelings or desires (including towards the patient), but a particular desire has installed itself in them that is stronger than all others. It is the desire that the patient's private and subjective truth be expressed and come into its own. The desire to make an absolute difference underpins, as it were, the desire to do good or to cure[5] that can be built

DOI: 10.4324/9781032698052-4

upon it. As such, the analyst's desire aims to surpass identification.[6] It is not the patient's resistance that impedes the psychoanalytic process. After all, this resistance is full of meaning, and both parties can learn a lot from it. Only the therapist's resistance can undermine the potential of a psychoanalytic undertaking. Lacan regards the 'desire of the analyst' as a purified or purged desire.[7] It does not yield to the most diverse and influential resistances inside and outside the consulting room and keeps the engine of the psychoanalytic process running until the end.

2 Curiosum

How is it possible that, barely five decades after the 1960s–1970s, psycho-analysis is considered an irrelevant and outdated curiosity by the current generation? Indeed, today, it has a huge image problem and has fallen into a not-so-splendid isolation.[8] Freud is – for starters – for many a *fraud*. He is sometimes referred to as a quack, then as a person with a cocaine addiction or an outright cheat or liar. To quote French President François Mitterand's provocative response to questions about his illegitimate child: '*Et alors?*' Was Richard Wagner a racist, Martin Heidegger a Nazi, Pablo Picasso a monster and Albert Einstein a womaniser? If so, does this detract from the quality of their work? Those who would be annoyed by such *ad hominem* attacks should – just to be precise – never forget that even within the psychoanalytic world, it is teeming with character assassinations against dissenters or apostates. In defiance of psychodynamically-inspired forms of treatment that found their way into evidence-based practice guidelines thanks to proven efficacy, psychoanalysis is routinely dismissed as not working and as a pseudoscience.[9] According to some, it is said to be more akin to a form of faith, arguing in catacombs over the exegesis of its gospel. Except among some diehards, however, it has entered a post-apostolic phase[10] and today it is characterised by pluralism and integration.We will see that the sometimes wildly divergent theorising is perhaps mostly the consequence of the increased breadth of its scope.[11]

Many believe that psychoanalysis is only for capitalist navel-gazers with luxury problems. However, research[12] shows that most patients only end up with psychoanalytic therapists after a (sometimes long calvary) road through previous short-term, symptom- and/or solution-focused mental help. As for the psychoanalysts themselves, Dutch novelist Harry Mulisch once mockingly said in an interview that its practitioners behave like contact-impaired intellectuals. Moreover, they wield an incomprehensible esoteric discourse[13] *Far from the madding crowd.*[14] It is a shortcoming from which several contemporary international psychoanalytic bestsellers such as Adam Phillips, Stephen Gross, Darian Leader or, in our part of the world, Paul Verhaeghe, seem to be able to escape with great success.

3 Stirb und Werde

With a nod to Mark Twain, Freud once called reports of his death greatly exaggerated. Or at least he has risen several times like a phoenix from his ashes. In a way, everyone speaks a little Freudian these days (though not always correctly). A subtitle of one of the books in the *Current Psycho-analytics* series[15] calls psychoanalysis alive and kicking despite its troubling disappearance. It may not be in crisis, but it mostly struggles with a stubbornly lousy reputation. By definition, it probably cannot or will never belong to the mainstream or the establishment's hegemony. Will its trademark always be a semi-clandestine existence on the cutting edge? A radicalisation of speech and subject characterises it and invites whoever ventures into it to produce their exception. It is not the blows due to pharmacotherapy or behavioural therapy or from protocolised managed care that cause its apoplexy. Instead, its problem may be that it is no longer perceived as a pertinent, *avant-garde* theory. It shows signs of gerontocracy and atherosclerosis, locking itself into a rhetoric that no longer appeals to today's youth. Especially on the shop floor of the psychiatric setting, it needs to live up to its relevance and pertinence permanently, also by engaging constructively and self-critically in dialogue with other disciplines and forms of mental health care.[16]

Psychoanalysis overplayed its hand somewhat over various psychopathologies (e.g. autism and psychosis).[17] For a long time, it made illegitimate claims of therapeutic monopoly. It is used to invoke authority arguments and refer to canonical texts. It often expressed itself too disparagingly about various other forms of mental health care and, according to Nobel laureate Eric Kandel, haughtily failed to produce scientific evidence.[18] Although, of course, lack of evidence is not evidence of lack. Psychiatry and psychology are beginning to return from a biological and behavioural reductionism; neuroscience recognises and even demonstrates that (especially early) life experiences have their plastic influence on neurophysiology and anatomy; behavioural therapy takes feelings and the therapeutic relationship more into account, and with cognitive science fully recognising the importance of the (at least descriptive) unconscious, the climate is possibly suitable for some comeback.

4 Psychoanalytic Trinity

Freud's psychoanalysis has been called an ancient art but a new science. Indeed, the rationality of psychoanalysis is linked to the fact that it transcends the pragmatic empiricism of a mere technique to distil from this practice a method and a theory: the science of the unconscious. To begin with, the term 'psychoanalysis' classically has several meanings. First, it is a scientific research tool. Indeed, according to James Strachey, Freud's invention of free association introduced a research method par excellence for unconscious processes. In this respect, free association can be considered the equivalent of the microscope for histology, the radio telescope for astronomy or functional magnetic imaging for neuropsychology. There are, of course, significant differences. For example, learning about tissue, stars or the brain does not change their nature. In contrast, a different 'view' of what goes on psychically creates a critical distance that can bring about psychic change almost as a matter of course. Moreover, the psychic naturally involves something fundamentally invisible. This applies *a fortiori* to the unconscious. How could you use a torch to get to know the darkness?

Psychoanalysis, secondly, is a particular form of treatment. Free association allows the unconscious to speak, and all kinds of pop-ups (GE: '*Einfälle*') contribute to understanding and interpreting its formations, such as the dream, the parapraxis, the joke, acting out, the transference and the symptom. After more than a century, psychoanalytic treatment has long ceased to be limited to the traditional cure on the couch. With a particular focus on transference and resistance characterising its approach, contemporary practice extends to the most diverse psychopathology and treatment settings. Its focus has gradually moved to the facilitation or development of mental capacities or processes, adding to the ongoing importance it has traditionally attributed to interpreting and understanding mental contents and conflicts.

Third, psychoanalysis is the science of the unconscious. Before Freud, the unconscious could also be found in rudimentary form in the work of Arthur Schopenhauer and Friedrich Nietzsche. For example, with his statement '*Es denkt in mir*', the latter anticipated the *Es* that Freud incorporated into his structural Id–Ego–Superego model after his topographical model of unconscious, preconscious and conscious. Freud's predecessors, however, approached this unconscious philosophically or phenomenologically. They did not subject it to systematic and scientific investigation, nor did they attempt to distil the laws of the passions from it. Of course, all sciences (chronologically starting with mathematics and astronomy) have detached themselves from philosophy. Today, they rely on sufficiently experimentally confirmed (at least explanatory and preferably also predictive) knowledge for this independence.

5 Psychoanalysis and the Clinical Situation

Freud was awarded the Goethe Prize in 1930 because his psychology 'has not only upended and enriched medical science but also the ideas of artists and pastors, historians and educators'.[19] Indeed, psychoanalysis believes it has something to say about very diverse human domains. However, its *core business* is and remains, of course, clinical practice. In response to the rule of free association, the patient is invited to speak their mind, to speak in a 'draft' form and to leave censorship behind. This allows them to experience while speaking and speak while experiencing, while the analyst listens with poised attention with a twilight sense or third ear. As the sessions progress, the psychoanalyst evolves into one of the main characters in the patient's history. This history gradually plays out more and more *in* the consulting room. This creates a unique opportunity to find out what patients' feelings and relationships are about. Together, they can also write a different or better outcome than would otherwise be the case. This is serious work, of course, but it also has something of play to it. The therapist does not just listen; they are a participatory co-player in this highly intimate enterprise. In doing so, they must be curious, wanting to understand the patient's mind and heart and build a meaningful relationship. They play a part in the patient's story while trying to provide necessary subtitles, footnotes, peripheral comments and translation.

The relationship that develops is determined by the needs and inclinations of the patient, and it simultaneously lends itself to research from which both parties can learn. It is not so much the taciturn analyst behind the couch but the psychoanalytic play therapist, the clinical or group psychotherapist, who is the model. After all, the therapist has to venture onto the floor, enter into a sufficiently natural relationship and at the same time continuously maintain a reflective, symbolising, mentalising and interpretative thinking mode. Their interventions are between interpretive cutting-edge technology and symbolising development aid, about deconstruction or construction. The analyst must go for *it*, even if necessary by untracked paths, and not be someone 'who disdains to adapt himself even in technique to the idiosyncrasies of the individual.'[20]

Without realising it, we are, as it were, possessed by our history. Either we tell our history or our history tells us. *That* mums and dads are critical to our psychology is something everyone would reasonably assume. To beginners and outsiders, it is unbelievable *how* important they are.[21] Our feelings and sensitivities are determined by what we have made of our history. All that exists has a past; many animals have a memory, but only humans have (or instead write) their history. This is never objective, always subjective, coloured and distorted. It is not static but dynamic. It is essentially fictional and evolutionary. It is also constantly edited from a present remembering context.

In therapy, the patient gradually becomes aware of the invisible glasses of transference. They realise that their history, fears and fantasies colour their view of themselves, others and the world. The analyst, in turn, is loved, hated, envied, desired, scorned, avoided, mocked or criticised. Meanwhile, that analyst maintains their serenity and continues to play their role professionally. This is sometimes compared to that of the court jester: the only mouth out of which His Majesty (in this case, the Ego) accepts less pleasant truths. However, you never know in advance how things will turn out. What hurdles will be overcome, how and when?[22] The speaking space is a kind of theatre without ever two identical performances.[23] It is mainly a matter of tuning in. This makes the work – however tricky – interesting, stimulating and/or challenging. It is probably one of the reasons why many psychoanalytic therapists continue to work with undiminished enthusiasm well beyond their rightful retirement age.[24]

A psychoanalytic characteristic is also an ethic focused on absolute difference. The patient is led to find or become themselves as much as possible. The therapist is not a silent figure shrouded in anonymity. They are not a person without qualities, but (a fortiori) in clinical psychotherapy, they retain their liveliness. Meanwhile, they relentlessly try to maintain a reflective, symbolising and mentalising mode of thought. Especially when working in a clinical psychotherapeutic setting, they draw from the entire psy- repertoire. They sometimes employ a master, then a university, but typically and primarily an analytic discourse. The analyst's desire that characterises the latter provides the pivot, at times, around which the engine of the psychoanalytic process keeps turning. In clinical psychotherapy, everyone is invited to think for themselves and speak on their behalf. Sapere aude or 'dare to think' from Kant becomes, more specifically, dare to think aloud. Under the rule of free association, coercive freedom seeks to bring the patient to full speech. I quote Tristan Tzara from the Dadaist Cabaret Voltaire: la pensée se fait dans la bouche.[25] Thought is (only) formed in the mouth.

Not only is there integration between psychiatry, psychotherapy, and psychoanalysis, but within the latter, there is also integration between different theoretical perspectives. Paraphrasing Picasso: 'Tous les yeux d'une femme sur le même tableau.' All of a woman's eyes are on the same canvas. Thus, clinical psychotherapy combines cubism and perspectivism. The unconscious and hidden histories feature live on stage. In the form of lateral transfers,[26] all sorts of things unfold a world of now two-dimensional and thus caricatural and more nuanced and three-dimensional inner objects. The entire thing can be considered a game. It's not a game without boundaries but (on the contrary) with boundaries and with boundaries. Paraphrasing Friedrich Schiller: is man ever more authentically himself than when he is at play?[27]

6 Nonspecific

Psychotherapy research shows the importance of the so-called 'non-specific therapeutic factors'[28] in any psychotherapy. They weigh heavily and are effective regardless of the theoretical model used by the therapist. For instance, almost half of the psychotherapeutic effect is related to support, the quality of the therapeutic relationship, empathy and 'belief' in the therapist/therapist.[29] Authors such as Melanie Klein, Donald Winnicott and Wilfred Bion are credited with exploring the psychopathological field beyond neurosis as well as the in-fans (Lat. non-speaking) in the patient.[30] They have thus analysed the psychogenetic and psychodynamic foundations of the nonspecific factors that play an essential role in any therapeutic enterprise. In addition, from actual observation, the developmentalists (René Spitz, Margaret Mahler, Daniel Stern, Robert Emde) have also produced much research data that shed light on what happens in the first stage of life. Integrating all their insights and concepts ensures that psychoanalysis has as many words about the nonspecific therapeutic factors as the Inuits have for snow.

For example, empathy is crucial in mental help, but from a psychoanalytic point of view, Lacan warns against being too understanding.[31] Against emotional understanding, which he exposes as illusory, he promotes rationalism. What private laws exactly underlie what sometimes escapes empathy and understanding? Psychic phenomena cannot be adequately analysed through affective identification with the person but only through the synchronic and diachronic contextualisable signifier in the patient's speech (Lacanian: the signifier chain). The symbolic order is characterised by the fact that there is no fixed connection between the signifier and the signified. This is most clearly expressed in dream analysis, where meaning cannot be obtained in advance from some dream lexicon.[32] Dream language can only be translated considering the subtext produced in the psychoanalytic space and the context within which it occurs. The attachment patterns recorded in procedural memory function as a *sols key* for the stave. They set the affective tone within which signifiers resonate that can only be interpreted diachronically in the context of life history and synchronously in the context of the 'total transference situation'.

From the first contact, there is a nonspecific or generic and a specific agenda. The nonspecific has to do with building a secure relationship, which is, after all, a necessary condition for an important therapeutic agent within any therapeutic encounter. The patient needs to feel understood and sometimes even carried, which presupposes an analogue of the primary maternal preoccupation in the therapist's mind and heart.[33] The extra-uterine mother is exceptionally attuned to her child's vital and categorical affections at the end of/just after pregnancy, helping to contain and symbolise them in a back-and-forth mirroring and marking. Winnicott's detailed description of one of his analyses shows a need for *holding and interpretation*. Even non-interpretive moments (the so-called 'moments of meeting' that can be emotionally unparalleled)[34] can only occur with positive acceptance, truthful engagement and empathetic alignment.

7 Specific

Clinically, the specifically psychoanalytic agenda mainly concerns detecting what repeats itself in history. From neuroscience, about repetition, we also remember the specific operating principles of implicit, procedural memory from our first years. It is not an anecdotal or autobiographical story (-fragment) but is expressed very differently. In the case of so-called 'memories in feeling', feelings that occur are a form of memory. When the patient is invited to return in time based on these feelings, he is sometimes catapulted through a wormhole into a distant past. Implicit memory also enters the scene through action and interaction that time and again appears to bear the imprint of deep-rooted patterns. Thinking of Freud (for whom memory was the antidote to repetition), they should be made explicit as much as possible. What rhymes also, especially in the incongruous? The patient is led to look at themselves and wonder about certain initially self-evident things so that they can first find the strange and incomprehensible in themselves and then try to analyse and work on it as best they can. What is repeated must be remembered. Remembering, repeating and last but not least, working through is the message. As in a fugue, problems keep repeating themselves in variations on the theme until they have been sufficiently recounted to make way for new melodies.

According to Freud, only those who use the (specific) concepts of transference and resistance may call themselves psychoanalysts. In a first summary explanation, transference is the invisible lens of our history and our fantasies through which we view reality. Resistance is the fact that, in many ways, we 'don't want to know' precisely and want things to change as long as we don't have to change ourselves! The only person who welcomes change is a wet baby. Within these broad lines, it is up to each psychoanalyst to give their own answers and bear responsibility. In more contemporary terms, the psychoanalyst works through relationship and interpretation. The relationship is the bearer and matrix of the psychoanalytic process. Specific emotional or interactional patterns can (or will) repeat within the therapeutic relationship. This therapeutic relationship can also offer a healing experience that can still be internalised.

To return to basics: for Freud, psychoanalysis is primarily about *The Mind in Conflict*.[35] To begin with, there is conflict between conscious and unconscious, between a part that likes to show itself and a part that is hidden, between something repressing and repressed. But conflict is also ubiquitous in other ways. Between conflicting feelings or impulses, between different attachments, between desires and norms and values, between the latter and so on. But even within the constantly evolving science of psychoanalysis, conflict (or even schism) is predominant. Different figures occupy different positions and move between several extremes. I list a few tension relations. There is the one between nature and culture, between focusing primarily on constitution or disposition or primarily on the environment. There is the one between those who give the most significant weight to the impact of the inner vs that of the outer world. Some adopt a defect model rather than a conflict model of psychological pathology. Some see problems as developmental disorders, and others as a more or less phantasmatic distortion of experiences with others. Some aim at construction rather than deconstruction and reconstruction with therapy. Some pursue a musical inspiration of the patient, while others focus on analytical interpretation. And all this with the therapist sometimes posing as a kind of better parent and thus offering a therapeutic or healing experience. Then again, the therapist may act like a surgeon carefully trying to separate the healthy from the sick, the benign from the malignant tissue, or sometimes there is even the therapist as poet or mystic, as conceived, for example, by the late Wilfred Bion.

Of course, the psychotherapist should adapt the technique and methodology to the patient rather than selecting or formatting patients to their preference. It is not 'one size fits all'. Technique and methodology should be tailored to the patient and the moment. Fortunately, psychoanalysis has now developed several viewpoints and methods to describe and work on the field of the human mind. Today, it is a container ship that can accommodate the most diverse cargo in its hold. The greater the repertoire it contains, the better it can match the, after all, highly variable clinical requirements.

8 Psychoanalysis and Psychiatry

The previous chapter discussed the ethical and epistemological differences between psychiatry and psychoanalysis. For instance, it showed that the former seeks to remove the symptom as a sign of disease, while the latter seeks to understand it. Psychotherapy focuses on norm and normality, while Joyce McDougall wrote a book in 1978 as a *Plea for a Measure of Abnormality.* We need to be neurotic enough to experience guilt and responsibility, perverse enough to enjoy, and psychotic enough to transform reality. In one of his introductory lectures, Freud talks about the crystal structure of our psyche. There are facets of every psychopathology within us. In this sense, nothing human is alien to us.[36] In a neologism, Tomas Geyskens speaks about us as humans, not only as polymorphic perverse but also as polymorphic pathological beings.

Like medicine (as an applied natural science), psychiatry refers to a generality, while psychoanalysis looks for the private laws underlying psycho-(patho)logy on the part of the patient. The analytical process proceeds experimentally and leads to evolving and increasingly precise hypotheses and theories about psychogenesis and psychodynamics. The various analytical concepts and complexes act as superimposed maps to get away from area and un-land. However, the map is never the area. The practised hiker focuses and looks with their own eyes.

Freud had many views on psychiatry that still hold (again) today. Now just as then, many psychiatrists know too little about psychoanalysis, and many psychoanalysts know too little about psychiatry. Psychiatry could not and cannot substantively explain the precise form of many psychopathological phenomena. It may demonstrate *that* a person develops symptoms but not *which* symptoms. It has no insight into the meaning of symptoms. Nevertheless, Gottfried Leibniz's *'Nil sine ratione'* (nothing without reason) is a classical scientific premise. It is Freud's merit to point out that even mundane and/or universal phenomena, such as the dream or the parapraxis, have a particular content or a precise meaning.

Medicine and behavioural therapy see humankind as reasonable beings. We may be misled by irrationality, but we firmly believe that we can get on the right path through the power of reason, by the 'right' thoughts or information. Implicitly, there is a therapeutic optimism: with the right pill or technique, all problems can be solved. In contrast, psychoanalysis has an essentially tragic view of the human condition. Between normality and abnormality, there is a continuum. We are not sure that we are the descendants of Adam and Eve, but we are the children of Narcissus and Oedipus. Ideas and ideologies may separate us, but our dreams and fears unite us.

This is entirely at odds with the implicit assumptions of the five (1980–2013) successive versions of the *Diagnostic and Statistical Manual of Mental Disorders* that have shrouded psychiatry in increasing obscurity over the past decades. In them, happiness and health are medicalised and reduced to the presence or absence of measurable complaints or symptoms. The exponential increase in diagnoses with each edition[37] is a treat for, if not the creation of, a wealthy Big Pharma because financial interests do steer and disturb science. The psychotherapeutic world must try to keep up by conducting small-scale research for which it can only obtain limited government funding and which, moreover, methodologically does not fit in at all with its purpose. One of the main difficulties is how one could objectify change in subjective experience. In his latest book on authority, Verhaeghe denounces the use of pseudo-figures on well-being. In it, the Likert scale widely used in human sciences is exposed once and for all as pure wet-fingeredness. How could we, *a fortiori*, measure the efficacy of psychoanalytic psychotherapy if, in its view, a disillusioned patient can sometimes be a 'success' and a satisfied one a failure?

The one-size-fits-all McDonaldisation of mental health care involves over-consumption of drugs (including in children) to cure double, triple and so on diagnoses piled up like Big Macs and offered as fast food. The emergence of psychopathology is linked, on the one hand, to a cerebral substrate that can finally be made visible and thus plausible by sophisticated technology. On the other hand, psychopathological aetiology is attributed to life events that are valid and scoreable for everyone. A minimum of respect for the always private and complex genesis of psychopathology[38] threatens to be definitively lost. Ahistoricism (Lacan) and decontextualisation (Verhaeghe) reign supreme. Psychoanalysis, on the other hand, is pre-eminently a science of the particular.

9 Psychoanalysis and Science

With his highly revered tutor Ernst Brücke, Freud had solid roots in his time's biological and natural science world. Through several publications, he initially tried to profile himself for a post as a neurophysiological researcher at the ultra-Catholic Vienna University. Not for nothing did Frank Sulloway call him a *Biologist of the Mind* in the title of one of his books.[39] Initially, Freud engaged scientifically in the fields of neuroanatomy and neurophysiology. With his 1895 project for a scientific psychology, he tried to lead psychology into the framework of the natural sciences. He hoped that chemistry would one day isolate the substances linked to sexuality and neurosis. He whole-heartedly endorsed Darwinian thought, and thermodynamic views such as the law of energy conservation can be found in many psychodynamic and drive-economic reflections. Together with Alfred Einstein and Ernst Mach, among others, he published a manifesto calling for scientific positivism banning all metaphysical formulations.

Freud did give psychoanalysis a special status as a science. Every science is based on observations and experiments through the medium of our psychic apparatus. But psychoanalysis *investigates* precisely this psychic apparatus and thus differs from most other sciences in that in it, the human mind is both subject and object of investigation. He was also aware that his new science was problematic. For instance, it can only work retrospectively, not predictively, and hardly lends itself to experimentation. However, if we define science as systematised and formulated knowledge, it may claim scientific status. In his theorising, Freud was sometimes quite adamant. He is often full of his ideas, generalising excessively, drawing from the rhetorical box to disarm the reader, and trying to convince them (or the patient).

While Freud drew significant inspiration from the natural sciences, Lacan problematises an overly naive extrapolation of the psychic from biology. According to him, Freudian references to these sciences should also be taken figuratively or metaphorically rather than literally. We should grasp the *precise* way biology intervenes in the psychic. With Jacques Lacan, we find a shift towards structuralism. Following the lead of linguist Ferdinand de Saussure and anthropologist Claude Levi-Strauss, psychoanalysis becomes the science of the subject (of the unconscious). This subject is mainly the effect of a pre-existing structure or even ideology that he calls (the desire and/or discourse of) the big Other. For Lacan, psychoanalysis is not only the science of the subject but also of the particular. Indeed, it searches 'experimentally' for psychic laws that apply (only) on account of this one and only person, whose one or only ground (-lessness) it tries to work on. Science seeks to close off access to knowledge by intuition. For Lacan, psychoanalysis is based on rational dialogue even when reason collides with the limit of madness. He would say like Polonius about Hamlet: 'Though this be madness, yet there is method in it.'[40]

Besides attachment research and infant research, neuroscience has become one of psychoanalysis's most essential touchstones. With our triple brain roughly consisting of the brain stem of reptiles, the limbic system of mammals and the specifically human neocortex, and our hemispheric lateralisation, there is also neuronally under our cranial pan a vat of contra-dictions where peace of mind struggles to thrive. The right hemispheric communication between the mother and her baby, the effect of stress on the hypothalamic–pituitary–adrenal axis and thus on resilience or immunity, implicit and explicit memory, fast and slow emotional responses, the neuro-plasticity and different rates of maturation of specific cerebral structures, the importance of priming and subliminal perception, and so on. All shed new light on long-established psychoanalytic concepts.

For example, there are things we do not want to know, but also things we *cannot* know. Many findings invite or challenge psychoanalysis to reflect on neuroscientific correlations. In particular, the relationship between prehistory and history deserves investigation. Some things are etched in our memory, but we cannot recount them. '*Saxa loquuntur*' quoted Freud. Stones can speak. Archaeologists refer to 'stones and bones' or other fragments based on which they reconstruct our prehistoric times. Natural scientific methods, such as DNA research or radiocarbon dating, can illuminate the matter. Similarly, psychoanalysis needs to consult neighbouring sciences or sources to reconstruct the ups and downs of our prehistory.

10 Between Science and Art?

Every right-minded psychiatrist is obliged to occupy an uncomfortable bifurcation between humanities and natural sciences. Moreover, as a *scientist-practitioner,* he moves between science and art or skill. For the psycho-analyst, this staggered position applies *a fortiori*. It has something of a craft, but, in a *bon mot* of Lacan, it also tries to fulfil its scientific vocation. Some see psychoanalysis, like art, as something that can be passed on but not taught.[41] After all, psychoanalysis would escape the criteria of objectivity on which science and education are based. Of course, Freud had great attention and respect for art (although this was not true for the creations of his con-temporaries). He flirted with Leonardo da Vinci as the *uomo universale* par excellence: artist, discoverer, inventor and scientist. He also found psychoanalysis indebted to poets and other artists for many of its insights.

Science presents truth under a form of abstraction. The abstract world of theory or algebraic formulas clarifies the diversity of phenomena. Art then presents truth in a very concrete form: the concrete one of Don Quixote, Faust, Othello or Anne Frank. The particular clarifies the general there. Art is the realm of private things resistant to concepts yet possessing the dimen-sion of the universal. It is, in the words of Jean Cocteau, science incarnate. For many readers, Freud's disease histories, for instance, have great literary value. In part, they read like novels, elevating the particularity of his patients to prototypical proportions. Even many who are not convinced of the scien-tific content of psychoanalysis appreciate the unmistakable style and rheto-rical arts of Freud's texts. The words of the French poet René Char certainly apply to Freud: *'l'homme de science cherche des preuves, l'artiste cherche des traces'*. The scientist seeks proof; the artist seeks traces.[42] In its practice, psychoanalysis might be more akin to a craft: between the science of traces and the art of tracking.

Notes

1 Bruno Bettelheim (1983 p 40).
2 Daniel Dennett (1995) on neo-Darwinism.
3 Size exists only in the Imaginary. Not in the Real or the Symbolic.
4 http://www.quotationspage.com/quote/457.html. This curiosity neuro-psycho-analytically probably rests on the SEEKING system, which is considered libidinal in the view of affective neuroscience (see extensively: Panksepp, 1998; Solms, 2021a and Kinet, 2023a).
5 Jacques Lacan (1986).
6 Moustapha Safouan (2005 p 68). Identifying is not becoming who you are but becoming like the psychotherapist. For me, Plato and Aristotle are exemplary. Although the latter spent 20 years schooling with the former, he went utterly his way afterwards.
7 About transference love: 'however highly he may prize love, he must prize even more highly the opportunity for helping the patient over a decisive stage in her life' (Freud, 1915b p. 170).
8 Peter Fonagy (2003a).
9 Thanks to Hans Eysenck (1985) and Karl Popper (1991).
10 Jacob Arlow (1982).
11 Analogous to the contradictions between the ultra-fast theory of relativity and the ultra-small quantum mechanics that do not affect the scientific status of physics.
12 See, e.g., Doidge et al. (1994).
13 Discourse is a concept introduced by Jacques Lacan (and later elaborated by, e.g. Michel Foucault in the form of his *epistèmè*) by which the speech of a particular collective is meant. It structures reality in terms of values and truths cf Lacans. 'The unconscious is the discourse of the big Other.'
14 Thomas Hardy (1874).
15 Jef Dehing (2007).
16 Currently convergence with cognitive psychology, developmental psychology, attachment research and neuroscience (Luyten et al., 2015).
17 Glen Gabbard states: 'The history of efforts to apply psychoanalytic or psycho-dynamic thinking to autism has been one of the disgraces of the field of psychiatry' (2014 p 385). On the other hand, see Cluckers et al. (2012) further in this book.
18 Eric Kandel (1998, 1999).
19 Sigmund Freud (1930a p 12).
20 Neville Symington (1986 p 193).
21 Psychoanalytically, it is about what we make of mum and dad throughout our journey.
22 Freud compares chess, whose beginning and endgame can be mapped, not the middle game.
23 See Glen Gabbard (2014 p 297) 'recall of a memory is more like a theatrical production'.
24 A notable example is Otto Kernberg, who retired at 95.
25 Tristan Tzara (1924).

26 Lateral transferences: not only directed at the therapist(s) but equally at fellow patients.

27 Friedrich Schiller (1796 p 58).

28 'The big four' (Hubble et al., 1999).

29 To avoid poor efficacy and drop-out, a flexible approach tailored to the patient is necessary (Cloitre, 2015). Differences in outcome also depend more on the therapist than on the therapy (McKay et al., 2006; Wampold and Imel (2015); van Os et al. (2019).

30 '*Infans*' as a term for the child who cannot (yet) speak instead of the more common infant or (Fr) *enfant*.

31 '*Gardez-vous de comprendre*': understanding can be an imaginary trap: The therapist feels the same (problem) as the patient.

32 In contrast with Joseph Campbell or James Frazer, for Claude Levi-Strauss, mythology consists of mythemes, just as language à la Roman Jacobson consists of phonemes. Their meaning can only be interpreted within their context.

33 Donald Winnicott (1956) states that the mother is generally in a state of grace at birth. Thanks to talent, education, experience, and analysis, the therapist can also be deemed extraordinarily gifted...

34 Daniel Stern (2004). I lyrically compare it to Michelangelo's ceiling fresco of the Sistine Chapel. They produce vital momentum and increased well-being because of the mutual connection. (Boston Change Process Study Group quoted by Allison and Fonagy, 2016 p. 283).

35 After Charles Brenner (1983).

36 Supplementing Terentius' *'humani nihil a me alienum puto'* with nothing *in*human is alien to me.

37 DSMI counted 60, DSMII 106, DSMIII 230, DSMIV 410 and DSMV 500 different disorders. See Frances (2013).

38 The 'complementary series'. Sigmund Freud (1916–1917).

39 Frank J. Sulloway (1979). Psychoanalysts sometimes do well to study publications by critics or dissenters rather than reject them a priori.

40 Shakespeare, *Hamlet*, Act 2, scene 2.

41 Psychoanalytic training proceeds essentially (as in art) by doing, in other words, as you learn to paint, sculpt, and play music...

42 'His (the psychoanalyst's) task is to make out what has been forgotten from the traces which it has left behind or; more correctly, to construct it' (Freud, 1937b p 258–259).

Chapter 4

Time and Mind
History and Petite Histoire

I Human Bestiality

In his *Discourse on Human Dignity* (considered today the manifesto of the Renaissance)[1] Giovanni Pico della Mirandola compares man to a chameleon. He is essentially a Protean. There is no such thing as human nature. Man can assume all forms according to the circumstances in which he finds himself. A few centuries later, Jean Jacques Rousseau wrote his *Discourse on Inequality*, [2] one of the founding texts of the Enlightenment. The animal is caught in its instinct, i.e. the logic of its genetic programme. Feed a pigeon meat and a cat grain, and they both die of hunger. They cannot free themselves from their herbivorous or carnivorous destinies. Man, on the other hand, is not one but two with nature. In this removal from nature or this *excess* rests precisely the freedom to which he (in a famous statement by Sartre)[3] is condemned. For example, in terms of love, sexuality and relationships, contemporary freedom of choice is downright dizzying. Historically, this is possibly unique.

Still, according to Rousseau, humankind has a double historicity. There is the historicity of the species, namely civilisation. An anthill, a flock of antelopes or starlings shows identical behaviour today as it did millennia ago. On the other hand, look at London, Paris or today's countryside. After barely a century, their societies have sometimes changed beyond recognition. There is also the historicity of the individual, namely education. A few minutes after a calf, a crocodile or a duck is born, it possesses the almost complete adult behavioural repertoire in a genetically programmed way. This is while a human is born in neoteny, i.e., utter physiological immaturity and absolute dependence.[4] We need about twenty-five years in the West to fully stand on two feet.

Humans are at once the inventor and author of our history. *Story* and *history* are the constant sum of our choices.[5] For Aristotle, man was a reasonable animal. Meanwhile, we know that some animals (with great apes at the forefront) possess great intelligence. Nor is sensibility a human prerogative. For instance, many more or less empathetic emotions come into

DOI: 10.4324/9781032698052-5

play in mammals. Even language may not make a qualitative difference, but rather a gradual one. But only humans have eaten from the tree of knowledge of good and evil.[6] We are moral beings, capable of both crime and holiness. That is precisely why, of all mortal beings, humans were the best remedy against boredom for the Olympian gods.[7] Unlike animals, humans can indeed commit bestialities. In French, this sounds more innocent: '*des bêtises*'. But in contrast to the animal, humans can also perfect themselves.

Human medicine and especially psychiatry are, therefore, not *veterinary* medicine. Nothing animal and certainly nothing mammalian is alien to us. We have much to learn from the biological and ethological. Yet this common ground is insufficient to enable us to follow humans in their often unfathomable paths. In the human, nature and culture, brain and mind meet. To understand them, there is a need for counting and recounting, cyphers and deciphering. On top of the double historicity, a dual causality is also at play.[8] There is the general (because of) natural causality. Appendicitis or cystitis produce the same symptoms Everywhere and Always. But in addition, there is private, say, psychological causality. Jacqueline only suffers from her lift phobia in the presence of bald men with beards. The reason is to be sought within her private, individual history.[9]

2 From Civilisation

After this brief anthropological excursion, we can reflect on the current *Zeitgeist*. Its main trademark is probably the postmodern condition with the end of Big Narratives. For many centuries and in solid ways, religious and secular ideologies have provided humans with structure and footing. The classical era was characterised by cosmic harmony. Everything and everyone had their proper place within this divine order. After Descartes' *cogito,* modernity made its appearance with methodical doubt. Authority arguments were thenceforth undercut by critical reason. Moreover, the cosmos turned out to be an infinite and disorienting space. To make matters worse, Nietzsche proclaimed the death of God and all (other) idols and ideals. He thus pioneered a postmodern deconstruction that brought about the contemporary fragmentation of man and his world.[10] The three Rs of tradition, namely routine, ritual and religion, remain only in the so-called developing world.[11] Symbolic order and the father function are said to be weakened. The once self-evident respect for authority figures such as teachers and train conductors is disappearing. There is a generalised scepticism towards any power and authority. It is forbidden to forbid, and it is obligatory to enjoy. At the same time, we have to invent more than ever, including ourselves. After all, the security of convention has given way to the uncertain adventure of invention. In all areas of life, the motto is: away with tradition, long live permanent revolution! Even industry, culture and the culture industry are dominated by the passion for innovation and the dictatorship of novelty.

The whole of the 20th century bore the stamp of deconstruction. Not only the mentioned deconstruction of religious and secular ideologies but also a deconstruction of beauty and figuration in the visual arts, deconstruction of harmony and melody in atonal music, deconstruction of plot and characters in the *Nouveau Roman*, etc. At the same time as this deconstruction, a universal competition has installed itself. It is globalised capitalism in which everything tries to measure itself against everything and everyone according to the new standard of benchmarking. It amounts to a second era of globalisation. This time, however, it is no longer dominated by the Enlightenment's faith in progress with its joint humanising project. Globalisation is purely about global Darwinism. More and more, better and faster, must be produced to survive as a species (of entrepreneurs, politicians, artists, hospitals, etc.). It is not just 'publish or perish' but more generally 'produce or perish'. Not according to a biological but a neoliberal-capitalist logic of survival of the fittest. Meanwhile, protocol and transparency refer to a utopia of complete mastery, social engineering, and risk reduction, behind which the subject and human lack disappear.

According to Heidegger, our world has become pre-eminently a world of technique and technology.[12] We are all caught in the hellish rhythm of its blind machine. The result is an uncontrollable rat race of growth and expansion without knowing why and where. There is a loss of meaning, purpose and destiny. We do experience being willlessly at the mercy of the merry-go-round. It escapes our control entirely. Nor is it so clear whether we benefit in any way. It may, but it may also not. Would we be happier with a larger television, higher pixels on our camera, yet faster working memory, internet connection and so on? We are in the grip of a runaway dynamic like a gyroscope that has to keep spinning on its axis at great speed or a cyclist who has to keep pedalling and thus move forward to avoid stopping or falling over. With his *Metabletica*, Dutch psychiatrist Jan Hendrik van den Berg[13] convincingly demonstrated that every age has and creates its mind. For instance, his standard work shows that the childhood that psychoanalysis is all about only appears as such in modern times. The myth of maternal love was placed in a cultural and historical context through Elisabeth Badinter's[14] study and thus lost its universal, 'natural' character. Michel Foucault[15] studied the changing cultural perception and treatment of a seemingly as common human phenomenon as madness.

3 To the Clinical Situation

With such well-researched studies on 'time and mind' in mind, we can only speculate on what the spirit of our time is. In psychiatric and clinical psychotherapeutic practice, shifts seem to be occurring within psychopathology. These are leading away from the classical[16] neurosis towards a more narcissistic[17] (in the sense of pre-oedipal) register of severe personality disorders,[18] acting-out behaviour[19] and substance abuse. Thereby, the psychoanalytic model of unconscious conflicts rooted in childhood is increasingly complemented by a defect model of psychopathology in which capacities essential for psychological well-being, such as basic security and trust, integration and mentalisation,[20] are said to have insufficiently developed.

From his earliest writings, Freud distinguished neurosis between actual neuroses and psychoneuroses.[21] Actual neuroses are characterised by an anxiety against which the subject cannot defend himself.[22] In psycho-neuroses, on the other hand, a whole arsenal of symptoms is developed as a more or less successful defence against anxiety. Consequently, the psychoneurotic fear is less overwhelming (traumatic) and is limited by this psychic or symbolic processing. In the case of actual neurosis, on the other hand, an unbound drive leads to various relatively nonspecific disturbances in physical and mental functioning. He describes the newly introduced nosological entities of anxiety neurosis and neurasthenia as the most critical actual neurotic manifestations of his time. The actual neurotic symptom, moreover, according to him, forms the core and, in a certain sense, is also a preliminary stage of the psychoneurotic symptom, which is a secondary, symbolic-imaginary elaboration of it.[23]

It is a distinction that can also be found elsewhere in his thinking. For instance, in *The Interpretation of Dreams,* he speaks of navel of the dream.[24] This resists the analytical labour of interpretation (the reversal of the displacements, condensations and other concealments typical of dream labour) and is, therefore, the fundamental core of our being in Lacanian terms.[25] When discussing symptom formation later in Dora's case study, he compares this process to the oyster forming a pearl around a grain of sand.[26] The drive springing from the somatic starts the root around which the symbolic 'construct', the (psychoneurotic) symptom, is formed. The mother (of pearl) plays a vital role in drive and trauma becoming bound to word and image representations. In a wink to René Descartes, not '*Je*' but 'Elle *pense, donc je suis*'.

Paul Verhaeghe[27] has pulled this somewhat disused distinction between actual neuroses and psychoneuroses from under the dust, giving it a modern twist. Neurosis, perversion and psychopathy in their clinical manifestation are situated between the two ends of a spectrum going from actual- to psychopathology. There is insufficient psychic processing of the Real, drive and trauma at the actual neurotic pole. Unbound energies, therefore, exert a disruptive effect on physical and psychosexual functioning. He situates severe (including borderline) personality disorders in this model on the actual pathological side of neurosis. They are the result of structural (the drive) and/ or accidental trauma (e.g. molestation or sexual abuse) that have been insufficiently processed and become 'bound'.[28] I return to this distinction. They both create an unbearable 'load' that the patient walks around with and wants to get *rid of* in all sorts of possible and impossible ways.

Fonagy and Target[29] make a similar distinction between mental representational disorders and mental process disorders. While classical psychoanalysis addresses conflicting intrapsychic *contents* in the former through free association and interpretation, in the latter, psychoanalytic work will have to focus more on facilitating mental processes, leading to construction and 'subject amplification', in which (*dixit* Verhaeghe) parental mirroring has to be redone.[30] Only in this way can a capacity for mentalisation develop in so-called 'early' disorders in connection with a more secure attachment. This is a necessary (yet insufficient) condition for subject development, just as a solid violin must first be built before it can find its tone.[31]

4 Primaeval Time

To clarify this further, we return briefly to the mythical primordial time of the infant. Both Freud[32] and Lacan[33] draw attention to the helplessness and physiological immaturity of the human child. In Winnicott's terms, the child's first period of life is indeed characterised by 'absolute dependence'.[34] Hence at a meeting of the British Psychoanalytic Society, his somewhat vehement exclamation 'There is no such thing as a baby!'[35] He alluded to the simultaneously manifest yet often misunderstood dependence on the 'primary maternal preoccupation'[36] of the mother. According to him, it is a state of grace that allows the mother to identify almost entirely with her child, without which the infant cannot develop optimally psychologically.[37]

The starting point of human development is an original painful or unpleasurable experience from our prehistoric times, a '*Schmerz*' resulting from a physiological need, distress or lack. Hunger and thirst are the primary forms. Freud understands this painful experience[38] as a quantitative tension accumulation whose stimuli breach the stimulus shield formed by the first big Other (usually the mother). Moreover, these stimuli come from within, so defence is impossible, and flight altogether (even motorically) is impossible.[39] The infant's reaction is prototypical and determines all its later interpersonal relationships. The helpless infant addresses the big Other through the cry, and the big Other must provide the 'specific action'[40] by which the inner discontent is lifted. Such intervention by the big Other will always consist of actions and words showing that the Other understands and responds to the child's appeal. The child receives from the big Other images and words for what is going on internally.

It is the basic form of drive and trauma where something cannot be worked on in the absence of an appropriate answer from the Other. This gives rise to automatic or traumatic anxiety,[41] which is attributed to and 'blamed' on the Other. Abandonment rage and depression are related to it. Indeed, when the big Other is missing, they are held responsible for perpetuating inner tension. In this way, arousal acquires an intersubjective as well as a psychosexual[42] dimension from the start. The need articulated in a cry becomes a demand. This demand finally (and beyond the need to be satisfied) becomes a demand for love. At the same time, the physical unpleasure, on the other hand, becomes a psychic suffering as soon as the big Other does not appear on the appeal. It is the primary form of drive and trauma in which something from the Real of the body (in the absence of an appropriate response from the big Other) is not worked on or 'bound'.

The human child is thrown into the world in absolute helplessness and physical immaturity. For its survival, it is, in the first instance, totally dependent on the care and protection, on the power and intervention of the big Other. With every need, stimulus or urge, the human child can only appeal to the Other through a cry (for help). On top of this dependence on the big Other, a second dependence superimposes itself. As soon as the big Other satisfies the need, protects against the stimulus or mediates against the arousal, they immediately make the human child dependent on the law of language. This law of language is characterised above all by installing a lack. For the word, by definition, establishes something present that is absent: *'le mot est déjà une présence faite d'absence'.* [43] Because of this double dependency, a complex interpenetration arises in our human primordial age between three things that are determinant for the further course of life:[44] firstly, one's natural disposition and drives; secondly, the attachment to and relationship with the first significant others (the big Other), and thirdly, their linguistic and (micro-) cultural response based on which the human child begins its historiography. By mirroring her child, the mother gives the child an illusion of security, mastery, and identity. Through these illusions, the reality characterised by puny and powerless helplessness is, as it were, covered under a cloak of love, and the dimension of hope can take root once and for all.

5 Demand and Answer

On the other hand, the human child's question will never be fully satisfied or answered. However much the big Other endeavours to bring about complete satisfaction, a lack will still arise this first time, a deficit. Moreover, the big Other also lacks something and longs for some Thing other than fully satisfying the child's needs! The human child needs two things to achieve optimal development. First, it needs sufficient mirroring and 'nourishment' to mature and endure frustration. If not, the absence of the breast is such an unbearable sensation that the child can only evacuate the bad (because absent) breast, that is, try to get rid of it in every possible and impossible way. If, on the other hand, the child has received sufficient mental nourishment from the big Other, thinking can arise: a thought for a no-thing.[45]

Equally and at the same time, on the other hand, the child needs sufficient lack and difference so that this dimension of thought and desire can open up. This is provided by the father, who, with his law, drives a wedge between mother and child. He thus protects the child from this all-powerful and devouring (first) big Other to which it would otherwise be defenceless. Indeed, absolute dependence is always also accompanied by a great fear, namely the fear of being devoured or sucked up by the big Other. Winnicott speaks of the 'fear of WOMAN' in this context[46] and, in a Lacanian view, it is the fear of loss of self and subject when we are at the mercy of the abyssal enjoyment of the big Other (*'la jouissance de l'Autre'*).[47]

To answer its arousal, the child turns to the first big Other. Together with a first drive regulation, it thereby arrives at a first dual and pre-oedipal mirror identity. Only when the register of the demand (for love) and separation is sufficiently digested and dissolved can separation anxiety give way to a *desire* for separation. This is made possible by the subsequent oedipal triangular relationship: the second big Other (usually the father) appears in front of the child, opening the dimension of difference between the child, the first Other and the second Other and creating a possibility of choice.[48] This will manifest itself, among other things, in male or female sexuation (the gender difference), based on which the earlier primordial time is retroactively 'phallicised'.

Whether and how the first big Other responds to the inner need of the human child will determine the foundations of the personality and especially its drive regulation and identity development. Indeed, a representative system consists of an image of self and others, crystallised around the child's experienced *'arousal'* or stimulation.[49] Depending on the theory, this involves an 'inner working model' (John Bowbly),[50] a cognitive scheme (Wilma Bucci),[51] a 'self–other–affect triad' (Otto Kernberg),[52] proto-narrative envelopes/schemes of togetherness (Daniel Stern),[53] a particular attachment pattern (Mary Main)[54] and so on, which (under the form of a primal transference)[55] determine our way of being-in-the-world.

In actual pathology, the problem is usually already situated at this level. The domain of the so-called nonspecific therapeutic factors plays a leading role in any form of psychotherapy. Positive acceptance, commitment, truthfulness, sustaining a trusting relationship and the professional role through good and bad days. We will see that this domain was conceptually, clinically and psychotherapeutically mapped mainly by Anglo-Saxon psychoanalysis (Klein, Winnicott and Bion). There is, however, something significant to reiterate in this context. After all, even if that first big Other *does* mediate sufficiently and responsively, the 'answer' always falls short. There is never a perfect match between arousal and answer. Something is always missed, and there is always something wrong. It is in that gap that the dimension of desire installs itself.[56] Hence, Freud states that it is as if our children have remained forever unsatisfied. To which we can add: and have become desiring: desiring for that something (or -Thing) lacking.

6 Losing our Mind

As a biopsy of contemporary society, let's take the front page of a quality newspaper that reads in bold letters: 'Nearly three million Belgians with brain disorders'.[57] Every so often, the media also report that the incidence of suicide and depression is on the rise.[58] In fact, according to the World Health Organisation, depression is the most significant health threat in the Western world. By selling a 19th-century view (mental illnesses are brain diseases)[59] as old wine in new bottles, the illusion is created that all this mental suffering belongs to the domain of medicine. Now, everyone is over the moon about scientific and technological medical advances. Sometimes with the aid of new joints, blood vessels or other parts, life expectancy in most Western countries has increased by about twenty years since World War II. Psychiatry also participated in these developments. Since the 1950s and 1960s, there has been the discovery and emergence of psychopharmaceuticals for major psychiatric disorders (depression, mania, schizophrenia and so on). Their efficacy was exhaustively scientifically proven. The quality of life of millions of psychiatric patients has risen very appreciably, thanks in part to the judicious use of these drugs. However, with this have come persistent misconceptions. First, there is a misconception about causality. It is not because aspirin helps against pain, fever and/or inflammation that these are *caused* (let alone purely and simply) by a lack of aspirin in our bodies. Nor is it because demonstrable imbalances occur in our brain's neurotransmission in psychiatric disorders that this is necessary, let alone a sufficient condition to explain psychopathology.

More generally, a pronounced medicalisation of happiness and well-being is underway. Biological-genetic determinism increasingly resembles an ideology. It is a discourse and a practice whose intentions and sources remain hidden from the public and whose own assumptions are still hardly questioned. The powerful and wealthy medical industry of the pharmaceutical, technology and 'managed care' lobby holds the strings behind the scenes and determines which scientific research is funded. An overriding medical model equates health with absence and illness with the presence of symptoms. The fact that symptoms are, by definition, surface phenomena of a more profound process is neglected. Deep, personal and/or existential suffering is reduced (like appendicitis) to a medical problem addressed by technicians who reduce the patient to a vessel of symptoms to be eradicated. All psychological suffering, in this view, is biologically based and can be eliminated by medication, thanks to which our adaptability and productivity are increased. Against this background, it is almost heretical to postulate that suffering makes us wiser and can open up new possibilities. To reach heaven with our branches, our roots must go as far as hell. Or perhaps we may refer to an aphorism by French moralist Cioran: '*C'est par la souffrance, par elle seule, qu'on cesse d'être une marionnette*'.[60]

The last century ended with the decade of the brain. Cognitive and neuroscience made great leaps forward, providing insights into memory, brain molecular biology and neuroplasticity. It can finally be shown that environmental factors influence the structure and function of the brain. Various functional brain imaging techniques (such as PET scans and MRI) have successfully visualised the brain's anatomy and functioning. The advantage is that the (by definition invisible) world of the psychic, thoughts, feelings and fantasies can be made visible and tangible. Psychiatry could finally sit at the table with its big brothers of natural science and have a say in honest and serious matters. After all, medicine has traditionally treated the psychic/invisible as a stepmother: what transcends the visible is, therefore, unreal.[61]

Medicine/psychiatry is a discipline of the eye, whereas psychoanalysis is a discipline of the ear. This increased and visualised neuroscientific knowledge leads to situating but not understanding psychic activity.[62] This, then, is the difficult question in the brain–mind dilemma.[63] There is a radical and unresolvable alterity between natural science and mental science, which the phenomenological psychiatrist Karl Jaspers translated into the distinction between explaining and understanding, between '*erklären*' and '*verstehen*'.[64] If causal relations are the object of the former, then intelligible coherences are the latter's object. The two psychologies are not mutually exclusive but overlap. However, it should be stated that explanatory or objective psychology works with objective data and, in consequence, leads to a psychology without a psyche. We are reminded of what the famous neurologist and best-selling author Oliver Sacks observes: 'Neuropsychology is admirable, but it excludes the psyche'.[65] It is the asymmetry between explaining and understanding that constitutes the central and foundational gap of psychiatry as well as of the subject.[66]

In an interview, Hungarian writer Gyorgy Konrad says (in the context of the war in former Yugoslavia) that nationality and identity do not exist for him. According to him, there is only a story and history. We will see that in Lacanian[67] terms, the imaginary (mirror) identity is purely illusory and presents us with the dreamed unity of the (ideal) image. Therefore, the imaginary domain is primarily the domain of resistance.[68] The Imaginary disregards the fact that the Real drives us, and the symbolic discourse of the big Other determines us. The question is whether the present age does not mean, besides the end of the Grand Narrative, the end of the *petite histoire*. The *ahistoricism* denounced by Lacan seems to be increasing rather than decreasing, absorbed as we are by the light speeds of current events. Everyone's subjectivity comes about in the ever-private encounter between nature and culture. A time without ears for this hidden and invisible history is synonymous with a time that loses its mind.

Notes

1 '*De hominis dignitate*' (1486). At the age of 23, Pico wrote a manifesto consisting of 900 theses on philosophy, religion, physics, etc.
2 Jean-Jacques Rousseau (1754).
3 In Sartre's terminology, the animal is *a being; it* is '*être*'. On the other hand, man is *nothing*, is '*néant*' and can *become* anything precisely because of that (Sartre, 1943).

4   Donald Winnicott (1960 p 46).
5   Sartre (1970) compares the animal to a letter opener in a famous example. Its design determines its entire existence. *'L'essence précède l'existence'*. Not so with humans: *'L'existence précède l'essence'*.
6   'Values are both external ("objective") and internal ("subjective"). As "external points of reference", they enable a good human life in particular circumstances' (Kienstra, 2020 p 253–259).
7   See the myth of Epimetheus and Prometheus in Plato's *Protagoras*.
8   André Green (1995a).
9   In natural causality, there is proportionality. Not so in the psychic, where some endure disaster unscathed while others are broken from a pea under mattresses.
10 Antoine Mooij (2002 p 17–21).
11 Peter Watson (2001 p 440).
12 Luc Ferry (2009). Also concerning (mental) health, person-centred *care* is giving way to disorder-centred *technique*.
13 See Jan Hendrik van den Berg's *Metabletica*: Historical Phenomenology of Cultural Phenomena (1960).
14 Elisabeth Badinter (1998).
15 Michel Foucault (1961).
16 From Freud's prewar Vienna.
17 Christopher Lasch (1979) and Erik Ceysens (2005).
18 Personality disorder is a durable pattern of inner experiences and behaviours that manifests in multiple life domains and leads to suffering or limitations in psychosocial functioning (Vermote 2000).
19 Reeling off unbearable and/or unthinkable mental contents in all sorts of possible and impossible ways.
20 When the roots are in yourself, you can settle anywhere. For mentalisation: see later in this book.
21 Sigmund Freud (1896).
22 Actual neuroses were divided by Freud into anxiety neurosis, neurasthenia and hypochondria. The second corresponds strikingly to chronic fatigue syndrome or fibromyalgia, in which a cluster of symptoms is promoted to a disorder/syndrome.
23 Sigmund Freud (1916–1917).
24 There is an opaque core in both the symptom and the dream. The navel is a trace of what is invisible and memorialises prehistoric separation. Literal separation from the placenta and-more generally-figurative separation from our mother nature. With Jacques Lacan, we will explain that at the logical and mythical moment of our entry into language, the (maternal) Thing is simultaneously killed and born.
25 Sigmund Freud (1900 p 609).
26 Sigmund Freud (1905b p 112).
27 Paul Verhaeghe (2002).
28 Paul Verhaeghe (1997). For a recent comprehensive review on borderline (diagnosis, etiology, treatment etc.) see Leichsenring et al. (2024).
29 Peter Fonagy & Mary Target (2003a).
30 Paul Verhaeghe (2002 p 258).
31 Cluckers & Meurs (2005 p 25).
32 Sigmund Freud (1923a).
33 Jacques Lacan (1949) in (1966 p 93–100).
34 Donald Winnicott, (1960 p 46).
35 Donald Winnicott (1952 p 99).
36 Donald Winnicott (1956).

37 Empathy plays an *essential role* in all forms of psychotherapy.
38 Sigmund Freud, '*The design*' (1895 p 4–11).
39 For details, see Paul Verhaeghe (ibidem p 133–137).
40 Sigmund Freud (1926a p 224–228).
41 Which other authors capture in other terms, e.g. Bion's 'nameless dread', Winnicott's 'primitive agony', etc. For further elaboration, see, e.g. Kinet, 2008.
42 On need satisfaction, pleasure grafts itself. She is polymorphically perverted from both sides.
43 Jacques Lacan (1953) in (1966 p 276).
44 See later in this book: the three Lacanian registers of the Real, the Imaginary and the Symbolic.
45 Wilfred Bion (1962 p 110–119).
46 Donald Winnicott (1950 p 252).
47 When discussing Lacanian *jouissance*, I will henceforth use the somewhat archaic term enjoyment. *Jouissance* can initially be defined pragmatically as the unconscious benefit that specific behaviour provides so that it persists even when it is no longer 'healthy' (or even harmful/lethal) (Evans, 2006 p 92; Lacan, 1986 p 209).
48 The child recognises himself in the mirror/other-equal. Making a difference requires a symbolic 'third'.
49 Peter Fonagy et al. (2002 p 36–37).
50 John Bowlby (1988).
51 Wilma Bucci (1997).
52 Otto Kernberg (1976).
53 See also the RIGs 'representations of interactions generalised' (Stern, 1985).
54 Main & Goldwyn (1995).
55 (Early) childhood relationships that are (distorted) from unconscious/implicit memory.
56 Philippe Van Haute (2000 p 102–108).
57 Front page of *De Morgen*, 3.05.05, where depression and anxiety disorders appear alongside, for example, brain tumours, migraine and multiple sclerosis. See Andlin-Sobocki et al. (2005).
58 Every year, 5% to 7% suffer from depression. 15% men and 20% women suffer from depression in the course of life, see Corveleyn, Luyten and Blatt (2005).
59 Wilhelm Griesinger: '*Geisteskrankheiten sind Gehirnkrankheiten*'. See Hoff & Hippius (2001).
60 Emil Cioran (1986). It is only by suffering that we cease to be a puppet on a string.
61 L. Heyde (2000 p 61): 'What transcends visibility – the free subjectivity itself, the secret of its being – becomes *unreal*.'
62 Andreas De Block and Paul Moyaert (2004 p 117).
63 David Chalmers calls correlating psychological symptoms to a neurological substrate/process the *easy* questions (1995).
64 Karl Jaspers (1913 p 253 ff).
65 Oliver Sacks (1984 p 164). For a detailed discussion of a neuropsychoanalysis that avoids this shortcoming (Kinet, 2022, 2023).
66 Erik Nieweg (2005a).
67 Jacques Lacan (1949) in (1966 p 93–100).
68 Frédéric Declercq (2000 p 16).

Chapter 5

A Moving Science
Conversation and Contradiction

I Medical Psychoanalysis?

In his technical writings between 1911 and 1915, Freud repeatedly refers to the doctor when discussing the psychoanalyst, thereby unquestioningly including the analytical work in medicine and psychiatry. To him, psychoanalysis is an empirical science:[1] it conducts experiments *in vivo* with a single person whose reactions to interpretations are tested against ever-evolving and refining pathogenetic hypotheses. He did complain that psychiatry and psychoanalysis did not know each other well enough. He took a different stance in 1926 when, on the occasion of a complaint against Theodor Reik, he made a comprehensive plea for the admission of non-medics to the psychoanalytic society.[2] In this context, he argues that the analyst has as much, if not more, to learn from literature, art and philosophy than they could draw on medical knowledge for their analytical work.[3] Psychoanalysis moves more and more to the level of philosophical anthropology, which is the foundation of the human sciences. The analyst becomes a pastoralist with a domain more extensive than the church and the consulting room combined.[4]

Meanwhile, in contrast to North American psychoanalysis (which, with Egopsychology,[5] has always remained a stronghold of predominantly medicalised psychoanalysis), particularly on our old continent, an increasing distance from the natural sciences emerged. There, psychoanalysis found more connection with the (more or less philosophically inclined) humanities. However pertinent Freud's arguments for lay analysis may be, this all resulted in a decreasing familiarity of its practitioners with psychiatry and (neuro-) biology. Moreover, the Lacanian movement, in particular, militantly opposed an overly naive biologism and an adaptationist ideology inherent to it. Jacques Lacan denounced the American 'managers of the soul'.[6] To him, their pursuit of happiness and belief in an autonomous and conflict-free Ego meant no more or less than a negation[7] of psychoanalysis. When invited to the United States, had Freud not compared psychoanalysis to bringing in the plague?[8] Was not the essentially subversive nature of drive and infantile

DOI: 10.4324/9781032698052-6

sexuality, for example, misunderstood and obscured by the blind spot that is the (American) Ego?

While in Europe, psychiatry was very much dominated by the nosologists (Emil Kraepelin, Eugen Bleuler, Kurt Schneider et al.) and the phenomenologists (Karl Jaspers, H.C. Rümke et al.), American psychiatry increasingly fell under the spell of this adaptation-oriented psychoanalysis. Even before World War II, it had been widely accepted as a treatment for neuroses. In the absence of a (neuro-) biological explanation and an effective treatment, it also went on to provide a pathogenetic theory for the psychoses. The 1950s were (in a nostalgic formulation by Wallerstein)[9] the 'halcyon days' of psychoanalysis in America. Medical schools recruited psychoanalysts to head the psychiatric department, psychodynamics was promoted as the model of explanation in psychiatry, and various forms of outpatient and residential psychoanalytic therapy emerged for the more severe forms of psychological suffering.[10] With some delay, similar developments also occurred in Europe in the 1960s and 1970s.

2 DSM

Meanwhile, however, the first psychopharmaceuticals had their spectacular premiere in the treatment of major psychiatric mood- and psychotic disorders. On the other hand, psychoanalytic forms of treatment were shown to be less effective for psychoses than supportive and structure-building ones.[11] The pathogenetic explanation for psychiatric disorders was increasingly being sought in disturbed neurotransmission in the brain, and drugs acting on this appeared to support this line of thought by their demonstrable efficacy. Biological psychiatry rapidly took the dominant place instead of psychodynamic psychiatry. Worldwide, the quality of life of psychiatric patients has improved considerably. Not insignificantly, effectiveness research sponsored by the pharmaceutical industry soon gave this discipline a highly scientific and 'medical' allure. All the more so as it contrasted sharply with the perceived illegitimacy of psychoanalysis. After all, the latter was characterised by unproven scientific claims and, on the contrary, relied mainly on authority arguments referring to charismatic figures. A virtually non-existent therapeutic effect in terms of schizophrenia treatment also seriously discredited its efficacy for neurotic disorders. Moreover, it failed to substantiate its basic concepts and effectiveness scientifically.[12]

Partly with a view to scientific research (in which 'homogeneity' of the studied target group is essential), the American Psychiatric Association drew up a *Diagnostic and Statistical Manual of Mental Disorders* at the end of the 1970s, which would further define psychiatry's profile. This DSM (now in its fifth edition) gives a descriptive account of certain disorders. Its diagnostics are a-theoretical and a-etiological. It categorically distinguishes entities and between normality and pathology.[13] This while, according to current clinical and empirical insights, a dimensional approach is more appropriate for psychopathology that is always multiconditional and situated on a continuum opposite normality.[14] Neuroses (the pre-eminent domain of classical psychoanalysis) have all but disappeared from the DSM.[15] The symptom as a symbolic construct and as an (unsuccessful) compromise for intrapsychic and childhood and adolescent conflicts also went up in smoke in the process. In its place have come various depressive, anxiety and personality disorders that appear out of nowhere, as it were, or are attributed to the *'endon'* [16] or scoreable life events.[17] In both cases, the patient is implicitly reduced to suffering passively. Nowhere are the precise pathogenetic mechanisms of these disorders addressed, despite the obvious therapeutic opportunities this would offer. That all this has to be understood in connection with life history also disappears from the agenda.

Compared to the former nosology, DSM classification is highly imprecise. Suppose the botanist stated that if *x* of the *y* following descriptive characteristics are fulfilled, a plant is a foxglove. This is how many psychiatric diagnoses are made according to DSM criteria. In use, this DSM finally leads to excesses of 'co-morbidity',[18] which is nevertheless more the rule than the exception about psychopathology.[19] Understanding the more profound, underlying coherence underlying the surface phenomena (that symptoms are, by definition) seems superfluous. This diagnostic bible is perfectly tailored to biological treatments because psychopharmaceuticals do not address disease states but symptoms. It is also tailored to (cognitive or other) behavioural therapy. After all, both focus on symptoms, the severity of which is assumed to be quantifiable by all kinds of tests and measuring instruments before and after treatment.[20] As a result, both also lend themselves perfectly to the *randomised controlled trials* (RCTs) promoted to be a *passe-partout,* as they have now become nearly the main criterion for assessing the scientific validity of a treatment.[21] However, all research indicates that dimensions not addressed in the RCT (such as patient and therapist characteristics, but especially the therapeutic relationship) are of the utmost importance for efficacy.[22]

Moreover, an increasing 'treatment-prevalence paradox' is occurring in contemporary mental health care: treatments have improved, and their availability has increased, but the prevalence of depression, for example, has not declined. There is 'fairly strong' evidence that this is due to two factors.[23] First the efficacy of RCT treatment is overestimated in day-to-day (not experimental but naturalistic) practice, which, after all, and second, is often characterised by complex, relapsing and chronic psychopathology. Partly due to the DSM, mental health care has come to regard mental problems as diagnosable disorders. EBP is guided by symptom reduction at the group level and should orient 'expert' treatment. This model is currently under debate. It might be disconnected from what the patient needs, it is blind to the trans-diagnostic nature of mental health problems, and it overestimates the importance of technical intervention compared to relational and ritual aspects of treatment. Last but not least, this model underestimates its applicability in moving from a collective-statistical to an individual-clinical logic.[24] After more than half a century of research and many thousands of RCT studies, the 'trillion-dollar brain drain' caused by mental problems is not remediated by the treatments offered today.[25]

3 The Human Factor

Psychoanalytic forms of treatment are more person- and experience-oriented than symptom- and behaviour-oriented. The particularity of each person's life story plays an essential role, and the methodology of the RCT is challenging to apply.[26] Psychoanalytic forms of treatment are characterised by a tragic view of the human condition that differs radically from the medical or behavioural therapeutic perspectives.[27] After all, in a sense, both medicine and behavioural therapy view humans as rational beings. Irrational schemas may mislead us, but it is believed that the power of reason and rationality can change us. Implicitly, this assumes a ready and clear distinction between rational and irrational, healthy and unhealthy, normal and abnormal. Another characteristic is great therapeutic optimism: with the 'right' pill or technique, the problem is solved. For psychoanalysis, on the other hand, there is essentially a continuum between normality and psychopathology. According to it, human beings will always be 'disturbed' by drive, conflict and frustration, which are an integral part of the human condition. What is a rational, healthy way to deal with the death of a loved one? Which of the 'fifty ways to leave your lover' is right?

The therapeutic process is not only about *Enlightenment* through reason and rationality (insight and interpretation) but also about what, since Franz Alexander,[28] has been called the corrective emotional experience or 'learning from experience'[29] in the psychoanalytic relationship.[30] The result of the hegemony of the medical and behavioural therapeutic model, meanwhile, is that much psychiatric professional literature is quietly bulging with tables and charts. They comprise the 'strength' of medicinal or behavioural therapeutic (symptom) treatment. Through these (natural) scientific views, they have effortlessly conquered the world of government and managed care (with their focus on social 'profit'). Indeed, evidence-based psychiatry (EBP), with its empirically supported treatments (EST), was born out of this practice. Sad is it when they are offered one-size-fits-all,[31] i.e. standardised and under the form of treatment protocols, to anyone with a specific 'diagnosis', i.e. disorder- and not patient-centred. This is the case with many short-term, 'solution-focused' (crisis) interventions. The outcome of this type of symptom-focused treatment is limited and transient, as has been amply demonstrated.[32] Well understood, however, such treatments should instead lead to integrating individual clinical experience and respect for increasingly private and complex therapeutic practice on the one hand with the best external scientific knowledge on the other. As such, they can help eliminate arbitrariness disguised as therapeutic freedom. The scientific prestige of psychiatry has risen sharply in recent decades thanks to convincing research. By thoughtfully factoring in the guidelines of an EBP, the danger of over-reaching and/or idiosyncratic practice can be avoided. In contrast, if applied automatically and uncritically, they will inevitably and dehumanisingly tyrannise the care and treatment to be always tailored.[33] Meanwhile, a lot of psychiatric and neurobiological findings often provide highly relevant data for psychoanalytic forms of treatment.[34]

4 Daughter of Science

Most commonly, 'science' refers to the rational experimentalism that became dominant in the 19th century. It is a body of knowledge organised by a coherent and orderly combination of fundamental concepts and explains empirically established phenomena. These phenomena are objects of possible experimentation, and a method is consistently employed that makes these phenomena comprehensible and testable in controlled reproduction. From this point of view, a death sentence on psychoanalysis as a science has already been pronounced countless times.[35] However, the question of whether psychoanalysis is a science *at all* depends entirely on its definition, and this definition is also currently highly controversial among scientists themselves.[36] If science is defined as an attempt to establish causal links between events, one may question whether the concept of causality can be applied to living beings with consciousness.[37] For some philosophers of science, the assumptions of psychoanalysis are neither confirmable nor falsifiable and, therefore, do not meet scientific requirements. However, if science is defined as knowledge derived from experimentation and measurability, psychoanalytic treatment forms[38] has provided abundant convincing effectiveness research[39] in recent years. If we restrict science to systematised and formulated knowledge, psychoanalysis can naturally and unquestioningly claim scientific status. Moreover, is it not an attitude that constantly questions everything and does not offer/seek certainty, 'grip' or reassurance, which is the most characteristic of the true scientist?

In the late 19th century, Wilhelm Dilthey[40] foregrounded the distinction between the human and natural sciences. In any case, psychiatry and psychoanalysis uncomfortably bestride[41] these two. The right, the exact, is the norm in the natural sciences. In a pointed formulation by Lacan, it is about bringing the measurable into the Real.[42] Nevertheless, with Harry Mülisch,[43] we can ask how best to grasp, for example, a crime against humanity like the Holocaust. By statistics about six million dead Jews or by the diary of that one girl, Anne Frank. By the logic of big numbers or the particularity of n = 1. According to Lacan, psychoanalysis is, at most, a daughter of science,[44] albeit with a scientific vocation. As a science of the unreasonable, it is based on rational dialogue even when reason clashes with the limits of madness.

Like any science worthy of the name, psychoanalysis is also in evolution. It is characterised by ever-advancing and changing insights in response to impasses. From generation to generation, psychological processes of individuation and separation come into play alongside scientific ones.[45] Unlike other sciences, psychoanalysis does not try to exclude subjectivity but to analyse it. No doubt Freud's Oedipus complex and the depressive position of Klein[46] and Lacan's Name-of-the-Father[47] have become theoretical cornerstone abstractions from their personal lives. Thousands of analysts with and after them have explored not only the unconscious of others but also that of themselves.[48] In doing so, they have often made it a matter of (scientific) honour and their desire as analysts to leave no blind spot untouched.

We must and can take much from our parents and other teachers. We cannot (and, thankfully, do not have to) experience everything ourselves. Within a (transference) love towards parent figures, we 'believe' to a certain extent in their experience and authority, with which we nurture ourselves. After more than a century of psychoanalysis and millions of pages of scientific publications (in its field alone), every analyst hesitantly tries to find their way through the largely accidental (because they are bound to time, space, language and culture) and all-too-limited encounters with and words from their psychoanalytic parents. Like any analysant,[49] however, they need to detach themself from these transference figures, find their way and find their answer to the confrontation with the Real/the *Thing-in-itself*. Achieving this requires moments when they have to leave the convention of their group/ association/the Establishment[50] and go beyond the level of identification (with their analyst 'parents').[51] However, even when they try to reach this point (which is always a point of anxiety), it remains – however paradoxically – a dream. It is the dream of ever fully waking up and grasping the immediacy of the Real: the dream of an absolute awakening.[52]

5 Unconscious Known

Psychoanalysis is a movement and a science, and these are, as said, two completely different things.[53] It is also a practice that sometimes has the character of surgical or archaeological exploration,[54] then again of a detective, and finally is to be regarded as a mystically poetic encounter with a sample size of 1 in psychoanalytic space. We will see that according to Lacan, the analyst takes the place of the object small a to keep the engine of free association running as the object-cause of their analysant's desire. Bion will argue that they must move into O without memory, desire or understanding to enable true transformation.[55] For both, this always and by definition means that both parties must leave the comfort of the known and familiar. Only thus do moments of invention, creation and truth become possible. However, while this pre-eminently analytical position is the indispensable essence and *primum movens* of its practice, it can rarely be reduced to this. In all psychoanalytic encounters, psychotherapeutic and psychoanalytic moments, psychoanalytic and master discourse, deconstruction and construction alternate. Therefore, psychoanalysis is neither the servant of psychiatry nor should it be reduced to a kind of esoteric quest for 'truth'. It is neither medicine nor philosophy. Grounded primarily in clinical practice and constant and critical dialogue with its surrounding sciences, it sheds light on the unconscious in psychological and psychopathological phenomena. Its ethics is not aimed at normalisation or moralisation but at human tragicomedy's mental or emotional processing. Insofar as it wishes to retain its significance within the field of psychotherapy, however, it must be sufficiently connected to psychiatry's prevailing scientific framework of thought and intervention.[56] If not, it risks falling into the corner of so-called alternative therapies.

Psychoanalysis does not only develop knowledge about the unconscious: psychodynamics, psychic causality, a psychotherapeutic method and technique, etc. It is, above all, a science of the singular situation that arises in every psychoanalytic encounter.[57] Furthermore, in this situation, the desire to know (however paradoxical) can be precisely at the service of the passion of ignorance. Indeed, in the realm of the psychic, it is paradoxically knowledge (about diagnosis, reason and so on) that 'drains' truth from the subject.[58] Instead, knowledge must be drained to leave room for an unconscious truth. This unconscious 'known' can only come into its own in the psychoanalytic situation and on behalf of both parties. When Robert Wallerstein[59] asks whether there is 'one psychoanalysis or many', we can answer: 'many' and as many as there are analysants and analysts. Freud said it literally: no golden rule fits all; each must find out in what private ways they can be saved.[60] Within the psychoanalytic space, community differences stop giving way to the 'absolute difference'[61] the analyst wants to make.

Wilfred Bion, in his theory of psychoanalytic technique, not only points to the fact that the analyst must move into O to be receptive to thoughts in search of a thinker. He also emphasises the role of the analyst's subjectivity and imagination reflected in his provisional understanding. Sometimes, he compares interpretation to second thoughts. Other times, he considers it an imaginary conjecture about missing pages in a book.[62] However, these suspicions and guesses are then prompted by prolonged listening (a trademark of any psychoanalytic work) and by opening up to the psychic and affective reality of the total transference situation.[63] In his clinical work with psychotic patients, he describes the confrontation with the rawness of the Real, with black holes, bizarre objects and a beta-screen of de-symbolised *débris*.[64] In a Bionian view, psychotics are the orphans of the Real[65] and contact with them is possible only if the analyst dares to venture (with them) into the un-land of O to tame wild thoughts there.[66] It is fair to say that 'typical Anglo-Saxon' empirical positivism somewhat gives way to an imaginary proliferation here.

Jacques Lacan, for his part, argues that we should approach the words of the analysant as Holy Scripture. Following Freud's example,[67] he gives great importance to a rigorous analysis of the signifier's laws. He fundamentally distrusts the (for him, imaginary) dimension of understanding.[68] Often, the Lacanian analyst will limit themself (especially in the first analysis phase) to rather 'dry' interventions, such as repetition and punctuation. According to him, the ideal position of the analyst is that of *le mort* in the game of bridge.[69] After all, the analyst should not make themselves present (e.g. in the form of more or less shrewd interpretations) but the big Other:[70] they merely let the analysant hear what – while thinking aloud – escaped their reasoning.[71] Well then, such views on psychoanalytic technique may well strike the cure in the neurotic patient, but in this, do we not recognise the sober view of the exact scientist?

Besides the Real and the Symbolic, we have the imaginary order. It is a dimension Bion honoured and seems reviled by Lacan.[72] The psychotherapeutic importance of this dimension is different depending on whether it is actual pathology vs psychopathology, with their respective need for construction and subject amplification[73] on the one hand and their need for deconstruction and interpretation on the other. In the first case, the problem is that the dam against the Real of drive and trauma has not yet been adequately formed, and drive and trauma are disruptive and overspilling. In the second case, the dam is so layered and rigid that, conversely, nostalgia arises for the surf and waves. According to American Bionian James Grotstein, the psychotic takes O (truth) for K (knowing), and the neurotic takes K (knowing) for O (truth).[74] In the next part of this book, we will explore in more detail what inspiration Freud and co. can offer to mediate and remedy the 'K.O.' of many psychiatric patients and thus enable truly psychoanalytic work.

Notes

1 Jaap Ubbels (2000 p 136).
2 Sigmund Freud (1926b).
3 He opposes medical studies for daughter Anna and encourages her towards lay analysis (Gay, 1989 p 397).
4 Willem Van Tilburg (2000 p 114) or Freud's letter to Oskar Pfister dated 25/11/1928: 'lay curers of souls who need not be doctors and should not be priests' (Grotjahn, 1963).
5 Anna Freud, Heinz Hartmann, Kris and Löwenstein considered the 'autonomous Ego' that would be naturally oriented towards adaptation. The American school is most in Freud's natural science line, see Neville Symington (1986, p 60).
6 Jacques Lacan (1955b) in (1966 p 403).
7 Jacques Lacan (ibidem p 416).
8 Jacques Lacan (1955b).
9 Robert Wallerstein (2002 p 1248).
10 Dixit Freud: In the eyes of Americans, 'analysis is nothing but one of the *servants* of psychiatry' (my italics) in Peter Gay (1989 p 572).
11 Gunderson et al. (1984).
12 Gunderson and Gabbard (1999) and Bornstein (2001) hold psychoanalysis responsible for its marginal position.
13 The descriptive, atheoretical, categorical, non-developmental and disorder-centred approach is at odds with psychoanalytic models, e.g. the Psychodynamic

Diagnostic Manual (2006) which is more theory-driven, more person- and development-centred (Blatt & Luyten, 2010) and strongly emphasises continuity between normality and pathology (McWilliams, 2011).

14 'DSM appears not to "carve nature at its joints" but rather introduces sharp distinctions where they do not, in reality, exist,' See Corveleyn, Luyten and Blatt (2005 p 254). Moreover, there is an inextricable link between symptomatology (axis I pathology) and personality (axis II pathology). For the reification caused by DSM, see Vanheule (2015).

15 Freud sees 3 main causes of neuroses. 1) the biological helplessness and dependence of the human child installs the earliest dangerous situations and triggers the lifelong need for love. 2) The fact that our sexuality proceeds phylogenetically in two times and that in the first period, infantile sexuality represents an internal danger, as it were. 3) that the 'Ego' can only defend itself by curtailing its activity and creating symptoms in exchange for the frustration of temper claims. (Freud, 1926a p 155–156).

16 As difficult to specify 'predisposition'.

17 Marriage, birth, divorce, death, then get a fixed (and supposedly for everyone) 'score'.

18 For example, 'major depression, recurrent with melancholy and without psychotic symptoms, dysthymic disorder mixed neurotic and abandonment type, posttraumatic stress disorder, sexual aversion, impulse control disorder unspecified and histrionic borderline personality.' Which (of course) should all be understood in interrelationship with (early) childhood experiences.

19 Westen et al. (2004) or Corveleyn, Luyten and Blatt (ibid p 8) and see infra.

20 Mattias Desmet (2018) is critical about the Likert scale, which only creates an illusion of objectivity that threatens to make psychology a pseudoscience. Moreover, psychoanalysts do employ very particular (and hardly measurable) objectives.

21 Patrick Luyten and Nicole Vliegen (2005) in their critique of the medical model and canonisation of impact research.

22 Corveleyn, Luyten and Blatt (ibid. p 122) and especially Flückiger et al. (2012), who did a meta-analysis of 200 studies and 14000 treatments.

23 Jacques Ormel et al. (2022, 2023).

24 Jim Van Os et al. (2019).

25 Falk Leichsensring et al. (2022).

26 Bergin & Garfield (1994) find that *all* psychotherapy (as a complex human and social situation) is hardly experimentally studyable…

27 Corveleyn, Luyten and Blatt (ibid. p 86–87).

28 Alexander & French (1946).

29 Wilfred Bion (1962b). Galatzer-Levy shows in a large study that lived insight is essential for psychoanalytic efficacy (2000).

30 Hubble et al. (1999 p 8) for whom *'the big four'* play a role in psychotherapeutic efficacy: 1) Characteristics of the patient and their environment (abilities, motivation, supportive or unsupportive environment), 2) Characteristics of the therapeutic relationship (support, commitment, empathy, solidity), 3) Placebo, hope and expectation; 'belief' in the therapist (=transference), 4) Theoretical model and technique. Their respective estimated importance is 40, 30, 15 and 15%. It does appear essential that a guiding theory is used.

31 See in relation to depression Corveleyn, Luyten and Blatt, (ibidem) or in relation to trauma Cloitre (2015).

32 Roth and Fonagy, (ibidem), Westen et al. (ibidem), Corveleyn, Luyten and Blatt (ibidem).

33 Guido Pieters (2000 p 125).
34 Glen Gabbard: 'Psychodynamic psychiatry is an approach to diagnosis and treatment characterised by a way of thinking about both patient and clinician that includes unconscious conflict, deficits and distortions of intrapsychic structures and internal object relations *that integrates these elements with contemporary findings from the neurosciences.*' (2014 p 4, my emphasis). The latter was discussed at length in my previous book (2022, 2023).
35 Sigmund Freud (1933 p 31) argues that American medics do not give psychoanalysis scientific status for lack of experimental evidence. He replies that they could raise the same against astronomy: experimenting with celestial bodies is very difficult...
36 There is far from unanimity; see Guido Pieters (1998).
37 Andre Green distinguishes between natural and cultural causality, the former being characterised by universal and the latter by private laws (1995).
38 This mainly concerns applied (often residentially offered) psychoanalysis, which lends itself better to scientific research because of its embedding in the institution and larger patient population.
39 Sandell et al. (2000), Bateman & Fonagy (2001), Leuzinger-Bohleber (2002). For a recent comprehensive overview of 298 RCTs of psychodynamic psychotherapies, see Lilliengren (2023).
40 Wilhelm Dilthey (1988).
41 See the saying, 'You can't ride two horses with one behind...'
42 Frédéric Declercq (2000 p 27): 'Science does not extract knowing from the Real but introduces knowing and measuring into the Real.'
43 In this essay, Harry Mülisch (1984) presents comparative reflections on science and art. According to him, they are similar in that they are both concerned with truth. The paradox in art is that through a product of the imagination, i.e. through something that is not true, we can still learn something about reality. The big difference between science and art is that a scientific law or theory describes the concrete-many of phenomena as the abstract- one. Laws and theories always represent the passage from the particular to the general, from the complex to the simple. $E = mc^2$. On the other hand, a work of art represents the concrete-many in the form of the concrete-one. Creating a work of art at no point has an abstract phase.
44 '*Fille de la science*' (daughter of science) in Moustapha Safouan (2005 p 105).
45 In an allusion to Margaret Mahler's (1975) individuation-separation process that is perhaps most fiercely expressed in the (adolescent) world of e.g. art, pop and fashion.
46 Phyllis Grosskurth (1987 p 216).
47 Elisabeth Roudinesco (1993).
48 See the humorous psychoanalytic rule: 'don't generalise based on one case, generalise based on two cases' in: Peter Gay (1989 p 365).
49 Lacanians write 'analysant' with t to stress their active contribution to the process.
50 A term often used by Wilfred Bion in connection with the opposition between '*genius*' and '*mystic*' on the one hand and '*the Establishment*' on the other, where the *mystic* is an exceptional individual/aspect of the self or an exceptional thought that disrupts the *status quo* of the Establishment and where this Establishment can be more or less growth-promoting (1970).
51 See Moustapha Safouan '*le franchissement du plan de l'identification*' (2005 p 68). This is explicitly different from Ego analysis, in which identification with the analyst is the finality of the cure. On the contrary, compare with Lacan's '*faites*

comme moi: n'imitez personne!' A remarkable conclusion of Sandell et al. (2000 p 941–942) is that identifications and ideals resulting from training become *detrimental* to the outcome of psychotherapy and psychoanalysis. The best treatment is that which happens in a dysfunctional (non-reducible singular?) manner.

52 '*Le rêve du réveil absolu*' in Antoine Mooij (2002 p 171).

53 Dixit Horacio Etchegoyen v Jacques-Alain Miller (ibid p 57): '*Distinguer ce qu'est la psychanalyse comme mouvement institutionnel d'avec ce qu'elle est comme discipline scientifique m'a coûté beaucoup d'efforts*'.

54 The various metaphors are by Freud himself, who also spoke of draining the Zuyderzee (which the Dutch almost succeeded in doing, see the unconscious without 'wetness' of the Anna Freudism long prevalent there).

55 For Wilfred Bion's O see (1965, 1970) and later in this book. This is clarified by e. g. Jan Cambien in (1999 p 169–177).

56 Willem Van Tilburg (2000 p 114).

57 Jacques Lacan (1960 in 1966 p 747).

58 Frédéric Declercq (2000 p 118).

59 Robert Wallerstein (1988).

60 'There is no golden rule which applies to everyone: every man must find out for himself in what particular fashion he can be saved' (Freud, 1930a, p 83).

61 Jacques Lacan (1973 p 248): '*Le désir de l'analyse n'est pas un désir pur. C'est un désir d'obtenir la différence absolue*'.

62 Wilfred Bion (1987 p 179).

63 Betty Joseph (1985), one of the most important (post)-Kleinian articles, shows that *everything* that happens during the session should be regarded as metaphorical (indicative of the infantile/unconscious), including the seemingly banal aspects. See Melanie Klein (1961), where she continued to analyse Dick's unconscious through his war coverage (drawn from daily WWII current events).

64 Consequence of what he calls 'excessive projective identification' in which there is no (symbolic) capacity for repression but unbearable and unthinkable psychic contents can only be evacuated and end up in (or under the skin of) the other (1970 p 13). See the Freudian '*Verwerfung*' or the Lacanian '*la forclusion*'.

65 Ludi van Bouwel (1998 p 38).

66 Wilfred Bion (1997).

67 See forgetting the name Signorelli (1901).

68 See '*gardez-vous de comprendre* (sic!)' in Jacques Lacan (1956) in '*Ecrits*' (1966 p 471).

69 Jacques Lacan (ibid. p 589).

70 Schokker & Schokker (2000 p 68).

71 That this technique does not prevent a warm '*prise en charge*' of the patient is abundantly clear from the testimony of a dozen of his analysants in Alain Didier-Weill (2001).

72 Colette Soler (2019) distinguishes between two types of unconscious. In doing so, she takes up Jacques Lacan's (2001) preface to his eleventh seminar. You have the first unconscious structured like a language: the symbolic unconscious with its signifier chain from which the subject derives its meaning. However, there is also a second unconscious. It is nonsensical and situated outside meaning: the core symptom as a somatic *jouissance* in which signifiers 'serve' to 'bind' them. See later in this book for a comparison with the Liquid Crystal Display.

73 A term introduced by Paul Verhaeghe (2002).

74 Quoted by Rudi Vermote (1998a p 68) with O = 'absolute Truth' and K = the passion he calls 'Knowledge'.

Part II

Psychoanalytic Principles

Chapter 6

Freud's Fountain
Open Mind, Open Work

1 Opening

Not many sciences have sprung from the mind of one individual. Leaving
Freud's cultural and scientific predecessors[1] aside for a moment, we may
consider the whole of psychoanalysis as the unique product of his creative
genius. He first used psychoanalysis as a term in 1896.[2] Over time, he gave
the term a threefold meaning: research method and science of the unconscious, a particular psychotherapeutic method (the classic couch cure) and a
set of theories derived from it about psychology and psychopathology. As
befits a full-blooded scientist, he always sought to unveil the truth no matter
how painful, hurtful or unbeneficial it was. He constantly fought against
illusions: his own and those of humanity.[3] For him, science was the reality
principle *par excellence*.[4] His attitude was characterised by the most objective
impartiality possible, 'like infinitesimal arithmetic'.[5] As a psychotherapeutic
method, psychoanalysis is essentially based on 'educated' guesses. Based on
the (admittedly subjective and not objective) data/material produced by the
patient in the consulting room, the analyst forms hypotheses tested through
interpretation. Their veracity is measured according to whether subsequent
(again: subjective) data confirm, specify or refute the working hypotheses.[6]
Time and again, he also critically revisited and adjusted his theorising and
did not even shy away from changing his paradigms.[7] In short, he persevered
with a rigorous scientific attitude with which he confronted the most diverse
human phenomena (including his feelings, dreams, and parapraxes).

As a new science, however, psychoanalysis was also his brainchild that could
only mature by the grace of a good father willing to take care of this child with
responsibility. He, therefore, tried to ensure that it could develop into independence while remaining and becoming itself. For him, then, psychoanalysis
was not only a science and a profession but also a movement.[8] After all, a
whole family grew out of this child, in which creativity and new ideas could
flourish, but in which he, as a spiritual father, determined how far one could
go without violating the family's identity. Viewed positively, he led the psychoanalytic movement as if it were a newly formed independent state, eager for

DOI: 10.4324/9781032698052-8

clear boundaries, standing up for its burgeoning sovereignty and looking after its influence and contacts with the rest of the world as best it could. If, a year before his death, he spoke of three impossible professions (the famous *edukieren, regieren*, and *psychanalysieren*),[9] we can say that psychoanalysis owes its survival to this triple task to which he devoted his entire life.

Of course, Freud didn't come out of nowhere. Vienna was the New York of his time. Enlightenment, scientific positivism, literary greats and philosophers like Schopenhauer and Nietzsche (who were already talking about the unconscious) were his intellectual breeding ground. Yet he especially deserves the dubious honour of having once and for all buried the widely held belief that humans are rational and ruled primarily by reason. He replaced this view with an idea that is still troubling today. Essentially, according to him, we are driven by unacceptable – and precisely for that reason repressed – aggressive, sexual and narcissistic forces that are inevitably at odds with our civilised selves. The primary basis of Freud's psychoanalytic theory is precisely this concept of the unconscious. It is the cornerstone of psychoanalysis. Repression is the mental process underlying its existence. After all, where in the mind is all that we have forgotten or do not want to know about and which we have banished from our conscious awareness and memory?

2 Open Mind, Open Work

Freud not only had an open mind but also produced an open work.[10] It is like a fountain of ideas from which many fruits sprouted during and after his lifetime. After him, psychoanalytic developments focused on various aspects or episodes of his thought. Sometimes, they were clarified; at other times, they were absolutised or simplified. I will go fast forward for a moment.[11] In the context of hysteria, he first developed an affect–trauma model. In his text on the psychotherapy of hysteria, the concepts of the unconscious, resistance, defence and transference emerge, and notions of the analytic attitude appear. Following his self-analysis and in *The Interpretation of Dreams*, he proposed his topographical model of unconscious–preconscious–conscious. He sees adult genital love as a conglomerate of childhood-rooted and polymorphous perverse partial drives[12] that develop in interaction with the environment. He introduced self-love or narcissism, which he saw in inverse proportion to love for others. Where he first divided the drives for self-preservation and the sexual drives, later came a distinction between eros and thanatos, life and death drives.[13] The latter is turned away to the outside and thus becomes a destructive drive. After age sixty, he arrived at the structural Id–Ego–Superego model of the mind. While he initially viewed anxiety as the result of repression, he would later conceive anxiety inversely as the cause of repression. Finally, in his final publications, Freud gave more importance to the vertical cleavages in our psyche than the horizontal ones. In other words, he was not afraid to change his paradigm several times based on new findings.

From early on, sexuality and the linguistic laws of the unconscious were central. Through narcissism, the focus shifted from the drive to the Ego and its objects. Destruction and aggression also became more prominent, and he became more cautious about the therapeutic claims of his psychoanalysis as a treatment. Towards the end of his life, he argued that a satisfactory result of psychoanalysis should meet only two requirements.[14] First, the patient must no longer suffer from their symptoms. They must have overcome their fears and inhibitions. Secondly, the analyst must be convinced that enough repressed material has become conscious, that much that was incomprehensible has found its explanation and that so much inner resistance has been overcome that a recurrence of pathological processes will no longer occur.

This is far less ambitious than the fantasy that the perfectly analysed patient would emerge one day. Indeed, conceptions of psychoanalysis are often very extreme. For some, psychoanalysis is pure quackery or popular delusion; others regard it as an all-powerful panacea. But psychoanalysis does not deliver some superman or superwoman. Freud may have talked in a famous metaphor about draining the Zuyderzee. Even after thorough analysis, there remains plenty of room for fluids on both sides of the bar.

3 1895

The birth of psychoanalysis took place sometime between 1892 and 1898. Indeed, it should be linked to the step-by-step establishment of the basic rule of free association.[15] Freud's technique came about largely intuitively and evolutionarily. In the process, as noted earlier, he gradually abandoned any material act. He started with hypnosis, then applied laying on of hands and finally limited himself to a purely mental act: listening and speaking. Free association has since emerged as a standard psychoanalytic research tool for the human mind. Thinking aloud unfiltered and thus allowing what you have never (yet) consciously thought provokes hitherto unknown dimensions of our subjectivity to appear. Some call the apparatus of free association the microscope or telescope of psychoanalysis. It provides a view of what goes on between our ears that cannot be obtained in any other way. All the more so because you tell your analyst things you would not reveal to anyone else, not to your parents, not to your partner, not to your best friend and – in a sense – not even to yourself. In Freud's classic psychoanalytic cure (patient on and therapist behind the couch), this happened even five to six times a week.

By now, psychoanalysis has been around for about five-quarters of a century. Most situate its actual birth in 1895 for several reasons. The *Studies on Hysteria* that Freud published with Joseph Breuer were published that year. Both Freud and his early followers[16] regard this publication as the starting point of psychoanalysis as a science of the unconscious and as a treatment. Hysteria enjoyed great interest at the time. After all, it was an enigmatic psychopathology whose origins were questioned, whether they were bodily or psychological. No anatomical lesions could be retained, and Freud's Parisian teacher Jean-Martin Charcot demonstrated in packed auditoriums how to use hypnosis to make its symptoms appear and disappear.[17] Hysterical patients (even then) caused a lot of irritation. Were they suffering, or were they simulants or comedians? The book results from ten years of clinical work and includes a detailed description of five patients. Freud's contribution to the psychotherapy of hysteria is clinically and theoretically a foundational text for psychoanalysis as it introduces not only free association, resistance and transference but also the symbolic meaning of symptoms.[18] Unlike Breuer, Freud insisted on the sexual aetiology of hysterical neurosis. He thought he had found the source of the Nile.[19]

1895 was also when he abandoned his project to ground psychology in the natural sciences. Under the guidance of Ernst Brücke and firmly rooted in the Helmholtz School of Physiology, Freud had already completed an international career as a neuroscientist by then.[20] He initially wanted to build psychology on scientific ground and base it on quantifiable data.[21] Without sufficient neuroscientific knowledge and technology, his project led to an impasse, so he did not want to publish this text.[22] He subsequently went on the meta- rather than neuropsychological tour[23] but counted on biology to solidify, correct or complement his hypotheses sooner or later.[24]

Finally, 1895 was the year he first extensively analysed one of his dreams. By this, I mean the dream about Irma's injection, with which he opens *The Interpretation of Dreams* and to which he returns again and again in the first four chapters of the work to illustrate his analytical theories. Finally, in 1896, after the death of his father and tormented by a variety of neurotic complaints, he began a self-analysis that would lay the basis for most of his subsequent ideas and concepts. On 14 Aug 1897, in a letter to Wilhelm Fliess, he wrote: 'The patient who concerns me most is myself'. There were three years of creative illness from which he would distil the laws of our unconscious and dream life, the Oedipus complex and a complete psychosexual developmental psychology.

4 The Unconscious

The Freudian unconscious is where desires, impulses and drives reside undisturbed by the realities of logic or time, nor by those of social norms and values.[25] It refers primarily to the existence of mental contents and processes whose existence we do not realise. On closer inspection, however, they constitute essential motivations for our strivings and behaviour. It is a domain of psychic *activity*. It is dynamic because it imposes itself on our mental life willy-nilly (hence, demonically). In addition, all kinds of automatisms and other repetitive patterns have also installed themselves (often from our early development) in our doings. Psychoanalysis clarifies why and how all these unconscious factors continue to assert their formative, if not distorting, influence throughout our lives. The contents of the unconscious are often experienced as painful, shameful, guilt-laden, frightening or forbidden. This, of course, is precisely why they were once repressed or banished from consciousness! However, this excluded material continues to influence our behaviour. After all, it is so emotionally charged that it must somehow express itself. It then appears in subtle, symbolic or hidden ways. For instance, dreams, slips of the tongue, jokes, and symptoms are all phenomena that Freud called the (veiled) return of the repressed.

Dreams, parapraxes and witticisms are, as a rule, one-off productions of the unconscious. We all know them, and we encounter them all the time. Take, for instance, the hundreds of slips of the tongue or mistakes (the German word *Fehlleistungen* is untranslatable because it is a contraction of failure and performance) that Freud analyses in his *Psychopathology of Everyday Life*. [26] We tend to think of them as meaningless, but on closer inspection, the form they take is always the expression of a conflict: something is kept away and/or replaced or distorted by a substitute. Similarly, dreams are more than the meaningless noise of nocturnal brain activity.[27] Nor are they otherworldly or superhuman messengers that can be interpreted by universal and/or cultural symbolic codes.[28] The dream is the creation of the dreamer and involves an organised mental activity characterised by laws all its own. Beneath the manifest dream are latent contents distorted by dream work, and these in return can be translated by psychoanalytical labour. Dream interpretation unravels what dream labour has woven. The dreamer's free associations and what takes place within the psychoanalytic process provide the sub-text and context, without which interpretation of the dream is impossible. More specifically, the dream is mainly about the veiled fulfilment of a frustrated or repressed desire.[29] The dream is the guardian of sleep. It dodges, as it were, both external and internal stimuli and thus ensures that we do not wake up.[30] The censorship on the edge of (pre-)conscious and unconscious may be less awake at night but remains active. Repressed sexual desires, in particular, are, according to Freud, the strongest motive for dream formation.[31] The regression associated with sleep also leads to a return of repressed infantile sexual scenarios.[32]

In his book,[33] Freud discusses as many as two hundred dreams, forty-seven of which are his own. The best known of the latter is the dream of Irma's injection, based on which he describes some typical dream mechanisms. There are (only) a handful of them. In the famous seventh chapter, he promotes them to the peculiar linguistics of the unconscious: condensation, displacement, inversion, imagery, symbolism, day's residues, dramatisation and secondary or final editing in which the dream is forged as much as possible into a coherent and understandable whole.[34] Here, he swaps his *Project*'s neuropsychological point of view for a metapsychological one.[35] Henceforth, he will thereby assume *mental* zones (Greek: *topos*) and forces that can explain the clinical phenomena. The dream censorship is introduced as a precursor to the later Superego; primary and secondary processes, thinking unconscious and conscious, respectively, are also distinguished. Freud remained true to his dream theory throughout the rest of his life and work. The dream as the royal road to the unconscious is and remains one of the most enduring foundations of his science. We can, therefore, whole-heartedly agree with French psychoanalyst Andre Green's statement that to date, 'post-Freudian contributions on dreams have been the least significant'.[36]

In this first period of the topographical (conscious–preconscious–uncon-scious) model, Freud conceives of the latter as highly linguistic. This is exemplified by *The Joke and its Relation to the Unconscious*. Further on in this book, it will become clear how much Lacan's return to Freud was mainly related to his thinking of this period.[37] After all, Lacan felt that his con-temporaries neglected the fundamental importance of man as a speaking being (Fr: *parlêtre*).[38] Together with their strong reservations about the therapeutic 'use' of countertransference, this linguistic approach probably constitutes the most essential feature of the Lacanian approach. It focuses mainly on neurosis and verbal communication, and it discounts less the theory and clinic of psychopathology where symbolising possibilities are limited or impaired.

5 Sexuality

Next to his book on dreams, *Three Treatises on the Theory of Sexuality* is probably Freud's most important work. After several reprints, it evolved from eighty to one hundred and twenty pages as it was updated each time in parallel with his developing thinking (e.g. about the Oedipus complex and the addition of the phallic phase).[39] To begin with, Freud arrives at a new taxonomy of perversions, which he subdivides as deviations in terms of the object and purpose of the sexual drive. They should be understood as a consequence of the stalling or derailing of our psychosexual development. In the process, the boundaries between normal and abnormal again become blurred. Briefly, perversion differs from neurosis because, in the former, a stereotypically perverse scenario is converted into behaviour. This often happens at the expense of sexual/genital intercourse in a narrower sense.[40] In neurosis, perverse elements operate mainly in fantasy and/or foreplay. Ideally, they spice up our sexual life by breaking (actually or in our fantasy)[41] the straightforward monotony of coitus.

Freud also expanded the importance and scope of sexuality forever. In length, he makes it begin (much earlier than assumed before him) as a poly-morphic perverse disposition in our childhood, in breadth because it comes to concern not only adult sexual behaviour but the entire household of pleasure and enjoyment. Indeed, it adds a premium of pleasure to various aspects of our lives.[42] He describes the oral, anal, phallic and genital phases, with successively different erogenous zones with their respective 'goals' taking precedence. In addition, the development of infantile drives chronologically includes sadistic and masochistic, exhibitionistic and voyeuristic components that are pleasurable. Only after puberty does a more or less stable alloy of partial drives emerge in each of us. Initially, autoerotic sexuality (characterised by self-gratification and organ pleasure) then gives way to object love. An ever-unique collage of infantile components and experiences gives everyone's sexual life a highly personal character. After all, a wide variety of positions are possible on (the statistics of) the Gauss curve.

The child at the mother's breast is the prototype of any subsequent love relationship, but only a whole, i.e., a non-partial object relationship, is considered typical of so-called genital love.[43] *Dixit* Freud, in all this, every newcomer to our planet is confronted with the Oedipus complex.[44] This core complex of neuroses leaves its mark on what is described because we never wholly escape incestuous influences.[45] In sum, on the psychosexual plane, our development revolves around the primacy of the phallus, while on the object-relational plane, it revolves around the Oedipus complex.

Around the same time, Freud analyses Dora's symptoms mainly in terms of this Oedipus complex and infantile sexuality.[46] These include her lips, thumb sucking and fellatio. This seems to revolve around the phallus of Dora's father. Still, on closer inspection, it turns out that (by deferred action) it refers instead to the nipple of Frau K. (to whom Dora harbours homosexual desires). The sessions are constantly about bodily sensations and their perception as they rise (according to Freud) from Dora's unconscious fantasies.[47] Mainly due to the object-relational modification of psychoanalytic views, such a detailed dissection of, say, sexual or masturbation fantasies is a lot less common nowadays.[48] In the earlier mother-child relationship, the distinction between self and object is unclear (yet). The analysis of transference and countertransference is done at the expense of explicitly discussing sexual content, possibly because of the fear of boundary loss or transgression. By a more traditional (firm and inflexible) Oedipal framework both partners of the psychoanalytic couple feel safer and more protected.

Freud's classical (sometimes somewhat authoritarian) technique has given way to a more egalitarian, cautious and subtle one today. In particular, what comes 'live on stage' within the psychoanalytic space is thereby understood as an enactment of the unconscious, history, and the characters in it. Thus, in the case study of Dora and even more so in his later technical writings, Freud further developed his core concept of transference.[49] It evolves from the *falsche Verknüphung'* of his early years to the main ally in the psychoanalytic process.[50] Many psychological experiences are relived not as belonging to the past but as applying in the here and now to the person of the doctor.[51] Transference is repetition that comes on the stage instead of memory. In the classical cure, a veritable transference neurosis develops over time: an artificial and analysis-provoked condition in which the problems eminently mature within the therapy room and must or can be worked on there.[52]

6 Self and Object

Another theoretical milestone in Freud's thinking is the introduction of narcissism.[53] It initially constitutes a phase, shuttled between autoerotic masturbation and object love. Just as Narcissus[54] falls in love with (an image of) himself, the child chooses themself as an object of love and thinks that all the world revolves around them. Freud speaks of His Majesty the Baby in this context.[55] He distinguishes between this primary and a later secondary narcissism, in which a withdrawal of libido occurs. Famously, Freud's comparison is with the amoeba that extends and retracts its pseudopodia, with the division of Ego-libido and object-libido (still) seen as at the expense of each other.[56] The origins of primary narcissism are later situated as early as the womb. It may not be object libido by then, but the subject and external world are not yet differentiated.[57]

In the choice of love objects, Freud would henceforth distinguish between narcissistic and anaclitic object choice. In reality, these are conceptual prototypes that occur in mixed forms, but where this or that preference typifies the subject in question. In the first, the object is chosen as an alter ego: the other person embodies the image of who I am, was or would like to be. In the second, the object is chosen on the model of our first nurturing figures. The later Ideal-Ego (not having and being led by ideals but wanting to *be* ideal) to which we continue to aspire is a substitute for the lost narcissism of our childhood in which we imagined ourselves perfect.[58] Henceforth, narcissism runs like an electric wire through the psychoanalytic world and its body of ideas.[59] Essentially, two poles can be distinguished in this: those who start from an initial undifferentiated, symbiotic state that the child outgrows and those who consider object relations (however primitive or partial) to have existed from the beginning and that narcissistic states should mainly be understood as defensive manoeuvres. A semantic shift is also emerging in this. The Ego (German: *Ich*) first meant the (conscious) person. Only in Freud's later thinking does it become an entity in its own right within our psychic apparatus. He does not use the term 'self', but this concept would become central to Heinz Kohut's views in the context of Egopsychology. It is then somewhat akin to Jacques Lacan's specular Self: the image we have of ourselves and through which we allow ourselves to be captivated.

Following Freud's reflections on mourning and melancholy, we see a more object-relational episode in his oeuvre. In mourning, we are aware of the loss and aware of *what* we have lost, but the melancholic cannot understand that/ what has been lost. In mourning, the world becomes poor and empty; in depression, this emptiness is within oneself. Ambivalent feelings complicate mourning work, and reproaches are directed at oneself instead of at the other. There is a rupture with the outside world and a folding back on and within oneself. In this process, the object is devoured in fantasy, and narcissistic identification occurs, where (in a famous formulation) the object's shadow falls on the Ego/self. There is a regression from love to the more original identification, and the subject directs hatred towards themself. Manifest/conscious self-reproaches can paradoxically be understood as latent/unconscious reproaches towards the other: *Klagen sind Anklagen.* Complaints are plaints in the old sense of the word. Further on, we will discuss how Melanie Klein continues this track of internalised object relations and relates it to what occurs in manic-depressive states.

7 Death Drive and Aggression

His theory of drives is undoubtedly one of Freud's psychoanalytic pillars. After an initial distinction between Ego drives (or drives of self-preservation) and sexual drives, as well as between libido directed towards the ego and the object, Freud takes a different path. The pleasure principle that characterised unconscious and primary process thinking mainly implies a desire to reduce unpleasure (tension).[60] In the clinical situation, after all, the patient wants to alleviate his suffering by seeking help from a therapist. To some extent, the reality principle is opposed to the pleasure principle because immediate gratification is postponed, and unpleasure can be tolerated as a necessary intermediate step towards a later experience of pleasure.[61] But there remained unanswered questions for Freud. How can we explain sadism and masochism, in which pleasure is found precisely in undergoing or causing pain? What about destructive phenomena such as drug abuse or suicidality? Some patients even seem addicted to their suffering or symptoms, or they keep reproducing traumatic experiences. What does that mean?

Repetition, of course, has traditionally been an essential factor in psychoanalysis. Repetition typifies the symptom. It plays a vital role in all transference phenomena. It contributes to learning and unlearning, and it is (also for this reason) necessary for 'working through': the logically last, most prolonged and most challenging phase of the psychoanalytic process. In both traumatic neurosis and child play, what was initially undergone passively is actively repeated (in an attempt to master and to symbolise). Indeed, with the new concept of repetition compulsion, Freud introduces repetition in a very different, demonic guise. A constructive working-through fails, and the *Ewige Wiederkehr des Gleichen* haunts us.[62] This compulsion to repeat responds to something more powerful than the pleasure principle, 'something that seems more primitive, more elementary, more instinctual than the pleasure principle which it overrides'.[63] By analogy with biological entropy, Freud postulates that this is a death drive seeking unbinding and a return to the inorganic state. It is the expression of an inertia inherent in organic life.[64]

Indeed, two contradictory processes exist in living organisms: constructive and binding and destructive and unbinding.[65]

Inner or outer excitations produce similar effects; they disrupt an economic equilibrium just as this happens in traumatic neurosis.[66] At this point, Freud primarily uses an economic conception of trauma. Unprepared for the dangerous situation and/or lacking a protective shield, the traumatised person faces a problem. How are they to master the large amounts of stimuli that invade or overwhelm them? How do they bind them to get rid of them?[67] It is one of the earliest functions of our psychic apparatus to bind excitations and thus replace primary process with secondary process thinking. Free energy is, therefore, converted into an admittedly tonic but also 'calm' energy level because of the bound charge. In this (chrono-) logic, the mastering of over-excitation is promoted to a more primitive function than the seeking of pleasure or the avoidance of unpleasure that follows. It is a logic that *precedes* the pleasure principle. Childhood play and post-traumatic nightmares obey the imperative of repetition and are not (yet) at the service of the wish-fulfilment principle, which comes into being only later.[68] The pleasure principle can establish its hegemony only when the life drive has triumphed over the death drive. If and only if eros prevails does aggression come to the Ego's service: destructive forces are no longer given free rein. The primary pursuit of mental life becomes reducing tension and obeying the Nirvana principle or constancy principle.[69] We can think of life as a constant succession of tensions disturbing the peace of mind. Being able to get rid of them is perceived as pleasurable, while the death drive exercises its efficacy mutely, silently.[70]

Freud tried to make his meta-psychological concepts of life and death drive more acceptable by replacing them with a phenomenological opposition between love and hate. Yet his speculations on the death drive were by no means enjoyed by everyone within the psychoanalytic world.[71] Melanie Klein, in particular, further embroidered on Freud's grief, melancholy, and the death drive. For her, the Ego defends itself from the beginning by deflecting internal destruction outwards under the form of sadism and/or projecting it onto the breast, which becomes aggressive and persecutory.[72] We will see that development for her revolves around decreasing splitting and increasing integration. Over time, the good may triumph over the bad and love over hate.

8 Ego, Anxiety and the Vertical

Since Freud's views on the relationship between the individual and the group are discussed later, it suffices here to discuss his later views regarding Ego, Id and anxiety. At sixty-six, he introduced his structural Id–Ego–Superego model in 1923. It does not replace the earlier topographic one but complements it. The same mental phenomena are described, but this time from the perspective of a metapsychologically assumed apparatus. Where the Ego originally denoted the conscious personality or individual, from 1923, it became a regulatory agent that sought to reconcile requirements of the Id, the Superego, and reality. On the one hand, the ego is a body ego: the psychic projection of a body surface. On the other hand, it is the precipitation of object-cathexes left behind. It is a conglomerate of object choices the Ego has identified with along life's journey. In our prehistoric times, loving an object and being like the object were still the same. In more technical terms, in that archaic phase, identification with the object and cathexis of the object could not yet be distinguished.[73]

The Ego is the seat of anxiety and mobilises defence mechanisms to repel or ward off this anxiety. When fear warns of danger from the outside world, the Ego (like that of many animals) defends itself by fight, flight, freezing and defeat/surrender. When danger comes from within, we draw on typically human (symbolic) defence mechanisms such as repression, regression, reaction formation, isolation, undoing, projection, introjection, turning against the self, reversal to the contrary and sublimation. They were mapped out by Freud's daughter, Anna. De facto, she introduced egopsychology (Heinz Hartmann, Ernst Kris, and Rudolph Loewenstein). This movement, especially popular in the Anglo-Saxon world, focuses on resistance and defence mechanisms and seeks to strengthen the Ego at the expense of the more classically psychoanalytic exploration of the unconscious (fantasy) life.

The Id or 'Es' was used by Friedrich Nietzsche and Georg Groddeck before Freud. It contains a seething pool of drives and instincts and lends itself more to neuro- and evolutionary biological approaches than the more textual unconscious.[74] Freud initially saw the Superego as a remnant of the Oedipus complex. It represents the set of prohibitions, commandments, norms and values that reside in our inner self via the culture carriers (parents and parental figures). For example, in Melanie Klein, the (maternal) Superego also has more primitive, pre-oedipal roots and a more cruel, sadistic, and/or punitive character.

Freud's thinking also made an actual reversal about anxiety. First, he saw anxiety as unsatisfied libido discharged randomly. In this view, libido and anxiety relate to each other like wine and vinegar.[75] Henceforth, however, he would distinguish three types of anxiety. *Real-Angst* is fear of a real danger. Automatic (or traumatic) fear overwhelms the helpless Ego. The latter produces signal anxiety so that it can react to an imminent threat in time to avoid the previous traumatic fear situation. Anxiety leads to repression and not vice versa. The Ego also forms symptoms to avoid anxiety.[76] Safety considerations guide the Ego.[77]

Anxiety emerges, not least in response to (impending) separation and loss.[78] Object relations theory and developmental psychology, in particular, pay a lot of attention to separation anxiety and attribute great importance to it.[79] For Melanie Klein, however, the former is a fear of destruction or annihilation, which for her is caused by the inner workings of the death drive that is projected onto or into the external world. Every child inevitably goes through moments of separation or abandonment. This can take the guise of persecutory anxiety (absence of the good object = presence of the bad object) or depressive anxiety. In the latter case, the child fears destroying or damaging the good object and is filled with reparative tendencies.

To conclude this concise account of Freud's evolving thinking, he adds to the horizontal fault lines in the psyche some vertical ones. Indeed, from 1924 until his death, he produced several articles in which denial of reality and/or splitting of the Ego play an essential role. They are important in distinguishing neurosis, psychosis and perversion. *Verneinung* implies the refusal to acknowledge a desire that, although it reached the conscious, is immediately denied. 'I am not angry'. 'It's not about my mother'.[80] The disavowal (*Verleugnung*) is instead the refusal to acknowledge a perception because it was perceived as too traumatic (e.g., the mother and the woman being castrated).[81] In the rejection of psychosis, the rejected part of reality constantly imposes itself on our mind, just as the repressed urge does in neurosis.[82] In this case, the Ego avoids collapse by distorting itself, encapsulating pieces of its unity and sometimes even bringing about a splitting or division of itself.[83]

9 Sagrada Familia

It is clear by now that Freud's psychoanalysis is an ongoing work. It is still under construction, like Antoni Gaudi's *Sagrada Familia* cathedral in Barcelona. Many theoretical and technical developments occurred during and after Freud, some distinct from his original *démarche* and views. More importance began to be given to interpersonal processes and the environment's role. The emphasis came to lie on social rather than sexual causes of psychopathology. Are we primarily pleasure-seeking, or are we instead looking for love objects? Different insights are emerging regarding the therapeutic enterprise's method, focus and finality. There is also a shift in emphasis from pathological to normal development. Finally, the radius of action of psychoanalytic forms of therapy is extended far beyond Freud's neuroses. The emphasis here shifts from interpretation to relationship and mental contents to mental processes. As a result, other problems have come under the microscope, which has yielded many different viewpoints and/or techniques.

American psychoanalyst Fred Pine talked in 1988 about four psychologies in force within psychoanalysis at the time: those of the drive, the Ego, the object and the self.[84] Drive psychology deals with impulses, desires, fantasies, defence mechanisms and conflicts. Ego psychology focuses on adaptation: whether and to what extent the pleasure principle gives way to the reality principle and illusion to reality. What is the state of the Ego functions? Can it regulate drives and affects, can it tolerate the inevitable frustrations of life, can it control emerging impulses? Anna Freud developed a comprehensive theory of normal and abnormal development. Erik Erikson's epigenetic theory distinguishes not so much drive stages as successive psychosocial developmental tasks throughout our life course.[85]

For object-relations theory, it is not the drive or the Ego that are central, but the relationships with others. It focuses on the largely pieced-together inner images and dramas that revolve around the earliest relationships with our parents, siblings or significant others. They can be embodied in conscious and unconscious memories that come live on stage in current relationships and within therapy. More than other movements, she focuses on borderline and psychotic problems. According to her, both development and treatment occur within an interpersonal matrix. Melanie Klein concentrates mainly on the unconscious *phantasy* (as a mental correlate of the drive) and attributes great importance to the death drive. Many other British psychoanalysts[86] also pay great attention to pre-oedipal development but mainly discuss the influence of the early environment. They often understand psychopathology as a deficit rather than a conflict.

For self-psychology, it is not so much internalised as external relationships that help develop and maintain self-worth and self-cohesion.[87] In this view, the need for affirmation remains. So is the fact that we continue to need others to mirror us or whom we can idealise. This narcissistic developmental line runs parallel to the psychosexual one. Its needs must be understood and even met where the other person fulfils the role of self-object. Sexual or aggressive acting out is understood by self-psychology as a product of breakdown. They are attempts to restore an inner coherence and harmony of a vulnerable self.[88] An important starting point is that we need sufficient self-empathic responsiveness throughout our lives because of our meaningful environment.

Fred Pine does leave out other and later psychologies. Jacques Lacan's took place outside his field of vision. Developmental and attachment theory, relational psychoanalysis, and neuropsychoanalysis developed mainly later.

10 Lacan and Later

In his famous *retour à Freud*, Lacan turned away from the egopsychology predominant in the United States and its conceptions of the autonomous, allegedly conflict-free Ego. He mainly returns to the early Freud, who read and understood the unconscious as a text. He adds to the overly imaginary derailments of most post-Freudians, both the symbolism of man as a figure of speech and the insistent tics of the Real. Indeed, by extending Freud's natural scientific (thermodynamic, physicochemical, neuroanatomical) frame of reference with a linguistic[89] frame of mind, he allowed himself to boast of having made '*Jardin à la française*' of Freud's at times confusing and/or inconsistent theory.[90] This will be further elaborated and explained in due course. Worldwide, the psychoanalytic world today falls into two major 'blocks', by the way. The International Psychoanalytical Association, founded during Freud's lifetime on Sandor Ferenczi's initiative, covers almost all currents or authors, according to its *International Journal*. On the other hand, there is the World Association of Psychoanalysis (*Association Mondiale de Psychanalyse*), which only saw life at the end of the last century and is explicitly to exclusively Lacanian in nature.

After the state of affairs from Fred Pine's time, developmental psychology and attachment theory, and relational or intersubjective psychoanalysis came into focus. Psychoanalysis always adopted a developmental perspective, but this was reconstructed from psychoanalytic work with adult patients. The more recent developmental perspective is based on empirical and observational (naturalistic or experimental) research with children. It bridges the gap between egopsychology and object relations theory. It demonstrates that psychological development occurs within an interpersonal matrix.[91] Whereas Margaret Mahler still described an initial autistic phase that precedes the symbiotic one, the findings of, for example, Daniel Stern, Beatrice Beebe or Edward Tronick contradict this. The baby responds specifically to the mother from the very beginning of its life. When she is insufficiently responsive, the baby becomes upset in no time. Stern meticulously describes how the self gradually forms in joint venture with the first caregivers.[92] Thus, ego- and self-psychology are also empirically linked. Daniel Stern's conclusion: 'We need the eyes of others to form and hold ourselves together.'[93] The human mind is interactive and not monadic but inherently social. Development and therapeutic processes spleen intersubjectively from the beginning.[94]

John Bowlby's attachment theory also draws on empirical research and stresses our evolutionary continuity with other mammals.[95] Attachment is an innate and biologically based system that motivates us to seek closeness and support from others, especially when in distress. After all, we need security to survive. Secondarily, attachment strategies may develop across two dimensions: fear and avoidance.[96] Attachment occurs independently of genetic influences but is passed on transgenerationally. It remains relatively stable over time, although it may change throughout life. Insecure attachment leads to general vulnerability to mental disorders.[97] Attachment theory and research can rely on a great deal of natural scientific evidence, and this prestige makes psychoanalysis that acknowledges it more scientifically and socially acceptable.

After the *relational turn*, which was particularly prevalent in the United States, relational or intersubjective psychoanalysis took off. It assumes the therapist's subjectivity partly colours every psychoanalytic encounter or process. The truth at stake in psychoanalysis results from a co-construction because of the two parties within the psychoanalytic couple. They do not apply a one-person but a two-person psychology. For them, psychoanalysis also does not need to be defined by any particular psychological or personality theory, developmental model or clinical theory. Their tenors state that psychoanalysis aims to unfold, clarify and transform the patient's subjective world.[98] This relational perspective transcends the various psychoanalytic approaches and is (like that of self-psychology) relevant to any psychotherapeutic situation.[99] It contributes to a more egalitarian than authoritarian approach, where the analyst's vision never precedes the patient's subjective perspective.[100] It also contributes to immediate intervention by the therapist if or when a break in the process occurs or is imminent.[101]

Neuropsychoanalysis[102] runs through all these latest developments. It seizes the technological advances of, for example, brain imaging and molecular processes, cognitive science and artificial intelligence to pick up the thread with the natural sciences psychology of Freud's *Project for a Scientific Psychology*. In particular, it provides an alternative to often highly hypothetical or speculative (meta-) psychological models. Whether and to what extent this neuropsychoanalysis can also contribute to concrete practice is debated. It can teach us how the human mind works (in general), but how does this one patient's mind work? In the terminology suggested earlier, its approach is nomothetic and explanatory rather than ideographic and understanding.[103] I have discussed the pros and cons of Freudian and Lacanian neuropsychoanalytic approaches at length before and elsewhere.[104] Here and now, therefore, I briefly go over the most *clinically relevant* ones.

To begin with, there is a distinction between explicit/narrative and implicit/procedural memory. We can recount the former; the latter is expressed only as repeated (inter-) action. Second, establishing first object relations/attachment is correlated with neuroscientific findings.[105] Third, Jaak Panksepp introduced the seven different instinctive systems that 'clash' with each other, as well as the clear distinction between sexuality and care/attachment.[106] Fourth, the (libidinal) SEEKING system is put forward. It animates our psycho-social-cultural life like a 'goad without a goal'. Fifth, we share the PLAY system with mammals. The *as-if* nature of play implies a dimension of 'training' that serves multiple developmental purposes. Sixth, reference may be made to the action of reconsolidation whereby the memory trace becomes labile/reaches awareness and where automatic driver programs can be rewritten. Finally and not least, the dopaminergic 'incentive salience' alias *jouissance* obtained by a given activity can continue even when it no longer provides 'utility' or goes beyond the pleasure principle/adaptation.[107]

All these views illuminate their facet of psychology and psychopathology. Depending on the patient or the moment, this or that perspective is more relevant. That, of course, is precisely the intention of this book. We must constantly be able to tap from different vessels. After more than a hundred years, psychoanalysis has become something of a patchwork. The psychoanalytic field is theoretically fragmented. Some call this pluralism, others feral.[108] Unfortunately, the various post-Freudian currents are often somewhat hostile towards each other. They dispute each other's principles that – they state – would stray from 'true' psychoanalysis. According to its critics, the psychoanalytic movement sometimes behaves more like a church than a scientific community. It prefers to rely on revelation and authority arguments rather than the empirical research tradition (that likes to test hypotheses rather than necessarily confirm them). All psychoanalysts 'believe' in the unconscious, but this unconscious takes different forms with them, and their practices, rituals and ceremonies also differ. There is a different liturgy, teaching and formation based on various canonical texts. The latter are commented on and explained by scribes who try to protect true doctrine from heresy. Here and there, this or that is banished or burned (figuratively) at the stake. Fortunately, in recent decades (in the analogy used), an ecumenical movement is underway. It searches for *common ground*: a combination of nonspecific/generic and specific factors.

Notes

1 Henri Ellenberger (1970).
2 Peter Gay (1989 p 103).
3 Peter Gay (ibidem p 485).
4 'No, our science is not an illusion. But an illusion it would be to suppose that what science cannot give us we can get elsewhere' (1927c p 56).
5 Peter Gay (ibidem p 484).
6 I quote Freud (1937b p 263) in one of his last (technical) writings: 'an association which contains something similar or analogous to the content of the construction' (and I add: interpretation).
7 A term from Kuhn (1970) that applies to Freud's revolutionary turns in his theorising: for example, the abandonment of his *Neurotica* or the introduction of the death drive.
8 Sigmund Freud (1914a).
9 Sigmund Freud (1937a p 260).
10 Antonino Ferro calls Freud's work open (1996). Indeed, it certainly belongs to Umberto Eco's *Opera Aperta* (1962/1989).
11 First an extreme fast forward and afterwards fast forward for the rest of this chapter on Freuds legacy.
12 Oral, anal, phallic, genital, sadistic/masochistic, exhibitionistic/voyeuristic.
13 I quote Freud on the fundamental importance psychoanalysis attributes to the *sexual* drive (1917e p 138): 'Unintelligent opposition accuses us of one-sidedness in our estimate of the sexual instincts. "Human beings have other interests besides sexual ones," they say. We have not forgotten or denied this for a moment. Our one-sidedness is like that of the chemist, who traces all compounds back to the force of chemical attraction. He does not deny the force of gravity; he leaves that to the physicist to deal with.' Later in Freud's work, there is a fundamental opposition between life drives (Eros), conceived as a tendency towards cohesion and unity, and death drives (Thanatos), undoing connections and destroying things. These life-and-death drives are never found in a pure state. They are always mixed/fused in differing proportions. Were it not for this fusion with erotism, the death drive would elude our perceptions since it is itself mute/silent (Freud 1930b p 120).
14 Sigmund Freud (1937a).
15 Anna O spoke of a talking cure (1895b p 30), symptoms being 'talked away' (ibid. p 35), and Emmy von N requested Freud to let her speak ('let her tell what she had to say') (ibid. p 63).
16 Ernest Jones (1953); James Strachey (1955).

17 Joseph Breuer was a very well-known Viennese doctor with an intellectually sophisticated and wealthy clientele. He was friends with Franz Brentano and Johannes Brahms, among others. Freud was apprenticed in Paris to Charcot (1885–1886) and in Nancy to Hippolyte Bernheim (1889). The former promoted hysteria to a separate nosological entity: a functional (and thus not organically induced) disorder where the neurological failure did not correspond to a neuroanatomical logic after all. While Charcot used hypnosis purely for demonstration, for Bernheim, it was a therapeutic tool; Bernheim also attributed its efficacy not to a mysterious magnetism but to suggestion as an actual *verbal* condition. She counts as spectacular proof of the power of words. Language serves as a substitute for action (ibid. p 8).

18 On this symbolic meaning: 'what unites the affect, and its reflex is often some ridiculous play upon words or associations by sound' (ibid. p 209).

19 Not that Freud was set up with this sexual aetiology. After all, he considered them 'a sort of insult' (ibid. p 260)

20 Four of the twenty-four volumes of his collected work deal with neurological topics. See the *Revised Standard Edition* currently being edited by Mark Solms.

21 Ibid. p 295.

22 Nevertheless, this text can be considered visionary. For instance, he argues that neurons function according to the inertial principle and want to eliminate energetic excess. Conscious, secondary process thinking responds to a constancy principle, the Ego is physiologically characterised by bound energy, mnemic connections arise between *arousal/unpleasure* and response/specific intervention in which something in the external world changes (p 318) and an affective dimension of positive and aggressive feelings *pari passu* with satisfaction or frustration arises and so on. All this is 'translated' by Solms into contemporary neuroscientific terms.

23 Metapsychologically, he assumed non-empirically observable mental forces/agencies/devices to explain clinical phenomena.

24 For example, Freud predicts: 'it is probable that sometime in the future there will be a bio-analysis' (Freud, 1933c p 229) as well as the possibility of psychotropic pharmacotherapy: 'the future may teach us to exercise a direct influence, by mean of particular chemical substances, on the amounts of energy and their distribution in the mental apparatus. It may be that there are still undreamt-of possibilities of therapy' (Freud, 1940 p 182).

25 Building on statements made by Secretary of State Donald Rumsfeld following the Iraq war, Slavoj Žižek (2014) adds an amusing but pertinent definition of the unconscious. Rumsfeld speaks of *known knowns, known unknowns, unknown unknowns*. The unconscious is then an *unknown known*.

26 Sigmund Freud (1901a). It is Freud's most popular and widely read book. During his lifetime, it reached ten printings. It makes it straightforward to laymen that 'the borderline between the normal and the abnormal in nervous matters is fluid.' (Ibid. p 278).

27 In my earlier book on neuropsychoanalysis, I elaborated extensively on Mark Solms' refutation of the activation-synthesis hypothesis (Kinet, 2023a). The latter regards the dream as meaningless noise, in which you can 'read' anything and everything at will afterwards (as in tea leaves), and in this sense, was a mockery of Freud's dream theory.

28 The dream does not come from 'higher powers, daemonic and divine' (Freud, 1901b p 633).

29 'The reason for dreaming is indeed to fulfil a wish' in his letter to Wilhelm Fliess dated 23/09/1895. It is about the 'disguised fulfilment of a suppressed or repressed wish' (Freud, 1900 p 160).

30 Sigmund Freud (1900 p 678).
31 Ibid. p 682.
32 In the dream, a twofold regression occurs: in time/developmental history in which a primitive narcissism comes to the fore again and a topographical regression characterised by the hallucinatory satisfaction of wishes/desires (Freud, 1917d p 223).
33 *On the Dream* (which Freud wrote in 1901b) is much shorter, precise and didactic than his *The Interpretation of Dreams* (see Anzieu, 1975)
34 Condensation, of course, touches on overdetermination. Dramatisation refers to what a theatre director does with the text. Freud distinguishes universal and individual symbols. They are ubiquitous to symbolise persons, body parts (especially the genitalia) or erotic activity (Freud, 1900 p 683).
35 With his metapsychology, Freud leaves the clinical and descriptive level and tries to develop generally valid models of the efficacy of our human mind. The fact that his technical writings cover only a tiny part of his entire work shows that psychoanalysis is fundamentally more/different from a collection of techniques (as, for instance, in dentistry). A good understanding of how the psyche (generally and in virtue of this one case) works is necessary. Free after Karl Marx: nothing so practical as a good theory. In particular, the unconscious drive and the principles of psychic functioning and repression only received a thorough metapsychological elaboration between 1915 and 1917.
36 Andre Green (1972 p 179).
37 The return to Freud is a return to the *meaning* of Freud (Lacan, 1955b p 405).
38 They abandoned 'the foundation of speech' (Lacan, 1953 p 243, 2004 p 37).
39 Addition of libidinbal phases in 1915 and phallic phase in 1923.
40 Perversion and neurosis are each other's (photographic) negative (Freud, 1905a p 165).
41 Because human *psychosexuality* is about our most intimate but also most complex life. It is about body and mind in their mutual relationship, inner world and outer world, the subject- and object-side of the other and ourselves and, last but not least, the crucial role and meaning of our fantasies. See most recently Kinet (2023c).
42 Whereby sexual activity attaches itself to functions serving the purpose of self-preservation (ibid. p 182).
43 Ibid. p 222 and 199, respectively.
44 More on the Oedipus complex later in this book.
45 Ibid. p 228.
46 Sigmund Freud (1905b).
47 This classical (sometimes somewhat authoritarian) technique has given way to a more egalitarian one, where what repeatedly comes live on stage within the psychoanalytic space is carefully and subtly understood as an *enactment* of history and unconscious.
48 See the following chapters.
49 Despite all the theoretical changes and innovations within psychoanalysis, Freud's technical recommendations remain guiding. That Freud himself was not always that Freudian has since become clear (Lohser & Newton, 1996; Gabbard, 2014 p 104).
50 Transference is not the most significant obstacle but the most potent ally (Freud, 1905b p 117).
51 Ibid. p 116.
52 Transference neurosis as an artificial illness (Freud, 1914a p 154).
53 It is not so sure that we are the children of Adam and Eve. What is certain is that we are descendants of Narcissus and Oedipus. For humans, Narcissus may

also be more important than Prometheus. After all, the discovery of the Self is more profound than that of fire.

54 In Ovid's *Metamorphoses,* Narcissus does not realise he is falling in love with a (mirror) image of himself. This imaginary/specularity of narcissism is elaborated especially by Jacques Lacan in his publications on the mirror stage, and it is (as will be shown below and Bionian said) a vertex from which all relationships can be viewed.

55 Sigmund Freud (1914c p 91).

56 Ibid. p 75, 76.

57 Laplanche & Pontalis (1967 p 338).

58 Sigmund Freud (1914c p 94).

59 Mark Kinet (2005d).

60 Sigmund Freud (1920 p 7).

61 Ibid. p 10.

62 Ibid. p 21 and 22, respectively.

63 Ibid. p 23. See also Levine (2020).

64 Ibid. p 36.

65 Ibid. p 49.

66 Ibid. p 34.

67 Ibid. p 29–31.

68 Ibid. p 33.

69 It is only in (1924a) that Freud clarifies the confusion. The Nirvana principle is indicative of the death drive, while the pleasure principle is a requirement of libido.

70 The death drive operates in silence, 'unobtrusively' (ibid. p 63).

71 Thus, Freud states at the end of his life that the death drive was not accepted, even among psychoanalysts (Freud, 1937a p 244). In a 1952 letter to colleague Money Kyrle, Donald Winnicott calls Freud's introduction of the death drive his possibly only blunder (Rodman, 1987 p 42). On the other hand, see Green et al. (1986) and (2007).

72 '...instead of dying, killing' (Segal, 1979 p 20).

73 Sigmund Freud (1923a p 29).

74 This Id is discussed extensively in my previous book (2023). I mention neuropsychoanalytic founding father Mark Solms' Es, so I keep it concise here.

75 Related 'as vinegar is to wine (1905a p 224).

76 Freud (1926a p 108–109) but also in lesson 32 of his new introductory lectures (1933).

77 'Considerations of safety govern the ego' (Freud, 1940 p 199).

78 Freud (1926b p 130). From affective neuroscience, we share two fear systems with mammals: FEAR and PANIC/GRIEF. They are capitalised because they are easily distinguishable neuroaffective and behavioural circuits. The first system is mobilised by real danger, and the second by separation (Panksepp, 1998 in Kinet, 2023).

79 While (see later in this book) with Lacanians, the main focus remains on castration anxiety.

80 '...you ask who this person in the dream can be. It's not my mother. We amend this to "so it *is* his mother"' (1925h p 235).

81 Sigmund Freud (1925h).

82 Sigmund Freud (1924th p 186).

83 Sigmund Freud (1927th p 152–153).

84 Fred Pine (1998).

85 Erik Erikson (1950).

86   Ronald Fairbairn, Michael Balint, Donald Winnicott.
87   Heinz Kohut (1971, 1977, 1984).
88   Baker & Baker (1987 p 5).
89   Richard Rorty (1967) in philosophy: linguistics becoming the central auxiliary science that comes to define philosophy both in English (Wittgenstein, Carnap, Ryle) and French (Ricoeur, Derrida, Barthes, Lacan)...
90   Frédéric Declercq (2000 p 15).
91   Blatt & Levy (2003). The importance of emotional attunement in the development of affect regulation is also confirmed from neuroscientific perspectives (Schore, 1994).
92   Successively, there is an emergent or body self, a core self, a subjective self, a verbal/categorical self and a narrative self.
93   Daniel Stern (2004 p 107).
94   Daniel Stern (1985) and Beatrice Beebe (2005).
95   There is the trilogy on attachment and loss (Bowlby, 1969, 1973, 1980) and how Bowlby applies attachment theory to psychotherapy (1988).
96   Cassidy & Shaver (2008).
97   De Klyen & Greenberg (2008).
98   Stolorow, Brandchaft, & Atwood (1987 p. 10).
99   Aron (1996).
100 Glen Gabbard (1997 p 50).
101 Luyten et al. call this 'embracing the elephant in the room'. It involves immediacy and monitoring the therapeutic relationship during the session. Focusing on this is a crucial aspect of psychodynamic therapy, significantly during conflicts or fractures and to increase the effectiveness of therapeutic intervention. Hill et al. (2008) and Muran et al. (2009).
102 For a detailed discussion of neuropsychoanalysis, I refer again to Kinet (2023).
103 I return here to the opposition between objectivity, predictability and explanation of the natural sciences and subjectivity, unpredictability and description of the humanities. The nomothetic/automaton model determines the former: what determinate laws or forces are at work so that we can predict and control. The *ideographic/tuchè* model is the accidental 'knock on the door' of the Real around which the dream/nightmare forms. It is the domain of the arbitrary, morality and subjectivity (see, for example, Verhaeghe, 2002).
104 Kinet (2010, 2022, 2023).
105 Alan Schore (1994).
106 Jaak Panksepp (1998).
107 Which is important in order to understand (especially posttraumatic) repetition compulsion; see Ariane Bazan (2016); Bazan & Detandt (2013).
108 Fonagy & Target (2003).

Chapter 7

To the Motherland

A Psychoanalytic Exodus

I Serious Play

Freud developed the psychoanalytic cure as a method of investigating the unconscious and as a therapy for adult neurosis. He never worked analytically with children himself. However, he did manage to convey psychoanalytically inspired insights and parenting attitudes via little Hans' father[1] to combat a phobia. In this context, he argued that it is a misunderstanding to think that 'bad' urges are strengthened by making them conscious; after all, psychoanalysis merely replaces unconscious repression with deliberate control/suppression.[2] In doing so, he unwittingly foreshadowed the discussions that would arise between his daughter, Anna Freud and Melanie Klein around the psychoanalysis of children: Is *pur sang* psychoanalytic work with them at all possible?

Guided by two fundamental psychoanalytic principles (namely that the main task of analysis is the exploration of the unconscious and that the analysis of transference and resistance are the appropriate means to this end), Melanie Klein[3] gradually and experimentally developed her play technique.[4] The child is received several times a week in a furnished playroom and offered simple toys (figures, blocks, trains and cars, houses, etc.), water, and drawing and painting utensils. The child stages their inner world in free play, and this play is, for Klein, the equivalent of the adult's free association. She analyses the material the play produces as a dream and sees similar mechanisms of concealment at work there as in dream work: symbolisation, displacement, condensation and so on.[5] This is accompanied by sometimes violent feelings in the transference, which is often frightening because aggressive inner objects appear on stage, which can only be 'tamed' by an active interpretation and giving of words.

This research method allowed Melanie Klein to explore the pre-oedipal phase in young, often severely disturbed children who could not yet speak (sufficiently). In her psychotherapeutic work, she was particularly struck by the pervasiveness of aggressive and destructive forces that are very frightening for the child. Oedipal elements were found to be present much earlier than

DOI: 10.4324/9781032698052-9

expected.[6] There was a primitive morality characterised by the fear of cruel, punitive guilt or a vengeful (inner or outer) persecutor. Under various pre-genital[7] guises, sadism largely determined the play. Object relations and a weak Ego in varying integration states were present much earlier than expected. The Ego and the object are still very fragmentary at first, however.

While Freud exposed the child in the adult, Klein discovered the infant in the child. In its earliest development, it appears to go through two con-stellations of anxieties and defence mechanisms. They are not stages but possible positions from which we can face the world. In the schizoid-para-noid stage, annihilation anxiety/aggression is deflected or projected towards the outside world. Persecutory anxiety and splitting (good and evil, love and hate), denial and projective identification dominate. The main 'concern' is about one's survival and well-being. In the next depressive position, the fear of having damaged or destroyed the object prevails, and an anxious pursuit of reparation dominates.[8] Aptly, this distinction is reflected, for example, in the experience of melancholy versus more neurotic depression. In the former, the patient bombards themself with scathing accusations and recriminations. A cruel/sadistic Superego inwardly rages against the self. This psychody-namic is destructive. After all, neither the person involved nor their object(s) benefit. In the more neurotic depression, guilt leads to remorse and repara-tion. The person concerned yearns for the 'lost' good[9] and puts most of their energy into repairing as much of the damage caused as possible.[10]

We know that Freud regarded the joke, the parapraxis, the dream and the symptom as spontaneous unconscious formations. He added a therapeutic *artefact*, namely free association. Klein takes credit for fully recognising children's play as a formation of their unconscious. Not only the verbal expression that characterises free association but also the manipulation, (inter-) action and dramatisation that belong to play turn out to be therapeutically valuable gateways to the unconscious. With the child, they even take over the prominent place of the dream as *the* royal road to the unconscious. Here, the therapist, for their part, does not sit safely out of sight and behind the couch but needs to engage in the play as a participating observer. With the pre-genital sadistic child as director, they may have to crawl on all fours, be put in the corner of the room or be bombarded with all kinds of material or immaterial (words, emotions) projectiles. The ability to combine a certain spontaneity with professional detachment and to keep reflecting on what goes on in the playroom (as an externalisation of the unconscious) is severely tested. Moreover, to determine the explosives of the negative transference, an active TNT technique ('tackling of the negative transference') is needed.

All this has proved very inspiring for the technique of psychoanalytic work with adults whose psychopathology is rooted in the archaic layers of their early childhood development. Even then, they often cannot speak and/or symbolise adequately. They evacuate unbearable and unthinkable contents, for instance, through substance abuse, acting out behaviour or by getting on someone else's nerves/system and/or crawling under someone else's skin in all kinds of possible and impossible ways. The infernal reality that may underlie such phenomena comes to life on stage in play therapy. At the same time, in talking to adults, it is often harder to discern through the psychotherapeutic encounter. Moreover, it has entered adults' implicit, procedural memory domain and must be understood and translated from the affective reality of the total transference-countertransference situation.[11]

Indeed, decades before neurobiological memory research, Melanie Klein already spoke of 'memories in feeling',[12] which, unlike narrative, anecdotal memories, do not come from explicit, autobiographical memory. From the circumstantial evidence and the emotionality offered by the psychoanalytic encounter, symbolisation, construction, or subject amplification should be done in addition to interpretation.[13] In this sense, the clinical psychotherapeutic (semi-)residential milieu proposed further has much more in common with the playroom than the consulting room. Action, interaction and manipulation as forms of acting out and enactment are performed daily around the clock. The treatment team members cannot stay out of the play either and often have difficulty maintaining a sufficiently reflective attitude. The play therapist's necessary flexibility can serve as an exemplary model here.[14]

2 Hell's Angel

Freud had already been shocked by his description of the polymorphous, perverse, infantile sexuality through which the child was snatched from the realm of angels. Klein additionally detected in the infant the presence of oral- and anal-sadistic destructiveness. Indeed, from her descriptions of what goes on in the playroom, a threatening and sadistic universe appears where an apocalyptic struggle occurs between love and hate, good and evil.[15] From such findings, she resolutely promotes the dualism between life and death drive introduced by Freud[16] to the cornerstone of her theory. In doing so, she attaches great importance to the constitutional origin of these drives. She retains the idea of the death drive (whether in the form of envy or not),[17] which is also responsible for the demonically destructive that can lurk in the unconscious.[18]

For her, mental life is mainly determined by drives and the accompanying unconscious phantasy from which the environment is constantly interpreted and distorted. Note that this phantasy is understood entirely differently from Freud or Lacan. With Freud, phantasy is like a refuge, a treasure island of the pleasure principle. For Klein, phantasy is not an island in psychic functioning but a mainland under the sea, a continuously present 'mental processing'.[19] It revolves mainly around (parts of) one's own body and that of one's parents, often in sexually or aggressively coloured interaction. For her, phantasy is the mental correlate, the psychic representative of the drive,[20] and this drive is not pleasure- but object-seeking for her.[21] For her, the mental life is not only determined by what is external, for example, by language and (the desire of) the Other as with Lacan or by the key figures of childhood as with many (post-) Freudians.[22] Her theory is distinctly intrapsychic. Reality is always seen through the glasses of phantasy, and what is internalised from the external world is always a phantasmatically distorted 'environment'.[23]

Since psychoanalysis seeks to bring the subject to the point where they take full responsibility for what happens to them, we could, in a way, consider this Kleinian view as fundamentalist. After all, it drives the formulation 'life is what you make of it yourself' to the top. At the same time, her conceived schizoid-paranoid position of the first months of life makes the persistence with which people place the cause of their problems outside themselves understandable. The 'evil' is then externalised until sufficient psychic and mental capacity is present to become aware of (an inner) evil and mourn for it. In the first case, there is radical extremism (black-and-white, good-evil, love-hate) in the approach to reality; in the second, there is more room for mildness, nuance and mixed feelings. Once this Cape of Good Hope[24] is passed, the way to a more neurotic level is open, and the subject has a more integrated view of themself and significant others.

About Oedipus complex and gender difference, she also goes against Freud's phallocentrism. The reason why the girl turns away from the mother has nothing to do with the feeling of being castrated but with the weaning of the breast,[25] causing her to turn to the penis orally. In the second instance, this passive-receptive aim 'sinks' to the lower-lying multi-lipped mouth. Against the penis envy that Freud attributes to the woman, Klein, on the other hand, posits a womb envy. The boy first goes through a 'femininity' phase and will later (narcissistically) overvalue his penis and develop a competitive urge to 'make it' culturally, financially or socially.[26] The Kleinian contribution also offers valuable insights for understanding the dark inner world in which some patients with severe psychiatric problems[27] are trapped. Indeed, while Freud thought that the Superego emerged only after the Oedipus complex as a precipitation of (mainly paternal) commands and prohibitions, according to Klein, the infant is terrorised even earlier by a more primitive and maternal Superego that can be destructive. It is, after all, the projected product of pre-genital sadism that reigns supreme in that phase, the (raging) charge of which for Klein is not in the least constitutionally determined.

It makes it understandable that the psyche of the infant can be bombarded in traumatising ways despite the good-enough concerns of the parents and that this can lead to the most severe psychopathology. Both the crying baby and ADHD problems from child psychiatry are some well-known and visible examples of potentially maddening temper (and) tantrums. Among adults, Gerald Adler[28] draws attention to an almost invariable sense of badness and unworthiness that he believes characterises the most severe personality disorders. Of course, this extreme badness is the result of the -as mentioned above- primitive, punitive, even persecutory maternal Superego. From an egopsychological tradition, Otto Kernberg[29] is indebted primarily to Klein's insights in designing his concept of the borderline personality organisation. According to him, the borderline exhibits identity diffusion: they have an unintegrated[30] image of themself and other. Moreover, whereas in neurosis, the Ego has higher defence mechanisms at its disposal, such as repression, reaction formation, rationalisation and the like, the borderline can only appeal to (more reality-distorting) primitive defence mechanisms, such as splitting, denial and projective identification[31] for protection from (in post-Kleinian terminology) 'psychotic' anxieties.[32]

Melanie Klein's views often raise a lot of critical concerns among non-Kleinians. These include her overemphasis on an innate and destructively understood death drive, the absolutisation of the inner phantasy world at the expense of recognising the importance of actual experiences with key figures,[33] with her focus on the (early) mother–child relationship with relative disregard for the role of the father and the actual Oedipus and castration complex. Her impersonal and 'cold' jargon, in which pathological-sounding concepts are used to describe general human phenomena of early childhood, also evokes much resistance and sometimes even annoyance.[34] Finally, her very active (and, to some outsiders, almost persecutory) technique of early and deep interpretations in a syncretistic language offends many psychoanalysts.[35] However, Kleinians remained on board the British psychoanalytic ship despite such hard-to-digest talking points. Nor did – for that matter – Heinz Kohut's later Self Psychology cause a schism within the International Society, as Jacques Lacan's school and practice would.

While admiring the clinical genius of *Madame Klein*, Lacan denounced her 'muddy' thinking.[36] According to him, she did not see clearly in the different statuses of the Real, the Symbolic and the Imaginary, not in the narcissistic-imaginary nature of the Ego, nor the peculiarity of psychic (as opposed to external) reality. Her conceptions of phantasy imply an imaginary colonisation of the maternal body for him. She also hardly considers the posteriority that characterises a psychoanalytically understood pathogenesis.[37] Melanie Klein has indeed, in many respects, moved far away from 'classical' Freudian psychoanalysis.[38] On the other hand, this led her to enrich the entire field of child and adult psychiatry in a groundbreaking way with her technical and theoretical innovations.

3 The Bizarre

We say that certain human phenomena, such as behaviours, statements or 'creations', are bizarre. By this (dis-) qualification, we mean that we find them frighteningly incomprehensible. Quite a few clinicians like Hanna

Segal, Ronald Britton, Betty Joseph, Susan Isaacs, Donald Meltzer or Herbert Rosenfeld, following in Melanie Klein's footsteps, have continued pioneering work into the furthest, most exotic and 'untreatable' corners of psychopathology.[39] In the process, they, too, have sometimes developed new insights and concepts that have made the inner dynamics of the more serious psychiatric disorders more comprehensible. All this contributes to a more profound and humane contact with the patient down to their most bizarre strangeness. In the meantime, however, there was the emergence of psychopharmaceuticals that provide effective symptom-oriented treatment for both major (psychotic or otherwise) mood disorders and psychoses (schizophrenic or otherwise). The decisive importance of biological factors in their pathogenesis is now widely recognised. Consequently, the psychoanalytic approach has modestly distanced itself from its former, illegitimate (because entirely unproven scientifically) and exclusive leading role in their 'treatment'.[40] Necessary (in this case biological) conditions, however, are by no means sufficient conditions for the emergence of this kind of psychopathology. Nor are the form and content of its symptomatology elucidated. While Freud himself never treated psychotics psychoanalytically, since then, quite a few psychoanalysts have drawn remarkable conclusions from their psychotherapeutic work with these patients, which comprises pathogenesis, psychodynamics and psychotherapeutic technique.[41] For a proper understanding of the psychotic experience, these insights remain indispensable today. Thus, alongside the biological, psycho-educational and rehabilitative medical-psychiatric approach, the psychoanalytic approach to psychosis retains its unique value.[42] Indeed, it has sustained attention to the particularity of the subject and its history and is willing to be an apprentice in this subject without prejudice. The analytic therapist is then a second-in-command:[43] a privileged witness who offers the psychotic patient a space to think and who is someone who does not know 'it' for the psychotic and who does not want to 'enjoy' them.[44]

Wilfred Bion is undoubtedly the most critical 'follower' of and innovator after Klein. Moreover, he left a firm (post-) Kleinian imprint on the entire South American continent through his emigration and educational input.[45] First, he developed his theory of psychosis in close connection with a theory of (the birth of) thinking.[46] In psychosis, according to him, mental life is entirely dominated by the death drive, hatred and envy towards inner and external reality. It is the 'attacks on linking' that characterise a Kleinian-understood death drive. There are massive fears of destruction, and the psychotic uses their senses not only to perceive but also as channels to evacuate unbearable content.[47] They then find themself in a world of bizarre objects, consisting of things (*Ding-an-sich*) and fragments of the Ego and Superego.[48]

This has to do with a low tolerance for frustration that results from an interplay between constitutional vulnerability (such as the innate tendency towards destructiveness) and difficulties in contact with the first parental figures (see Lacan's first and second big Other).[49] Indeed, the infant needs their digestive (detoxifying and digesting) or (in Bion's terms) *containment* function to develop psychic integrity and thinking. This 'containment' means, for example, that the mother is receptive to the unbearable and unthinkable content in the child and responds appropriately. Her capacity for reverie enables her to put her *alpha function* at the service of her baby.[50] It is an ability that, on the one hand, is similar to the suspended or free-floating attention that Freud prescribes for the analyst (which Joseph Sandler[51] extends to a 'free-floating responsiveness'). On the other hand, it bears similarities to Winnicott's 'primary maternal preoccupation', about which more later.

Only thanks to an appropriate presence and absence of gratification (the breast), on the one hand, and maternal containment, on the other, can the infant form a 'contact barrier'[52] that consists precisely of these alpha elements.[53] In a similar vein, Didier Anzieu introduces the '*Moi-Peau*':[54] a skin-ego that must develop in the first period of life in its triple function of enclosure (creating an inner space), of barrier (to protect against) and of a filter on which the first representations find their deposit. All this makes later condensations and displacements and the symbolic-imaginary of dream and symptom formation possible. When this process does not occur sufficiently, a 'nameless terror/dread' arises.[55] In the absence of sufficient containment, excessive projective identification and fragmentation occur in the psychotic.[56] Here, unbearable contents are split off, evacuated and end up (in the absence of a 'receptive' big Other) on a beta screen (a projection screen).[57] There is a reversal of the alpha function whereby the words, thoughts and meaningful actions provided by the mother, for example, are not used by the infant but are (oral-cannibalistically) destroyed and projected onto this 'beta-screen' to create a mess (*debris*)[58] of de-symbolised elements and bizarre and haunting *Ding-an-sich*-like objects.[59]

4 Protomental

From his work with psychotics and with groups, Bion introduced the term the protomental[60] to refer to a hypothetical and undifferentiated level of symbolic experience at the edge of the somatic and the psychic, consisting of bodily sensations, images, rudimentary feelings and primitive thoughts. As an analyst, Bion[61] wanted to understand everything in the session: a simple growl from the patient and his most elaborate thought. He assumed that much intrapsychic and interpersonal communication occurs at the preverbal level, where thinking and feeling remain partially undeveloped and separate. He stressed that emotional exploration and communication are frustrating and produce pain and uncertainty. A fundamental inner conflict occurs between one element that tries to tolerate, develop and integrate thoughts and feelings and another element that tries to avoid frustration. However, to free themself from 'the bondage of inarticulation' (the constriction of what remains unspoken), the patient must be willing 'to suffer the process of thinking'.[62]

From the point of view of the psychoanalyst, this involves both conscious and unconscious systems, creating a multiple, 'binocular'[63] perspective. The alpha function of the analyst ensures that raw experience (in Bion's terms, beta elements) is mentalised into conscious and unconscious thoughts. The alpha function transforms beta elements into symbols, nameable effects or feelings, and emotional thoughts of increasing complexity. Again, it is the function of containment exercised by the mother when she attunes herself in reverie to her child's needs. The child who is prey to unthinkable and unbearable content makes the mother feel and experience certain things through (a communicatively understood) projective identification. If open to this, she can grasp and translate these contents into a digestible and symbolisable form. This function models what the psychoanalyst must do in 'early' disorders. Indeed, such processes are essential for developing mentalisation and comprehension in infants and patients. The alpha function becomes internalised and then part of what he calls 'the normal part of the personality'.[64] On the contrary, the psychotic part of the personality[65] defends itself against emotional experience. The processes of mental linking are attacked by this psychotic part when integration causes mental pain. The activated drives persist undeveloped as beta elements and are denied, dissociated, evacuated, projected and acted out. Emotions remain 'stuck' as concrete entities and become unavailable for alpha function.

5 Passion and Pas-Science

Bion[66] introduced the concept of passion to describe the continuous integration process (rather than inhibition or evacuation) of primary emotions. He defined passion as the component derived from *Love, Hate* and *Knowledge*. It represents for him an emotion experienced with intensity and warmth but without any suggestion of violence, and it is radically different from the passion in the Lacanian perspective.[67] Bionian passion adds strength, intimacy and warmth to communicating with others. A person capable of passion grows in mental sophistication, emotional maturity and warmth while their violent potential diminishes. Bion[68] advocates a mystical attitude for the analyst. This is characterised by an experience of unity and immediate contact with reality as it is and by the use of intuition.[69] It provides knowledge beyond words that could bring about powerful transformation.[70] This mystical attitude requires '*negative capability*'.[71] There should be no enervating search for facts and reasonableness but, on the contrary, a 'suspension of belief and disbelief'.

In Simon Vestdijk's terms,[72] a kind of 'twilight sense' comes into play, thanks to which a fleeting glimpse of the *Thing* can be caught: the sensed but not immediately knowable reality behind sensory reality. In other words, the (messianic) thoughts in which Bion is most interested are *not* logical or rational but occur without *memory, desire and understanding.* [73] The psychoanalyst must be able to change from knowledge to experience and from K to O, from 'Knowledge' to 'Absolute Truth'.[74] Indeed, only being 'in O'[75] in this way, according to Bion, increases receptivity to thought. Only this experience can substantially change or (in his terms) transform the individual, not least because it is a way to tune into the wavelength of the total transference situation,[76] allowing the analyst to strike the right affective and emotional tone in his interventions.[77]

Oscillating, according to Bion, the patient moves between the schizoid-paranoid and depressive position and between incoherence and coherence, while the analyst moves simultaneously between 'patience' and 'security'.[78] There are times when they can listen at ease, and there are when they must be able to endure pain, anxiety and frustration and be prepared to suffer with the patient. Concerning 'patience', Lacan would probably speak of the point of anxiety where the analysant and analyst come into close contact with the Real. These are moments of *'pas-science'* (non-known and non-science). This contrasts with episodes of 'security' that are more about *'la sécurité de la science'*. Here, of course, the sense of security is provided by science only insofar as it is regarded as gospel, as *'savoir établi'.*[79] As such, it differs from true scientificity, which is instead characterised by permanent wonder and an open mind!

For those exposed to the traumatic or Real, the illusion of understanding and the (pseudo-) mastery of the Ego may be necessary to be (psychically) born and/or survive. Construction, subject amplification and mentalisation are at work to restore or help establish thinking, identity and integrity. Of course, psychoanalytic psychotherapy, thus understood, follows, in a sense, a more illusory path than the classical cure. In the neurotic, there is more of a longing for the Real. Here, a kind of nostalgia for *the Real Thing* prevails, but it does so in a conflictual manner. It is conflicting because the neurotic guards themself in all sorts of ways against enjoying the object they supposedly long for...[80]

6 Discussions

While Melanie Klein saw the baby as an almost solipsistic (because its world is fantasised together) monad, Wilfred Bion gives a more interactive and intersubjective interpretation of the psyche's birth.[81] While her technique emphasised translation and interpretation of play and enactment, Bion's technique focuses on being together ('in O') with the patient, the 'containment' and 'at-one-ment'[82] as a deep empathic attunement to his unbearable truth. International Bion authority Rudi Vermote makes a simultaneously poetic and pertinent analogy. He compares Freud's model to mechanics (drives, dynamics, resistances). Melanie Klein's can be called electric with positive and negative split units, while Bion's resembles contemporary physics, which is dominated by large empty spaces and the uncertainty principle.[83]

All the mentioned extensions of the technique are now part of the mainstream of the 'classical' International Psychoanalytical Association.[84] In a Kleinian perspective, we think of an early and more systematic interpretation of negative transference, with more emphasis on the total transference situation as the enactment of the unconscious, attunement to affect and focusing on inner object relations (which are the internalised precipitate of what we *have made* of significant others). From a Bionian perspective, we think of the container-contained model in which the analyst primarily contributes to developing thought and mental processes. They set themself up as concave a mirror as possible. Also, they do their metabolising and detoxifying work by digesting and translating projective identification, thus laying the foundation for psychoanalytic work in a narrower sense. For a lot of serious psychiatric problems, there is also the need for (intensive) care. For a proper psychoanalytic understanding of this challenge, the experience and thoughts of Donald Winnicott are indispensable.

The Second World War had not only caused a massive psychoanalytic Exodus (to mainly English-speaking regions) but certainly, in the UK, it created orphaned children and sundered families. Sensitivity and attention to child psychology increased enormously. Wartime nurseries were established to look after children's proper upbringing and development.[85] Observational research by psychoanalytically trained people shot up in many areas. John Bowlby began large-scale research on attachment and loss, culminating in his famous trilogy, about which more below. Such was the background to the sometimes fierce *Controversial Discussions* (1942–1944) that arose within the British Psychoanalytic Association, and that would lead in 1946 to the 'compromise' of three factions within the British Association: the Kleinians, the (Anna) Freudians and the so-called Middle group.[86]

Melanie Klein had been in the UK for some time, and she had already gathered many followers around her when the Freud family emigrated to London. Daughter Anna Freud mainly followed Freud's structural model, paid much attention to the fate of the Ego and adopted a pedagogical and adaptive developmental perspective. Melanie Klein elaborated on the pregenital life drive; she embraced the death drive, also took more into account the vertical cleavages of the psyche and combined the rigorous psychoanalytic method with a more flexible and child-appropriate technique in her play therapy. As the main figurehead of the *Independents* of the *Middle group*, Donald Winnicott put Kleinian emphases on the one hand, but by taking much more account of the environment, he de facto introduced a *two-person psychology*. He laid the foundations for later self- and relational psychoanalysis. He was not a theoretical system builder like Freud, Klein or Lacan but more of an artist/player. He adapted to the clinical situation each time and was not very concerned about framing his findings in a bigger picture.[87] He also did not create a school, but his contributions proved to bridge many psychoanalytic gaps. He made a difference in several areas: the importance of the relational environment, a distinct view of aggression and destructiveness, new ideas related to illusion and transitional phenomena and implications for psychoanalytic practice.[88]

Melanie Klein based her theorisation on intensive play therapy with severely disturbed children despite their tender age. In this way, she reconstructed a hallucinatory early childhood inner world. On the other hand, Winnicott developed his ideas mainly from paediatric practice with more normal mothers and their babies and interacting with them. In doing so, he had a keen eye for play and creativity, for him decisive signs of mental health. From this very different experience,[89] he doubted the innate nature of the death drive and its derivatives: hatred and envy.[90] Rather, he saw them as reactive products, namely as the result of disorders or deficiencies in the environment.[91]

7 Dependency

For Klein, the baby was highly differentiated from birth. According to her, the baby has imagination and an Ego from the beginning. The inner world largely precedes the outer world, just as projection precedes introjection. For her, what the child internalises is always and inevitably tainted by projection. She emphasises the temper with its attendant phantasy life at the expense of a relative disregard for the impact of the environment and external reality. In contrast, Donald Winnicott explicitly pushes the environment to the fore. For Winnicott, the mother and her baby are primarily a duality. 'There is no such thing as a baby'![92] There is only a being in absolute dependence. It can only continue to exist ('going on being') by the grace of the 'primary maternal preoccupation'[93] of the matrixial mother. If the mother is (not perfect but) good enough, she creates a 'continuity of being' in the child.[94] It is essentially an experience of fusion. The mother then first adapts herself almost wholly to the child's needs. She offers gratification (e.g. the breast, warmth, holding) where and when the child wants to create them (in a hallucinatory wish-fulfilment). She responds to her child's spontaneous gestures with good attunement ('mutuality'). In this way, the child is nurtured with an illusion of imaginary omnipotence that allows them to experience divine or majestic moments and to be somewhat the creator of the world.[95]

If the period of total dependence goes 'well enough', the child can develop a True Self from the core of its being and its centre of gravity. It can rely on a safe background figure and surrender to peace and quiet (the *incommunicado* Self[96]) in a state of un-integration[97] in the mother's presence.[98] For Winnicott, all these experiences are necessary (but insufficient) conditions for being creative, relaxing and enjoying oneself later on. When too significant disturbances occur during this first time of absolute dependence, the baby feels its survival is threatened ('threat of annihilation') and stands in mortal fear ('unthinkable anxiety').[99] Only then does Winnicott's thinking come closer to Klein's negative and altogether more pathological-sounding views of hate and sadism or the schizoid-paranoid position.

What often appears to the outside world, in retrospect, as hatred and sadism, Winnicott sees instead as unintentional 'ruthlessness'.[100] The 'ruthlessness' is the inevitable correlate of an all-consuming pleasure for life.[101] It is the 'mouth-love' in which the devouring is still an integral part of love.[102] Indeed, in love, the child only takes the feelings of the other into account in the later 'stage of concern',[103] when it becomes aware of its dependence (previously disregarded by imaginary illusion). Concern and anxiety are then (favourable and not pathological) alternative terms for Klein's 'fears' from the depressive position. For both Klein and Winnicott, the child becomes aware of an inner evil only in the second stage. It comes to an awareness of the damage that was and can be done by this evil only at a later stage, and only from then does it try to do or make good towards the other.

Underlying their very different to even contrapuntal concepts and language then is a common idea, namely that the child recognises the fact of its dependence only after a prior period of omnipotent narcissism.[104] After all, as James Grotstein notes, we are not the creator of heaven and earth and are incapable of separating day and night, the sea and the land, the good and the bad breast.[105] Klein's schizoid-paranoid narcissism, however, looks sickly and dreary because, to her, it is motivated by mortal fear and death drive. Winnicott's narcissism is like a gift from heaven, a gift from the mother, a shining germ cell[106] from which all later creativity will develop.[107]

8 The Transitional Space

In its first years, the infant evolves from absolute through relative dependence to independence ('towards independence').[108] From birth, the child is thereby surrounded and guided by the (environment-)mother and by mother-tongue. The environment-mother (with her 'holding, handling and taking care')[109] first adapts almost entirely to her child's needs and then applies frustrations in a dosed manner. In doing so, she tries to keep pace with the child's ability to tolerate these frustrations. On the other hand, this ability develops precisely thanks to the mother's *containing* and mentalising activity. After all, the ambient mother is buzzing with language.[110] All the child's experiences are embedded in a *basso continuo* of murmurs, where it is not so important what is said but that and how it is said. It is language (not only or so much in its *meaning-value* but) in its sound-value, as an affective-existential instrument. The mother mirrors, modulates and imitates.[111] By attuning to her child's affective tone ('affect attunement')[112] she provides vital and categorical affects[113] with image, sound and rhythm. She provides 'moments of meeting'[114] and contributes to ongoing meaning-making. The mother doses illusion and disillusion; in Winnicott's words she opens a 'transitional space'.[115]

This transitional space is the register of the imaginary and imagination opened by the mother, who allows her child to detach from her gradually. It is (in a Lacanian preview) the mother who obeys the law of the No and the Name of the Father, thus installing a distance based on the impossible Real and the Symbolic forbidden. She oscillates between two positions: between being something the baby can find and make actual in an omnipotent way and being itself waiting to be found. Indeed, at this stage, the child 'creates' itself a subjective object that Winnicott calls a transitional object.[116] There are the material transitional objects (a bedspread, a toy, a bear)[117] and the temporary/immaterial objects (sounds, songs, verses) to which the child can cling.

The transitional object is an object that appears when the child needs it so that the child has the feeling of having created it. It is an object that is simultaneously discovered and invented by the child, which is only possible by the grace of the environment that provides it.[118] It is an object that is neither internal nor external, simultaneously mediates and symbolises the mother's presence and absence, and protects the child (mainly) from (depressive) anxieties. It is an object that comes into being at the time of separation from the mother. It represents the transition from a state of fusion with the mother to a state of coming into a relationship with the mother as something/someone outside, as being- and distinct and distinguished. It is, after all, a temporary and transient object. It is not repressed, nor is it in some sense lost. It simply loses meaning as it is dispersed and diluted into the broader space of play, playfulness and culture.

For Winnicott, the transitional space that unfolds is, in summary, the play space in which the child comes to a symbolic-imaginary (and not omnipotent) mastering of the Real of presence and absence, of drive and trauma. For him, this capacity for play and creativity is essential for psychological health. For him, it also makes up the essence of psychotherapy, which is mainly about two people playing together.[119] Christopher Bollas[120] uses the term 'playwork' to describe the back and forth of work and play, of reflection and experience that plays a role in any psychoanalysis.[121]

9 The Holding Environment

In the first years of life, the child is totally and later relatively dependent on its environment. When psychopathology takes root in these periods, Winnicott considers deep regression to be therapeutically necessary to reconnect with the core of the True Self and to restart blocked ('frozen')[122] development. This requires a holding environment[123] that provides the care and support needed.

The need for this care and support certainly applies to all patients who (have to) receive residential treatment. After all, they have major psychotic and/or mood pathology, have serious personality problems and/or have often ended up in a more or less life-threatening crisis state. They then need the safety, care and protection provided by a continuously available nursing function (the environment mother). We point out in this context that 'nursing' and 'nurturing' as typical nursing terms are the same terms used to describe the 'primary maternal preoccupation' towards her baby.

With all these problems, the patient (like the infant) needs us to accommodate certain illusions. For example, the illusion that the caregiver possesses healing qualities and knowledge is powerful, can offer protection, and can satisfy basic needs. This creates an idealising transference that we need to leave intact in the first place. We need not interpret it but accept and respect it. After all, the hungry and needy baby in the patient needs our more or less intensive care. They also need mirroring and affirmation, holding and structure. By providing such a holding and facilitating environment, environmental deficits from the phase of absolute dependency can be repaired. Narcissistic hurts can be repaired in a combined work of 'panser' (anointing) and 'penser' (thinking),[124] and support is a necessary but insufficient condition for psychotherapeutic work to begin. The change process occurs partly because we allow the patient to use us.[125] Without putting much effort into this, we will gradually disillusion the patient during the psychotherapeutic process.

Donald Winnicott has since become a pivotal figure in 20th-century psychoanalysis, and his lasting influence on psychotherapeutic theory is almost as significant as that of Freud. Although he did not explicitly distance himself from Freudian orthodoxy, many of his theoretical and technical innovations are at odds with it. Not least because he implicitly adopted a two-person psychology and thus pioneered the later self-psychology and relational school. In this context, it seems appropriate to refer to the thinking of Heinz Kohut in connection with the treatment of narcissistic pathology in adults, as it has very striking similarities with Winnicott's thinking. He, too, emphasises the positive aspects of narcissism related to creativity, a sense of humour and wisdom. Across the narcissistic line, for him, psychological growth is the result of two contrasting processes: empathic mirroring and optimal frustration. For him, pathology corresponds to the defect model and would result from empathic deficits and/or traumatic disconnection of the mother–child duality, resulting in 'nameless preverbal aggression'. His concern is not so much with inner object representations and object relations but with external ties that we need to develop and maintain self-worth and coherence of the self. This involves, on the one hand, patients with a grandiose-exhibitionist self who need affirmation or admiration or, conversely, patients with a weak sense of self in whom fragmentation is imminent. This narcissistic lineage persists throughout our lives (parallel to that of object love). We continue to need the other to fulfil the role of self-object.[126] Sexual and aggressive acting out behaviour are understood as degradation products in this self-psychological view. Watching over and caring for narcissistic balance is also promoted to a continuous focus in any sustained psychotherapeutic process.

Winnicott and Kohut face similar criticisms from various psychoanalytic quarters. There is in their work a disregard for the sexual, the drive, the conflictual and the Oedipal. Technically, they both emphasise empathy, the gratification of pre-oedipal needs (safety, warmth, mirroring, caring, etc.) and corrective emotional experience. They made a substantial contribution to psychoanalytically inspired supportive psychotherapy and to better understand (so to speak, the chemical composition of) nonspecific factors that play an essential role in all mental help.[127]

10 Attachment

Concerning attachment, I would like to start with a quote from Freud: 'Just as the Id is only after pleasure, so considerations of safety control the Ego. The Ego has charged itself with the task of self-preservation, which the Id seems to neglect'.[128] These considerations of security are mainly addressed in attachment theory. It is the joint work of John Bowlby and Mary Ainsworth.[129] To this end, they drew on findings and concepts derived from developmental psychology, ethology and psychoanalysis.[130]

John Bowlby pioneered attachment research on thousands of children after WWII. He distinguished between two completely different issues. There is, on the one hand, the dependence the child exhibits towards 'primary caretakers' who are responsible for satisfying its various physiological needs. After all, the human child comes into the world immature and still needs a lot of extra-uterine care and growth (including of the brain) to function independently. However, attachment is something completely different. It arises towards figures who pay attention to and tune into the child's inner world and interact with it (e.g. playfully). To these persons, the child becomes attached. Love is said to be attachment-based, while pleasure has different evolutionary roots. We now know they are located in a different (neuronal) circuit in which oxytocin and testosterone play a leading role.[131] Attachment and sexual behaviour constitute two systems.[132] They are activated separately and directed to different objects, and the developmental stages within which fixation or imprinting occurs are different,[133] even though there are many links between them. That one is intertwined with the other is evidenced, for example, by the honeymoon of romantic infatuation that is strong enough to cement a strong bond.[134]

Attachment theory revolutionised thinking about the mother–child relationship and the consequences of separation, deficit and loss. Mary Ainsworth also succeeded in testing Bowlby's ideas empirically and experimentally, and she provided two additions. First, the concept of the attachment figure as a secure base from which the child can explore the world. Second, the idea of maternal 'sensitivity'. This ability allows her to read her infant's signals and plays a crucial role in developing the resulting attachment pattern.[135]

Besides studying medicine and psychiatry at Cambridge, John Bowlby volunteered with behaviourally disturbed adolescents. He also took training at the British Psychoanalytic Institute and was in analysis with Joan Rivière, who was closely associated with Melanie Klein. Bowlby, incidentally, subsequently also went into supervision with Klein. Although he acknowledges both of their object-relational influence, Bowlby had strong reservations about Klein's child analysis. He disagreed with the causal importance she attached to the inner at the expense of the outer world. Through his work at the London Child Guidance Clinic, he believed that actual family experiences played a much more fundamental role than childlike phantasy life. He sympathised with the object-relational theories of Ronald Fairbairn and Donald Winnicott, but he developed his ideas independently of them.

A detailed examination of forty-four cases allowed him to relate their problems to a history of deficits or ruptures in the mother–child relationship.[136] As an expert on affective neglect, he was asked by the World Health Organisation to report on the mental health of homeless children in post-war Europe. It allowed him to draw inspiration from numerous social workers and researchers worldwide, including, for example, René Spitz.[137] The report was written in six months, was translated into 14 languages and reached a circulation of 400,000 copies as *Maternal Care and Mental Health* in the English-language paperback edition.

Looking at this report from a contemporary perspective, it is notable that Bowlby still used the terminology of traditional psychoanalysis (love object, libidinal ties, Ego and Superego), but his conclusions were almost heretical.[138] For instance, he (like René Spitz) used embryology as a metaphor for the role of the mother in child development.[139] Bowlby presented his first official attachment-theoretical views in the form of three now-classic articles in London for the *British Psychoanalytic Society.*[140] They met with significant criticism there, so he would henceforth deliver and publish his further work only outside the psychoanalytic world.[141]

New methodological traces by Mary Ainsworth on attachment patterns in the *Strange Situation Test*, as well as Mary Main's *Adult Attachment Interview,* were embroidered on Bowlby. They both demonstrate the cross-cultural relevance and recognisability of different attachment patterns. Without their contributions to developmental and clinical psychology, Bowlby would probably never have been as influential today. Peter Fonagy, in particular, continues this paradigmatic line with his ideas related to mentalisation. He sees attachment and mentalising as correlative. They are also (independently of genetics) transmitted trans-generationally unless psychotherapy breaks this fatal chain reaction.[142]

11 Empirical

The *Strange Situation Test* [143] focuses on the child's reunion behaviour after separation from the mother. In a secure attachment, the child is briefly upset after separation from the mother but happy to see her again. It seeks closeness, feels comforted, and resumes play and exploration effortlessly. In avoidant attachment, the child reacts indifferently to the mother's return. It does not distinguish between a mother and a stranger. Reunion is avoided, and the child flees into the environment and play, as it were. In ambivalent attachment, the child is angry and emotionally overwhelmed and confused; love and hate fight for the upper hand, and the child does not come to play. Later, a fourth pattern is added by Mary Main, namely the disorganised type where the child goes in all directions at once. There is then no coherent strategy.

The four patterns described can also be found in the *Adult Attachment Interview*.[144] This is a half-hour tape-recorded interview in which more of the (linguistic, among other things) form than the content is analysed. The attachment pattern derived from it is then found to predict their child's attachment.[145] Autonomous and securely attached individuals will validate their past intimate relationships. They bring a coherent narrative, are cooperative, recognise the importance of past relationships and can distance themselves from positive and negative experiences. The dismissive tend to denigrate or idealise. They minimise or deny the importance of past relationships. They have a poor memory, tell short stories and emphasise mainly their strengths. The preoccupied are confused and overwhelmed, seemingly still entangled in early attachment experiences. There is much anger, and their narrative is somewhat incoherent or irrelevant. The disorganised have a manifest history of loss of attachment figures, neglect and/or trauma. There is disbelief towards their own reality, as it were.

Like the psychoanalytic, attachment theory is bipolar. Psychoanalysis is about love and hate, life drive and death drive, split and integration. Regarding attachment, the poles are closeness and avoidance, security and insecurity, attachment and loss. For psychoanalysis, it is about libido and the satisfaction of oral (and other pre-genital) urges. Attachment theory considers the search for security as the primary motive. After all, it is necessary for survival and essential in all our relationships. For Bowlby, it provides an empirical basis for object relation theory, and sex is simply a 'signpost to the object'.[146]

Since the 1950s, various psychoanalysts have studied deficits in the early mother–child relationship. Depending on the author, these include 'silent trauma' (Hoffer, 1952), 'cumulative trauma' (Khan, 1963) or 'neglect trauma' (Bowlby, 1973). Infant research (e.g. Beatrice Beebe, Daniel Stern, Colin Trevarthen or Edward Tronick)[147] also provided much additional data on the nature and importance of this first period of life. Fundamental assumptions such as Klein's early Ego, Winniocott's primary maternal preoccupation, and Kohut's mirroring found their correlation in empirically validated theories such as Colin Trevarthen's primary intersubjectivity, Daniel Stern's cross-modal affect attunement or the micro-analysis of video-recorded communication between the mother and her baby. Sometimes, objective observations and subjective descriptions come at odds. For instance, Freud's classic auto-erotic phase, Margaret Mahler's autistic-symbiotic phase, Thomas Ogden's autistic-contiguous phase, as well as an initial (allegedly primarily narcissistic) state of defective differentiation between subject and object are repeatedly contradicted.[148]

12 Development Aid

Obviously, after Freud, most authors shifted their attention to the pre-oedipal mother–child relationship and to psychopathology rooted in that first stage of life. However, while Melanie Klein still developed a play technique in which the interpretive processing and analysis of transference and resistance remained central, quite a few other authors emphasised the importance of an attentive, caring and supportive presence. Sandor Ferenczi, Michael Balint,[149] John Bowlby, Donald Winnicott, and Heinz Kohut theorised the more securing, supporting and/or empathetic components they felt analytic work in 'early' disorders should contain. Inspiration is the archaic mother: the mother-muse or the womb mother from whom the infant must, in some sense, *receive* enough to grow.

It was discussed earlier that the DSM's descriptive, a-theoretical, categorical, static and non-developmental disorder-centred approach is complemented by a psychodynamic, developmental and person-centred one.[150] With Otto Kernberg, it is founded on more or less mature levels of personality organisation, but with Sidney Blatt, it is more qualitative.[151] Here, he distinguishes between relationship/attachment/connection problems versus self-definition or identity problems. They each exhibit prototypical conflict and defence patterns as attempts to install and maintain relationships and self-definition.

Indeed, a thorough study of theorisation and empirical research shows that in much psychopathology, a dichotomy can be found between an introjective/autonomous and an anaclitic/sociotropic line of development.[152] The anaclitic line leads to increasingly mature, complex, and mutually satisfying relationships, and the introjective one leads to the development of a stable, realistic, and (predominantly) positive self-image and identity. Psychopathology can be seen as the overemphasis of one lineage versus the neglect (or defensive avoidance) of the other. The anaclitic/sociotropic group is more characterised by feelings of loneliness, helplessness, separation and separation anxiety. They have covetous and dependent traits, are clingy, long for care and protection and have dual, undifferentiated relationships with others that primarily serve to meet all kinds of needs. In contrast, the introjective/ autonomous group is characterised mainly by self-criticism and feelings of shame, guilt, worthlessness or fear of disapproval. There is exaggerated conscientiousness and perfectionism. These patients feel unloved rather than unlovable. Instead, they are aloof and cool, strive for control and independence, and are perfectionists and competitive. Their relationships are more differentiated and triangulated, however.

Outcome research and meta-analyses suggest that the introjective group would benefit more from 'classical' analytic and interpretive work (like that of Freud, Klein and Kernberg). In contrast, the anaclitic group would initially need and benefit more from supportive psychotherapy and the building of a secure bond/attachment (along the lines of Ferenczi, Balint, Winnicott, Kohut). They can benefit from more classical, interpretive work only when these 'needs' have been met and something has been built up sufficiently.

The human child is born in total physiological and motor immaturity and thus thrown into the world in absolute dependence. Freud repeatedly points out that this biological dependence installs the first danger situations and creates the need to be loved, which will continue to play a significant role for the rest of human life. Whether it is primary object love (Balint),[153] an innate tendency towards attachment (Bowlby),[154] the vital importance of holding and primary maternal preoccupation (Winnicott), alpha-function and containment (Bion), mirroring by the mother (Kohut) or mentalisation (Fonagy), most post-Freudians emphasise the essential role that the psychoanalyst also has to play as a development object and as a development helper.

Pathology is understood according to a defect model rather than a conflict model. It leads to actual rather than psychopathology, to mental process disorders rather than to mental representational[155] disorders. After all, psychic life is determined as much by the search for (the connection with) an object as by the search for pleasure/avoidance of un-pleasure. It depends more on satisfying needs than being driven by the order of desire. Because of the analyst, it is as much about construction and subject amplification as it is about interpretation and reconstruction. In this view, psychoanalysis took on a more 'parental' character. The post-Freudians above also paid relatively little attention to love and eroticism. Some, therefore, even speak of a specific 'flight from the erotic'.[156] Already according to Freud, love and sexuality belong to two different domains.[157] The word 'love' cannot be used in connection with the relationship between drive and object but must be reserved for that between the Ego and the object. Michael Balint considered the biological connection between mother and child as the basis for primary object love.[158] Balint's primary love foreshadowed Bowlby's evolutionarily understandable need for secure attachment. John Bowlby reproached Freudian drive theory for being trapped in orality.[159] However, in this so-called 'disagreement', are not the Ego- or self-preservation drives and sexual drives confused?

Meanwhile, psychoanalysts from the attachment tradition did return somewhat to infantile sexuality.[160] In doing so, Mary Target and Peter Fonagy proposed a model that integrates their views on mentalisation and developmental psychology with the thinking of Jean Laplanche, which will be introduced in the next chapter.[161] In Mary Target's words, the mother's seductiveness thereby sexualises her baby's arousal.[162] For his part, Peter Fonagy speculates that the internalisation of an incongruent response to frustration lends to the psychosexual core its unique interplay of urgency and incongruity.[163] Rudi Vermote also frequently quotes Fonagy's witticism, namely that we may all be functioning at borderline levels sexually.[164]

Also, everyone knows that development aid does not benefit from patron-isation, indoctrination or colonialism. Until there is proof to the contrary, we can assume that those involved have tried to make the best of it with their (too) limited resources and that we have to draw from their creativity and learn respectfully from them. Any development aid, therefore, will always be accompanied by a careful analysis of the why and how of any difficulties or deficits that arise. Nor can psychosexuality and emancipation be reduced to a mere matter of natural maturation or good-enough material or spiritual nourishment. A well-understood subjectification requires misunderstanding and faltering in addition to alignment and harmony. Nor does our sub-jectification come about without the necessary 'harshness' and negativity.[165] These result, among other things, from the clash with law and/or language. It is an excellent opportunity to move from the Anglo-Saxon (and more empirical) to the continental (more rationalist) language. In doing so, we ascend again to Freud's neurosis, also as the human condition.

Notes

1 Sigmund Freud (1909). Oedipus complex and infantile sexuality get ample con-firmation in this case study.
2 Differences of opinion on this premise are primarily at the root of the difference between the two schools in child psychotherapy. The (Anna) Freudian school is reluctant to explore the unconscious of the Oedipus complex and transference. It favours a more educationally tinged and developmentally oriented intervention, where positive transference is encouraged and pursued (Anna Freud (1927 p 3–69). The Kleinian direction does analyse (negative) transference. Given its aggressive/destructive content, it is very frightening and pathogenic for the child and should be clearly distinguished from the external reality of the natural parents.
3 Hannah Segal (1964).
4 Melanie Klein (1955).
5 Melanie Klein (1926 p 134): 'We can only fully understand (play) if we approach the method Freud has evolved for unravelling dreams.'
6 'The boy's and the girl's sexual and emotional development from early infancy onwards includes genital sensations and trends, which constitute the first stages of the inverted and positive Oedipus complex; they are experienced under the primacy of the oral libido and mingle with urethral and anal desires and phantasies' (Klein, 1945 p 414).

7   Pre-genital and genital classically apply to the drive source, and development results from 'natural' maturation. In contrast, for Lacan, it is about the orifices around which the 'traffic' with the Other revolves.

8   Winnicott (1954a p 264) speaks of the 'capacity for concern' so that he changes Klein's pathological-sounding designation to a 'more ordinary recognisable feeling' (Phillips, 1988 p 107).

9   'I now propose to use for these feelings of sorrow and concern for the loved objects, the fears of losing them and the longing to regain them...the "pining" for the lost object.' (Klein, 1940 p 348).

10 'Manic' repair: denial of loss and guilt and omnipotently (e.g. with a flower or a kiss) conjuring it away. Depressive repair: acknowledging one's share, empathically responding to others' subjectivity and repairing with due time and effort.

11 Betty Joseph (1985).

12 Melanie Klein (1952 p 55) and (1957 p 180): 'The infant feels all this in much more primitive ways than language can express. When these pre-verbal emotions and phantasies are revived in the transference situation, they appear as "memories in feelings", as I would call them, and are reconstructed and put into words with the help of the analyst'.

13 Subject amplification is a term coined by Verhaeghe (2002a). How can the inner state of the patient and therapist make understandable what is going on in the interaction (Bateman & Fonagy, 2004 p 203)?

14 In clinical psychotherapy, non-verbal expressive therapies, such as plastic expression, dance or music therapy, are also offered as a type of work by a therapist/mother-muse.

15 (Klein, 1932 p 3): 'Along with the belief in the asexuality of the child has gone the belief in the "Paradise of Childhood"'.

16 Melanie Klein understands the death drive as an (aggressive) destructive drive, which contrasts sharply with other interpretations of the concept, such as Barbara Low's Nirwana principle or Lacan's *jouissance*.

17 In Klein's own words: 'I consider that envy is an oral-sadistic and anal-sadistic expression of destructive impulses operative from the beginning of life and that it has a constitutional basis' (1957 p 176–177). Again, Klein: 'Envy is the angry feeling that another person possesses and enjoys something desirable – the envious impulse being to take it away or to spoil it...it implies the subject's relation to one person only and goes back to the earliest exclusive relation with the mother....Jealousy is based on envy but involves a relation to at least two people; it is mainly concerned with love that the subject feels is his due and has been taken away or is in danger of being taken away'(1957 p 181).

18 Psalms (51, 7): 'I was born in wickedness, alas! My mother received me in decadence.'

19 Rudi Vermote (2005a p 70) further elaborated by Bion with his 'waking dream thought' or 'dream work alpha' (Bion, 1997 p 62). In his posthumous publication, Bion (p 38) speaks of an undersea continent that he believes produces the unconscious with its alpha function/dream labour (ibid. p 71).

20 Melanie Klein (1959 p 291).

21 Remind the wonderful pictures of the child sucking thumb even *in the womb* (and thus before it has had any 'contact' with the breast)! For Klein, there is always a phantasy accompanying the drive.

22 In contrast to the image created of her by John Bowlby and Donald Winnicott, for example (which still largely determines her reputation), Klein did attach importance to the external environment. See Klein (1935 p 285 or 1940 p 347).

23   Jan Cambien (1988) speaks of a Leibnizian monadology. See also the assessment by Bercherie (1988).

24   The depressive position differentiates between splitting and integration and opens the way to object constancy: the capacity for stability in relationships and commitments 'in good days and bad.'

25   According to Jacques Lacan (1938), humans are defined by three significant complexes (being symbolic structures instead of instincts): *le complexe de sevrage* (weaning), *le complexe d'intrusion* (another child breaking the monopoly on the Other) and *le complexe d'Oedipe.*

26   Melanie Klein (1928) and (1945).

27   It is now well established that in personality disorders and depression, two types can repeatedly be distinguished, and this is from both behavioural therapeutic and psychodynamic research: the introjective/autonomous/perfectionist and the anaclitic/dependent/sociotropic. It is also well established that the former benefits more from interpretation (Klein, Kernberg,...) and the latter more from a way of working that focuses on building a secure bond and relationship (Ferenczi, Balint, Winnicott, Kohut,...), see Corveleyn, Luyten and Blatt (2005 p 67–137). Rudi Vermote's (2005a) large-scale study also confirms these findings.

28   Gerald Adler (1979).

29   Otto Kernberg (1984b).

30   Caricatured or consisting of contradictory 'pieces': 'My father is sweet. He's a mixture of Hitler and Stalin'.

31   The latter mechanism remains controversial. It was introduced by Melanie Klein (1946) and is the process by which pieces of the self or the (inner) object are split off and denied and projected into an object in phantasy, after which this object is identified with this piece. See later in this book.

32   Kleinism focuses almost exclusively on the early mother-child relationship. In a Lacanian view, psychosis is the result of *'forclusion'*: in the first instance, excluding the father from the family structure and in the second instance, excluding the (Name of the) Father from the Symbolic order.

33   The Rustins (2016 p 87) identify these prejudices about Klein, but the difference with Winnicott is noticeable.

34   But her texts teem with clinical (especially case) material and are confirmed by contemporary research (Fonagy & Target, 2003 p 134).

35   Dixit Melanie Klein 'to find an analytic technique specially adapted to the child, which we find in play analysis...The difference between this method of analysis and that of adult analysis, however, is purely one of technique and not of principle (1932 p 14) or 'the analyst should not shy away from making a deep interpretation even at the start of the analysis' (ibid. p 24).

36   Philippe van Haute (2005).

37   He comments on Klein in two consecutive seminar years, namely 1953–1955 (1975a) and (1978).

38   For Klein's rebuttal see 1927 p 137: 'consistent interpretations, gradual solving of resistances and persistent tracing of the transference...constitute in children as in adults the correct analytic situation' or still: 'analysis is not in itself a gentle method: it cannot spare the patient any suffering, and this applies equally to children' (ibid. p 144).

39   The 1950s saw the rise of a creative object-relational generation within the British Association (Greenberg & Mitchell, 1983).

40   Psychoanalytic work with psychotics is something with which some psychoanalysts are quite daring to 'act out'. Bion: 'They wear psychotics in their hair' (1974 p 92ff).

41 For an excellent overview of Freudian, Lacanian and (post-) Kleinian approaches, Smet et al. (2003).
42 Rudi Vermote (1997).
43 Wilfred Bion (1967).
44 Colette Soler (1987 p 30).
45 Some internationally renowned analysts in Bion's 'line' include Leon Grinberg, Horacio Etchegoyen, James Grotstein, Andre Green, Antonio Ferro and, in my own country, Rudi Vermote.
46 Wilfred Bion (1967 p 93–109 and 110–119).
47 Ludi Van Bouwel (1998 p 30).
48 Rudi Vermote (2018): 'Delusions and hallucinations are evacuated beta elements forming bizarre objects as a conglomeration of evacuated beta elements with attacked and split-off ego functions'.
49 There are huge similarities between Bion and Lacan. Both started their theorising with psychosis, strove for mathematical notation, and had an obtuse style. Bion's O and Lacan's Real are related (and only came to take precedence towards the end of their lives and work). The big difference, of course, is their attitude towards the mystical. Bion strives for immediate contact with O, while for Lacan, we are banished from this nameless being and the (supposed) *jouissance* that accompanies it. At first, the child is trapped in the mother's desire, sharing an imaginary language from which the third is excluded. The latter liberates the child from this imaginary and opens the symbolic order (Vermote, 2018).
50 Alpha-function 'converts sense-data into alpha-elements and thus provides the psyche with the material for dream thoughts and hence the capacity to...be conscious or unconscious' (Bion, 1967 p 115). The omega function is the opposite: the parent bounces the child's feelings back unchanged (Williams, 1997).
51 Joseph Sandler (1987).
52 Wilfred Bion (1962 p 17–18).
53 ibidem (1962 p 26).
54 Didier Anzieu (1994) In dermatological terms, psychosis is characterised by exposed flesh (whether or not hidden under the chitin of an exoskeleton). There is 'thick skinned' and 'thin-skinned' (respectively difficult and easy to hurt) narcissism; in borderline, there are gaps in the skin, and the neurotic suffers (jokingly) from too many goose pimples. The (autistic) exoskeleton arises as a defence against a threatening Other, while the endoskeleton is the internalisation of a supportive Other see Wilfred Bion (1982 p 48).
55 Wilfred Bion (1967 p 166).
56 For both Freud and Lacan, psychosis is essentially the result of '*Verwerfung*' and '*forclusion*'. What is expelled from the symbolic returns from the Real (delusions and hallucinations). See Jacques Lacan (1981b p 3).
57 Ibidem p 52.
58 Wilfred Bion (1970 p 13).
59 I think of a patient (one element of a one-egg twin) who had the numbers 66 and the word Fahrenheit in her head as if they were splinters of the Real. The 66 was not a signifier for twinhood but a concretism, a '*symbolic equation*' à la Hanna Segal (1957).
60 On the protomental, see Wilfred Bion (1961 p 101, 1962 p 103).
61 Wilfred Bion (1997 p 10).
62 Wilfred Bion (1970 p 15).
63 For the binocular, see Wilfred Bion (1962 p. 53). For this paradoxical, meta-phorical way of thinking, see Ignacio Matte-Blanco (1975) and his simassy:

'simultaneous use of symmetrical and asymmetrical thinking'. See also Slavoj Žižek (2009b) or Jacques Lacan's 'Listening with two ears' (Lacan, 1966a p 471).

64   Wilfred Bion (1962).

65   Wilfred Bion (1967). The Lacanians have a structural diagnostics of neurosis, psychosis and perversion as three 'answers' to lack that are repressed, excluded and denied, respectively. All other post-Freudians adopt a dimensional diagnosis.

66   Wilfred Bion (1963).

67   Mark Kinet (2002a, b).

68   Wilfred Bion (1970).

69   Not by reason but *intuition* 'to detect a pattern that remains unaltered in widely differing contexts' (Bion 1970 p 92). Rudi Vermote (1994) contrasts the experience of the Sphinx with the conquering (wanting to know) of Oedipus in this context.

70   Beyond words or with a 'language of achievement' (which the poet would possess).

71   A term of the Romantic poet John Keats in ibidem (1970 p 125). Claudio Neri believes it is crucial in group psychotherapy (2009).

72   Simons Vestdijk (1960).

73   Wilfred Bion (1970 p 31). Or: 'Memory and desire are "illuminations" that destroy the value of the analyst's capacity for observation as leakage of light into the camera might destroy the value of the film being exposed (1970 p 69).

74   Wilfred Bion (1965 p 158). Rudi Vermote (2018) places a caesura at Bion's transition from transformations in K to transformations in O. The analyst must be in O, allowing it to bubble up from the infinite primordial soup, the first mental molecules.

75   O is the symbol for the unknown and unknowable, the ultimate reality or for thoughts without a thinker. 'when I use the letter, O, I mean it to indicate noumenon, the thing itself of which nobody can know anything' (Bion, 1974 p. 69).

76   Betty Joseph (1985).

77   In his discourse theory, Lacan similarly situates the position of the analyst in object small a.

78   Wilfred Bion (1970 p 124).

79   Jacques Lacan (1978 p 22–35).

80   See Lacan's '*La jouissance est interdite à qui parle comme tel*' because they intuitively sense that the enjoyment that lies beyond would drive them *mad*.

81   Bion exerted a significant influence on Rosenfeld, Segal, Money-Kyrle, Tustin and Meltzer (UK), Grotstein, Isaacs, Ogden and Eigen (US), Anzieu and Green (Fr) and Ferro, Neri, Civitarese (It) See Vermote (2018).

82   Wilfred Bion (1965 p 163). Religious terms (act of faith, mystic, messianic idea) are paramount in Bion's thought. Referring to Winnicott (good-enough mother) and Balint (basic fault), Jacques Lacan ventures a 'delirious moralism' (1959) in (1966 p 716). He might have accused Bion of a delirious *mysticism*.

83   Reading Bion (Vermote, 2018).

84   Otto Kernberg (1993) and (1999).

85   Midgley (2007).

86   King & Steiner (1991). The Kleinians circulated four articles. These were commented on in writing and then discussed in 11 meetings led by Londoners Ernest Jones and James Strachey.

87   His only comprehensive work was published posthumously and was (drive stages included) very Freudian (Winnicott, 1988).

88 Rustin & Rustin (2016). In this, he will be followed by Marion Milner, Masud Khan, Christopher Bollas, Adam Phillips, Andre Green and Thomas Ogden, among others.

89 Because based more on observation than reconstruction, cf. earlier note.

90 In a 1952 letter to fellow analyst Money-Kyrle, he calls Freud's introduction of the death drive 'perhaps his only blunder' (Rodman, 1987 p 42).

91 Donald Winnicott (1969a p 462–463).

92 Winnicott (1952 p 99).

93 Donald Winnicott (1956 p 303). 'During late pregnancy and early post-natal life, the facilitating environment achieves structured integration so that disintegration is a possibility and unintegration a resource (Phillips, 1988).

94 Donald Winnicott (1960 p 54).

95 Donald Winnicott (1968 p 101).

96 Donald Winnicott (1963b p 187–190).

97 Donald Winnicott (1962 p 61).

98 In the psychoanalytic space, being able to be 'silent' can have a healing meaning for the analysant. There is no need for persecutory interpretation. It is the feminine element in psychoanalysis, where *being* is more important than doing, cfr resp Donald Winnicott (1958 p 29–30) and (1971 p 80–81).

99 Donald Winnicott (1967 p 114) places the mother's traumatic 'absence' on an x + y + z time axis. At x, the mother is qualitatively present; after x + y, she can still help mentalise and contain her absence; after x + y + z, a rupture occurs in the baby's survival that leaves its mark and triggers primitive defence mechanisms.

100 Donald Winnicott (1945 p 154).

101 See Jean Bergeret's *violence fondamentale* (1988), the alternative to Freud's thanatos (Verbruggen, 1999 p 89).

102 Donald Winnicott (1939 p 88).

103 Donald Winnicott (1963).

104 Absolute dependence is both the 'fact of life' of the human condition and very frightening for those who ask for help and the help-giver. For Winnicott, it underlies the 'fear of WOMAN' (1950 p 252): the fear of loss of self and subject whereby we are in danger of disappearing (Lacanian-style: into the enjoyment of the big Other).

105 Jan Cambien (2005 p 28).

106 Simon Vestdijk (1960), from which all art and literature develop.

107 See Andre Green (1983).

108 Donald Winnicott (1960 p 46).

109 Bion's containment and Winnicott's holding are often confused/used inter-changeably. The containment is inner, and the holding is also externally obser-vable; containment focuses on integration, holding on growth (Symington, 1986).

110 The environment mother must be distinguished from the object-mother (1956a, 1963a). In the first stage, what the mother does (well) is in no way realised by the infant (1956 p 304): primary maternal preoccupation (1963b p 300–306).

111 Winnicott refers to Lacan's (1949) mirror stage: 'However Lacan does not think of the mirror in terms of the mother's face in the way that I wish to do here' (1971a p 111). Joyce McDougall (2003) recalls Winnicott's analytic space as a space for play and creativity, while she sees Jacques Lacan's as a space where the patient never feels (entirely) at ease. It will be discussed later that Winnicott's approach is mainly about mental processes, and Lacan's is primarily about mental contents.

112 Daniel Stern (1985).
113 Vital: the quantitative grounding of vitality, categorical: referring to feeling qualities.
114 Daniel Stern (1998).
115 Donald Winnicott (1951).
116 The transitional object: It is a matter of agreement between us and the baby that we will never ask: Did you come up with this? Or was it offered to you from outside? (Winnicott, 1971a p 12). The transitional object is protosymbolic; developmentally, it is situated between Hannah Segal's symbolic equation and a full-fledged symbol (Alvarez, 1996).
117 Famous example: Linus' blanket in Charles Schulz's *Peanuts*.
118 In my view, the only 'effective' interpretation also has the status of subjective/transitional object: it is a paradoxical object between analysant and analyst that is 'created' by the former and provided by the latter.
119 Donald Winnicott (1971b p 38).
120 Christopher Bollas (1993 p 46).
121 Friedrich Schiller (1796): Man is most authentically himself when he plays. From affective neuroscience, an independent (temperamental, behavioural and neurophysiological) PLAY system is confirmed (Panksepp, 1998; Kinet, 2023).
122 Donald Winnicott (1954 p 281).
123 Donald Winnicott, (ibidem p 285–286).
124 M. Monjauze (1999).
125 Donald Winnicott (1968a).
126 A nice example is the volleyball on which Chuck Noland/Tom Hanks draws a rudimentary face and which he calls 'Wilson' in Robert Zemeckis' feature film *Cast Away* (2000).
127 See, for example, H. Rockland (1989). Winnicott (1962 p 169): 'Psychoanalysis is not just a matter of interpreting the repressed unconscious it is rather the provision of a professional setting for trust, in which such work may take place (see also 1986 p 115) or Thomas Ogden (2001 p 301): 'Winnicott transforms psychoanalysis…into the facilitation of the patient's being alive'.
128 Sigmund Freud (1940 p 495). Neuropsychoanalytically, following Jaak Panksepp's affective neuroscience, an attachment instinct (called PANIC/GRIEF) is retained. Its main neuromodulator is beta-endorphin, which acts on mu-opioid receptors. Like any drive, PANIC/GRIEF makes 'demands upon the mind for work' in this case, reunion with the missed caregiver (Panksepp, 1998).
129 Mary Ainsworth & John Bowlby (1991).
130 Van Rosmalen et al. (2012).
131 Mark Solms (2021a).
132 Attachment and sexuality are closely linked but distinct behavioural systems (Fonagy, 2001 p 9–10).
133 John Bowlby (1988).
134 Helen Fisher (2004).
135 Bretherton (1992).
136 John Bowlby.
137 René Spitz (1945, 1946, 1965) published on hospitalism, the dangers of institutional care for children and anaclitic depression. He influenced John Bowlby and Harry Harlow (Van der Horst & Van der Veer, 2008). There are more than 30 references to Spitz in Bowlby's trilogy.
138 One of them is reported to have remarked: 'Bowlby? Give me Barrabas' (Grosskurth, 1987 in Van Rosmalen et al., 2012).

139 'If mental development is to proceed smoothly, it would appear necessary for the undifferentiated psyche to be exposed during certain critical periods to the influence of the psychic organiser – the mother'. (Bowlby, 1951 p. 53).
140 John Bowlby (1958, 1959 and 1960).
141 John Bowlby was judged too behavioural, relying on observations of children and rhesus monkeys. The inner world seemed to disappear from his thinking.
142 Peter Fonagy (2001).
143 Mary Ainsworth et al. (1978).
144 See aai_interview.pub (rrcstaff.com).
145 Mary Main (1996).
146 *Jouissance* (under the guise of dopaminergic 'incentive salience') ensures the historicisation of our subjectivity (Kinet, 2022, 2023).
147 Beebe & Lachmann (2002).
148 Daniel Stern (1985, 1988, 1994).
149 Sandor Ferenczi was Melanie Klein's first analyst. He focused on the mother–child relationship and transference-countertransference events, excelling in a meticulous discussion of childhood trauma (Kinet, 2023b). Michael Balint (1952, 1968) elaborated in his line. Like Bowlby, they were opposed to libido theory and inaugurated a relational psychoanalysis.
150 Luyten et al. (2015).
151 Sidney Blatt (2008).
152 See Luyten et al. (2005 p 67–137).
153 Michael Balint (1952).
154 John Bowlby (1988).
155 See later in this book.
156 Adam Phillips (1988 p 152). See also Andre Green (1995).
157 Sigmund Freud (1915a).
158 Michael Balint (1952).
159 John Bowlby (1958 p 350–373).
160 Target (2007), Fonagy (2008).
161 See the next chapter.
162 Mary Target (2007 p 520).
163 Peter Fonagy (2008 p 23).
164 Rudi Vermote (2011 p 69).
165 A double difference characterises language: between the words themselves and between the word and what is represented (Lacan, 1966a p 276). The symbolic order is founded on presence/absence, e.g. *fort/da* of the mother and of the phallus. It is binary/digital (as opposed to analogical) and it allows for infinite combinations. Moreover, binary language refers (also) to things that do not exist. By 'fighting' for common myths, ideologies, collective fantasies, etc, we 'liberate' ourselves from biology (Harari, 2011).

Chapter 8

The French Connection
The Language Difference

I Word and Deed

Freud ends his text on *Totem and Taboo* [1] with a quote from Goethe's *Faust*:[2] 'In the beginning was the deed'. In contrast, the Gospel of John begins with: 'In the beginning was the Word'.[3] A substantial disagreement between these two gentlemen seems to have occurred from the beginning. Yet they may both be right. It has to do with the difference between chronological and logical time.[4] In nature, the cause always comes before the effect. If *a* is the cause of *b*, *a* also comes before *b*. With humans, this chronology is not so evident. What do I do today when I know I will die tomorrow? Or what about yesterday's decision to marry tomorrow if I learned today that my partner cheated on me the day before yesterday? We have already pointed out that in symbolic (as opposed to real) determinedness, there is the afterwardsness of a history constantly being written and rewritten. In human affairs, time does not have a linear but a more complex course.

If we look at it chronologically, however, our phylogenetic and ontogenetic prehistory[5] was dominated by action and interaction. Language was nonexistent in the child (*in-fans*), and when language 'develops' in the child, it is initially analogical, non-lexical, and semiotic. It emerges in a *joint (ad-) venture* based on which a social bond/relationship with the big Other is formed. Julia Kristeva[6] distinguishes between (pre-oedipal) semiotic and (post-oedipal) symbolic language. In semiotic language, the child produces sounds or babbles in response to the *motherese* of the maternal environment.[7] There is a fluidity where environment and primary process merge, and language is still mainly a matter of imaginary mirroring, where it is not so important *what* but especially *that* something is said. The entry into symbolic language and its rules make a big difference because it is accompanied by the creation of 'law and order', which contributes to increasing mastery.[8] In her (Lacanian) view, this is also necessary for achieving a stable and separate (symbolic) identity (son of, brother of, nurse, Belgian). The previous semiotic period is retroactively written and edited. However, the symbolic

DOI: 10.4324/9781032698052-10

'government' formed by the paternal order is never safe from the possible revolutionary 'upheavals' of the semiotic order.[9] For Kristeva, the three semiotic primary forms that (can) subvert the symbolic order are madness, sanctity and poetry.[10]

Walter Schönau[11] makes a similar distinction between analogue and digital language.[12] Analogue language operates in the immediate, intuitive and bodily perception of non-verbal signs that both animals and small children possess. On this, a digital language superimposes itself in humans where the relationship between word and meaning becomes arbitrary, based on a symbolic convention. There is no longer a compelling link between word and meaning, nor do we ever find the 'right' word again. According to Schönau, analogue and digital language can be identified with Freud's primary and secondary process thinking.[13] Schönau shares Kristeva's view: according to him, too, the poet refuses to acknowledge that language and reality do not correspond. The poem arises due to/thanks to this refusal. It is as if the ink tries to free itself from the alphabet.[14]

(Language) development looks gradual and chronological for most post-Freudians. It seems a matter of development on the (biological) model of crops that mature with proper care and watering. Following his famous 'retour à Freud',[15] this is *not* the view of Jacques Lacan.[16] He ties in with the Freud of dreams, jokes and parapraxes.[17] It is the early Freud of an unconscious he conceived as distinctly textual (unlike his later Id). Lacan will give these Freudian premises a linguistic and philosophical turn. Henceforth, he chooses a distinctive path (especially conceptually and metapsychologically) that opens up many new horizons, specifically in the game of love, whose enigma riddles us all to some extent.

2 Lacan's Trinity

By way of introduction, I will first outline a framework using the Real, the Imaginary and the Symbolic register. Lacan introduced this original Trinity at the very time of his resignation from the International Psychoanalytical Association.[18] This is slightly different from Freud's Trinity of Id, Ego and Superego, but, as will be shown, there are some parallels.[19] Lacan's views and descriptions evolved throughout his life and work, but fundamentally, his RSI describes three mutually interactive orders within which the human mind functions. They can be considered conceptual spaces because every concrete phenomenon is ultimately located at an intersection of the three registers.

For Bion, the infant is born in O. In French, this sounds better: '*il nage dans l'O.*' He *swims* in O. For Freud, the infant starts in the Id, and his Ego and reality principle come to growth based on experience. For Lacan, *mutatis mutandis*, we begin from the Real.[20] Indeed, the baby's living body initially buzzes with a still meaningless temper.[21] A biologically grounded and bodily rooted action-tendency goes in different directions. It is aimed only at immediate gratification or pleasure. We will see that this Real of the living body remains a nameless core of *being* at the heart of our identity. It is the unimaginable and unmentionable remainder that neither image nor signifier can (fully) capture. Unlike the Imaginary and the Symbolic that do not cease to write themselves, the Real (of Thing, drive, and trauma) does not stop *not* writing itself.[22] At the same time, against its will, it continues to haunt our scenarios, our stories and our dreams. At least when it does not (in the form of a blind or stupid compulsion to repeat) put its 'demonic' stamp on our lives.

In a subsequent logical time, the Imaginary is at the forefront. That this concept evokes connotations of unreality and imagination is fortunately not accidental. It is the Realm of the Senses, and it therefore plays a leading role, for example, in love and the arts, which, after all, often start from the body. From eye to sun, eyebrows to clouds and further via nose, arm, foot, tree, table, seat and bed, they provide the terms by which we gradually explore and recognise our environment. Also, more or less poetic: life is the sound of a drinking dog, and death is a truck filled with pigs.

Through this sensory ground, illusion, fascination, and seduction form an affectively charged substrate on which more and more concepts are progressively built. The Imaginary, meanwhile, allows us to see something in its entirety and distinguish, for example, between inside and outside, similarity and difference. It is also the domain of feelings: sympathy and antipathy, love and hate, admiration and contempt, attraction and repulsion. The earlier temper penetrates affectively into all our fibres. Not least in our first (still imaginary) analogical or semiotic language called *lalangue* (En: *llanguage*) by the Lacanians. It is loaded with *jouissance*, as it were, and it underlies our symbolic language.[23]

The infant was initially not yet mediated by language, law or norm. In other words, it was not yet a socialised subject.[24] All kinds of interventions from the big Other try to answer and/or curb early childhood needs and drive claims. But certainly, for the drive, this always succeeds only partially. After all, the drive has to be explicitly distinguished from need. The latter (hunger, thirst and so on) can in principle be satisfied, but the drive draws its pleasure ('*jouissance*') purely from the (also linguistic) functions it motorises. Meanwhile, (micro-) cultural habits and customs are imparted to the child with the spoon or mother's milk. All limit or regulate the child's *jouissance*. In a traditional (patriarchal) view, it is the father who drives a wedge between mother and child. It is the wedge of the law (even when served by the mother). The child must increasingly seek pleasure and satisfaction in civilised ways. Along the way, it loses the immediacy of a maternal Thing that only seemed to contain blissful pleasure in retrospect. It will henceforth have to settle for the small things of life. Of course, with all this, we are entirely in the typically human Symbolic order.

3 Adaptation?

With his Trinity, Lacan disrupts an all-too-simple psychoanalysis aimed at adaptation. He lifts it off its hinges, as it were.[25] According to him, an unbridgeable gap between nature and culture arises in human beings. The original immediacy is lost,[26] and this causes a necessarily unfulfillable[27] and inappropriate longing for *the Real Thing*. We *are*, in a sense, this lack that makes us yearn. This longing is not for an object but a lack (-of-object).[28] Therefore, for him, human beings are essentially not harmonious but rather ruptured, gaping and divided. The law of man is the law of language.[29] Language and/or the Symbolic order are external and pre-existent and constitute the unnatural nature of man as a language animal or speaking being ('*parlêtre*').[30] In the psychoanalytic process, the journey also begins beyond the mirror (of the Imaginary), whose purpose was to cover the rupture, division and lack.

For Lacan, psychoanalysis that focuses on adaptation ignores the alienating implications of the Ego and has a naive conception of reality (which, as the Real, is never knowable and perceivable as such). For him, development is not a natural or (neuro-) biological process but also and especially something motorised by (the desire of) the Other.[31] Nor is it a linear process in time, but it is characterised by afterwardsness. Development is not a fluid process of gradual transitions, but is characterised by leaps/choices and the ever-appearing *creatio ex nihilo* in which the subject manifests itself. After all, this subject is the missing link that, in all evolutionary thought, is conspicuous by its absence.[32]

Humans are governed not only by an instinct[33] (as a fixed and innate relation to the object) but also by drives and complexes. These urges are characterised by the interchangeability of their object, as shown, among other things, by polymorphic infantile sexuality. The drive also does not reach its goal but circles around it, and the final way the drive constellation organises itself inevitably has something of a surrealist collage.[34] There is no final synthesis or normality that would result from a natural developmental process, such as so-called mature genital love.[35] There is only an ever-personal relationship that each subject assumes towards a lacking object (aka object small a) that he considers his Thing.[36] It follows from all this that psychoanalysis has nothing to gain from biological or psychological developments that reduce it to an adaptive ideology. Nor, in his view, should it be reduced to a kind of second-chance education in which infantile needs and frustrations are still to be met. Man is essentially (and à la Nietzsche) a *sick animal*.[37] He is fundamentally maladjusted, and there is an unbridgeable gap between man and the world.[38]

4 A Story of Language

Zooming in on all this, for Lacan, the fundamental characteristic of our humanity rests in language. Our language is an instrument that determines our perception. We think as we speak, and we talk as we think.[39] We come into the world as an organism with a particular biological constitution. Still, we are inscribed from birth with reflections that form the basis of our tension regulation and identity. Language also precedes us. It clothes our living body, and it thus provides the transition to being aware. We need others to clarify who we are, what we feel and how we should or may relate to ourselves and the outside world. We are surrounded by stories written (even earlier than us) by others, stories in which we may or may not want to recognise ourselves. Some words tell us something, others nothing. In an alternating play of identification and rejection (inward or outward), a story forms that we relate to and about ourselves. In this speaking out, we feel involved. After all, according to our feelings, our truth is reflected in it. In doing so, we act as if we are an in-dividual, someone of one piece. However, we fail to recognise that we are (in a happy term of Gilles Deleuze) *dividual*. [40] Indeed, we are divided between inner fissures and fault lines. As a vessel of contradictions, we are fatally a *contradictio sine qua non*.

The speaker and their language do not coincide, yet they invoke language to express themself. In a Lacanian view, we choose words from the lexicon of the big Other. We try to characterise our 'being' that way, but we never run out of words about ourselves. After all, what we say or tell never (quite) captures who or how we are. Also, part of our speaking concerns defences and making fables of ourselves and others. There are pieces of ourselves that we like and pieces that we want less. Also, although we produce an 'I' as a subject of the spoken, the subject of speaking itself remains constantly absent from our story.[41] It's a bit like a photographer who never appears in his pictures.

While the unconscious gradually acquired mystical connotations with Carl Gustav Jung or animal connotations with the behavioural sciences, for Lacan it consists essentially of symbolic elements. This unconscious is not a *sub-conscious* situated somewhere ('depth psychology') inside. It installs itself in an encounter with the big Other between skin and flesh (*'entre cuir et chair'*). Lacan finds that in this, he ties in with early Freud. Drawing on dream language, Freud concluded that the unconscious writes itself like a rebus: with imagery, displacement, condensation and so on. Hence, Lacan's famous slogan is that the unconscious is structured like a language.[42] In a dream, affect is not repressed but intrudes, coupled with other signifiers 'chosen' according to the mentioned linguistic laws. The dream has the structure of a rebus or Egyptian hieroglyphics, and *mutatis mutandis,* psychoanalysis discovered a kind of Rosetta stone by which the peculiar laws of the unconscious can be translated.[43]

Lacan, in turn, would interpret Freud using the logic of Ferdinand De Saussure.[44] This linguist distinguishes between the signifier and signified, sound image and concept. The signifier is material and/or acoustic[45] and it is this signifier (and not the meaning) that becomes the bearer of affective charge. The signifiers are linked in a signifier chain,[46] and there is a gap with the meaning that slips underneath in ever-changing ways.[47] Bridging this gap is a typically human achievement. A dog or a monkey may seem able (through months of Pavlovian training and practice) to acquire something of the language, but the human child naturally succeeds without any training.[48] It forms ideas and hypotheses based on likes and dislikes, presence and absence.[49] But the conscious and the unconscious emerge only when the child formulates their thoughts in language. This unconscious consists explicitly (not of affects nor meaning, but) of signifiers. For displacement buries the signifier but not the affect. As a result of repression, the affect begins to haunt the psyche, orphaned and meaningless. For example, anger, sadness or fear start looking for other signifiers to attach themselves.[50] The mechanisms by which this happens are not random but are determined by condensation and displacement, metaphor and metonymy. Respectively, signifiers are *selected* on the so-called paradigmatic axis and *combined* on the syntagmatic axis.[51]

5 The Ego as a Trap

It has come up several times before. Compared to other animals (primates included), the human child is born extremely immature (in '*neoteny*').[52] For example, it is motor uncoordinated and still has extremely poor proprioception. Around eight months, according to Lacan, it identifies with a total image or *Gestalt* as it appears in a (literal or figurative) mirror. It is an eminently human act of mirror-self-recognition.[53] The human child experiences it as a jubilant *Aha-Erlebnis* or an Eureka moment: I have found (an image of) myself! Indeed, the human child henceforth assumes and identifies itself with an image of itself: an image it likes. Behold, in a nutshell, the famous Lacanian mirror stage.[54] In this logical moment, a relationship is established between the organism and its reality. It is nothing less than an intellectual act in which an image is promoted to an idea or proto-symbol. Even beforehand, the child could recognise the other person in the mirror. It knew that the mirror image was not the natural person. Unlike the primate (who can attack its image as if it were a rival), the child effortlessly understood the unreality of its reflection: that is me, and that is not me. Yet, at a particular (logical) moment, the sight of the reflection leads to a triumphant moment of identity acquisition, self-awareness, and self-reflection.

This is all good, but without realising it sufficiently, all this simultaneously and paradoxically creates an inner division. It results from a narcissistic split between the subject and the object. As a subject, we are suddenly (by identifying with a mirror image) alienated from ourselves. This alienation is the starting point of untruths. Indeed, the mirror image is false or falsifying in many respects.[55] Purely visually, there is left-right and foreground-background inversion. Just try cutting your hair in front of the mirror! Above all, it is also a screen or canvas on which we can keep sticking signifiers. The subject in us thereby chooses words to write the story it invents about itself: I am David, I am wise, sporty, a good student and so on. Thus, we gradually fabricate a fictional (if not idealised) 'I' against which we pale as *true* subjects. Powerfully formulated, this (specular or imaginary) Ego is a trap.[56] The Ego we produce secures us, on the one hand, against the impotence and incoherence preceding it.[57] But it also grounds a typically human lie that we henceforth tell ourselves and others. In the process, we constantly choose and repress signifiers. In this process, we produce a smokescreen for the other and ourselves in which we, as a subject, simultaneously emerge as we disappear behind it.

In all this process, a third party comments, namely the big Other embodied by this or that parent figure who immerses the child in a bath of signifiers. By mirroring and marking, (s)he helps the child build self-esteem and meaning. With their 'Mummy, look! Daddy, look' the child constantly ascertains whether and how their inside and outside are being mirrored.[58] Parental figures tell us what we feel, why, and what we may or may not do with it. Meanwhile, we are fed inside a more extensive (e.g., family) story. We are similar to…, utterly different from… and so on. Right from infancy, we also manifest our own will. We resist, oppose and try (largely oppositional at first) to make our own choices.

According to Paul Verhaeghe,[59] our identity consists of two fundamental or existential axes: the axis of determinedness and the axis of our own (conscious and unconscious) choices. We do not choose where our cradle is, but we do 'choose' in which direction and to what extent we move away from it. Our identity emerges relative to the big Other towards whom we gradually attribute our place.[60] Verhaeghe speaks of four crucial relationships. There is a relationship towards sexual and gender differences. There is a relationship towards authority (which norms and values we may or may not adopt and later try to pass on ourselves). There is the relationship towards our neighbour alias, our (small) other-equals. Finally, there is the relationship towards ourselves, including our living body with its pain, pleasure and enjoyment. In the process, we constantly assign values to ourselves: right or wrong, good or bad. Words are values, and so the named relationships are never neutral. They are full of standards and judgements, commandments and prohibitions, approvals and disapprovals.

The Imaginary of the mirror stage referred to the realm of self and body image. The symbolic includes the language and conventional system of symbols by which we give meaning to our experiences. Drawing on both registers, the human subject produces a ceaseless stream of images and words, simultaneously revealing and concealing itself.[61] Internally, however, there is a primordial discordance constitutive of the human being,[62] and the symbolic-imaginary mirrors mainly bridge the Real of fragmentation.[63] From an infant, not yet differentiated from the other (cf Winnicott's environment mother), we evolve into a speaking being in relation to the object-mother or big Other. As a child in distress, we thereby continuously and necessarily appeal to its intervention based on which our tantrums and affections are responded to, fine-tuned and civilised.[64] The symbolic identity we acquire in this way differs from the imaginary one on which it was based. In the imaginary position, we imagined ourselves omnipotent and perfect. As the flip side of this narcissistic medal, we were filled with envy, rivalry and competition with the (ideal) image.[65] The symbolic order breaks this mirror relationship, and we 'gain' in lack, imperfection and limitations.

6 Thing and Object small a

Jacques Lacan is sometimes called *Jack-the-Lack*. His thinking is undoubtedly and surely centred around a lack, and it also revolves around very peculiar lost objects. In a flying start and to boot: the Real of the Thing (*-an-sich*) of noumenal immediacy is lost through its entry into the Imaginary and the Symbolic of language. We are irrevocably separated from it by a wall of culture.[66] On the other hand, this Thing arises (paradoxically) precisely as an effect of language.[67] After all, the word is not only the murder of the Thing, but this Thing is born ('*nachträglich*'/deferred action) precisely from the law of the word.[68] Without the law and/of language, the Thing is dead.[69] This (logical) moment when the Thing is simultaneously murdered and born brings a want-to-be, a '*manque-à-être*' in us. What remains of the Thing is a nostalgia for an absolute enjoyment that we never actually experienced as such.[70] We lose something we never possessed.[71] The Thing seems to be embodied by an object that Lacan calls the small a object. It is an imaginary object that, as it were, covers the *lack* of an object. Both the Thing and this object small a (as object-cause of desire) resist our ongoing attempts at symbolisation. They slip away from us repeatedly, remaining behind as a residue that cannot be articulated. Even though we have – following the example of the Dutch poet Hans Andreus[72] – 'spoken the world language and the solar language and the lunar language and the language of animals'.

Jacques Lacan considered the object small a to be his most important invention. It is a factor 'x': an unknown that gives a thoughtful rationale to numerous irrational phenomena. Translated to, say, love life, his abstract-looking algebra means concretely and clinically that the characteristic of the lover is that he is short of something without knowing what. He lacks something: the object small a. What characterises the lover is that they have something without knowing what, but seemingly, it is precisely what the lover lacks: the object small a. The other sees *something* in me which I do not possess, and wants *something* from me which I cannot give. The conscious desire is for an object, but the unconscious desire is caused by something that can be seen in a particular object, something that attracts: an object small a.[73] We do not know where the charismatic attraction is situated: an object is it a gesture, a look, a voice?[74] However, we believe that the loved one has a hidden treasure,[75] and this belief starts the engine of our desire. Why we love someone is impossible to say, and if we find a reason, it is only acceptable insofar as it is false at the same time.[76] The object small a is, therefore, radically (inter-) subjective.[77] Love is characterised precisely by this leap into the subjective, being, in short, the *fact* of the superiority of his beloved.[78] Love turns chance into necessity.[79] It turns a chance encounter into the we-have-been-born-for-each-other and love into a 'fateful' encounter.[80]

Paul Moyaert[81] calls the object small a a non-empirical object or an object without properties, to which we do not so much attach ourselves as become attached without knowing it or without wanting to. We are seized by something we do not understand. For example, we desire with (a) reason: particular qualities we imaginatively attribute to something or someone.[82] We find our partner beautiful, sweet, friendly, warm, cheerful, artistic, intelligent, etc. But this desire with (a) reason is embedded in a desire *without* (a) reason: because of nothing. The object small a is a negative quantity; it is a hole that any object can fill. It is the name of a void, of the elusive surplus, the mysterious *je-ne-sais-quoi* that sets our desire in motion and can cause someone to turn their life around in ways that are incomprehensible to others (and even themself).[83]

In the object small a is crystallised the rest of an original, total and fusional, but impossible (because irrevocably lost) enjoyment. It is a mythical enjoyment beyond the pleasure principle, which precedes the (phallic) pleasure principle, about which more below. Just as the unconscious exists only for those with an ear for it, the object small a also exists only for those with an eye for it. It can only be perceived while looking awry by desire. It does not exist objectively because it is nothing. Only subjectively does it take the form of something (x). It illustrates how someone can see in a woman/man *the* woman/man and how, in other words, love takes off as a product of the imagination. For Lacan, our love life and entire existence revolve around the object small a. It is located centrally in the three registers of the Real, the Symbolic and the Imaginary. It refers to the lost object from the Real; it was created *nachträglich* by the Symbolic (from which it escapes), and it belongs to the Imaginary because it contains a missing piece of our self so that its recovery could heal/make us whole again. It includes a supposed portion of *jouissance* that we sacrificed on the altar of language, and it embodies *the Real Thing* that can appear in all sorts of imaginary guises and to which we continue to aspire throughout our lives.[84]

7 Complexes

What the other post-Freudians dealt with a lot less are the Oedipus complex and (especially) the castration complex in their structuring influence on sexual identity and orientation.[85] Jacques Lacan also lifts *this* repression.

According to Freud, the castration complex is a psychic and complex experience that the child goes through unconsciously around the age of five and which is decisive for the formation of their sexual identity. It begins for the boy and the girl in the same way, namely, with the belief in the universality of the phallus. It also ends partly in the same way, namely through separation from the mother: for the boy out of castration anxiety, for the girl out of anger because of the feeling of being castrated (by her). Regarding the demise of the Oedipus complex,[86] Freud left much room for ambiguity. On the one hand, it is said to prey on repression and pass into the latent phase. On the other hand, it is stated that it goes down to its failure, the 'inner impossibility'.[87] It is even suggested that it disappears by analogy with baby teeth when it is time. Finally, it comes down to castration[88] and ideally even shatters for the boy so that it does not even exist in the unconscious anymore. All this while, in the girl's case, it would be more of an open-ended affair, with all the implications for the more flawed development of the Superego.[89]

In 1905, Freud[90] had already argued that it was only at puberty that a sharp distinction between masculinity and femininity was established. After the partial, polymorphic and auto-erotic/fantasmatic of the latent stage, only then is a sexual object sought for the first time. There is a new goal (penetration), and the genital erogenous zone is given priority. In 1923, Freud added to all this a pre-history of gender difference. Initially[91] the distinction was active versus passive; in the phallic phase[92] this becomes: phallic versus castrated and in puberty it becomes male versus female. He goes on to say that the man comes to represent the active-conquering pole and that he carries the penis. The woman 'chooses' the passive position and comes to value her vagina as home to the penis or its symbolic equivalent: the child.[93]

For Freud, the phallus has always remained pivotal in everything. Whereas for him, by contrast, the penis is no more than an anatomical organ, Lacan promotes the phallus as a psychoanalytic and, more specifically, a metapsychological concept. It has to do with the lack, which, for Lacan, has been structural and existential from the very beginning. From birth, the child expresses its need in a cry, an appeal. The child asks something of the other, but the question is never entirely answered. There is always and immediately a shortcoming, even though everyone is trying to install or restore the mirage of blissful unity. The (first) big Other (primarily the mother figure) cannot fill the lack. Lacan clarifies that and how this also applies in reverse. Probably, the mother is one of the first (proto-) concepts the baby forms. This allows it to hold on to her image even when she disappears from the picture.[94] There are two states: mother and non-mother. On this non-mother, secondly, grafts the image of the father.[95] After all, he is usually the mother's biggest distraction. The child has to go to bed because the father and mother go out to dinner. Or to bed together. Around this time, particular importance is attached to the second big Other.[96] This second big Other apparently 'has' or 'is' something that mother desires (more than me) and which, therefore, keeps her away from me. For that matter, what does a mother want? From me and/or from this Other?

8 Phallus

The Lacanian phallus is initially that indefinable 'something' around which her desire seems to revolve.[97] He becomes the signifier of the mother's desire. Her enigmatic and fickle desire acquires a reason or rationale. The mother's caprice gives way to a rule and a protective and anxiety-reducing regularity for the child. When the mother says: I have to wash, iron or go to work, she obeys laws and rules beyond her will and whim. She rules in (the) Name of the Father.

From now on, this Name-of-the-Father acts as a shield against her will and whim. He also causes mother to change shape. She evolves from a ruler to an authority figure. She is no longer above the law but is instead a servant of the law. As soon as the child accepts the metaphor as if the mother disappears from its sphere of influence for the father's sake, it enters a '*marché de dupes*'. We are all fooled because we know the father she invokes for custody is a fable, but it is a beneficial fable. After all, the child realises that even the father does not have or is not the phallus. That no one even is or has it. The phallus exists only in the Imaginary. He is *missing*, as it were, but he (like the object small a) seems to exist, and by so doing, he feeds (often against one's better judgment) the illusion that he can be (re)found.

I summarise and reiterate this – admittedly – complex matter. In its first years, the infant is at the mercy of the will and whim of the all-powerful mother,[98] on whose presence and absence it (vitally) depends. In the process, the child feels inadequate. It looks like it cannot fully satisfy the mother since she longs to be elsewhere ('*autre part*').[99] The phallus, for Lacan, is what the child thinks it lacks to fulfil the mother and be her all/phallus.[100] The penis (as an anatomical organ) is only the privileged mark of the phallus on the body.[101] Freud's primacy of the phallus takes on a much more abstract form with Lacan. It becomes the primacy of the signifier, with the phallus being the ultimate signifier. He is the signifier of lack,[102] the signifier of desire or the signifier of the Law.[103] It is the threshold beyond which a kind of oasis is situated: the mythical world of another enjoyment/the enjoyment of the big Other.

For Lacan, therefore, castration has nothing (any more) to do with the butcher or with bodily mutilation, but it defines itself as the separation between mother and child. It is the complex cut/*coup* that breaks the imaginary and narcissistic bond between mother and child, where the mother thinks she has the phallus and the child thinks she is her phallus. The phallus henceforth becomes that which both sexes can never have (enough) for each other (in the case of the male) or be (in the case of the female) to fill the lack of the big Other. The agent of this castration is the father, who represents the law of incest prohibition.[104]

9 Pleasure and Enjoyment

Freud held a relatively simple view of pleasure: there is pleasure as appetite and pleasure as satisfaction of 'desire'. For the psychism governed by the pleasure principle, a decrease in tension gives pleasure, and an increase in tension gives unpleasure. In this simple logic, pleasure is comparable, for example, to emptying the bladder so that tension can be discharged. Pleasure takes self-preservation and what is right or wrong into account. Phenomenologically, it is associated with the pleasant. Against it, however, there is an entirely different pleasure: that of intoxication and rapture, of enthusiasm, ecstasy and self-loss. It is a pleasure in which one is *full of* something. This is a kind of pleasure that is transgressive, that takes no account of the pleasure principle and that, moreover, is (partly) frightening.[105]

The pleasure principle is a variation of the law of incest. It creates distance and, at the same time, creates the desire to remove this distance.[106] This law says: enjoy as little as possible. It keeps the subject safe from the (maternal) Thing. After all, this incestuous Thing is a 'good' that is at the same time a '*Mal*'.[107] Viewed this way, the father is not a repressive agency. Instead, he has a protective function, for he answers the inner need that the unbearable pleasure crystallised in this Thing be made inaccessible.[108] After all, the drive-pleasure (*jouissance*) attached to it cannot be enjoyed. In turn, the phallus that becomes operative with the Oedipal keeps the subject from the grip of the devouring omnipotent mother.[109] Indeed, castration protects against *jouissance* as the enjoyment of the big Other.[110] With the pleasure (signified by the phallus), there is a limit, while *jouissance* is boundless: it leads the subject to death.[111]

From reading Freud, we could already see that humans possess a constant, never-realised aspiration, namely the attainment of an absolute and undivided happiness/enjoyment that can take several forms. The manifestation *par excellence* is that of the purely hypothetical enjoyment of consummated incest. This is incest as a mythical dream image that fascinates the Oedipal child and is, therefore, a mirage.[112] For Lacan, too, every subject cherishes this dream of unlimited enjoyment. It manifests itself repeatedly in particular objects or projects to which a special meaning is assigned as a function of a dreamed completion. However, its realisation is contradictory to our existence as linguistic beings. The closer we approach this pleasure, the more it turns into a nightmare.[113]

Ecstasy and passion (as conscious manifestations of *jouissance*) lead to a subjectless enjoyment,[114] a desire-without-subject[115] on the verge of self-destruction. They bring about a kind of enjoyment beyond the pleasure principle in which the Ego is unconcerned about itself, does not allow itself to be led by consequences or effects,[116] but, on the contrary, pursues its goal unconcerned, uninhibited and confidently. It does not look back, is absorbed in what it is doing, is blinded in its drive, is beside itself, ecstatic and goes to extremes.[117] It is the drive that has become flesh. A drive that has taken the reins and left the desiring subject behind. In this movement, the Ego and subject disappear and *being* takes over. Slavoj Žižek, therefore, calls jouissance the place of Dasein, and desire is a defence against this *jouissance*. [118]

In *The Sexual Mask*, Camille Paglia distinguished between two registers: an Apollonian and a Dionysian.[119] They come in handy to characterise the two mentioned forms of pleasure. The Dionysian pleasure is tension-inducing, and the subject engages in it incessantly. It is the symbiotic *jouissance*, the unlimited enjoyment of the big Other.[120] This pleasure lies beyond the (phallic) pleasure principle, beyond language and signifier, beyond the phallus and gender difference. It is an immediate pleasure. It knows only one law: *Jouis!* (Enjoy!). This enjoyment means the death of the subject as a subject. The subject disappears from the symbolic. There is a free flow of energy according to a primary process. The enjoyment is total; the merger increases tension and results in symbiosis, where the subject disappears into the Other, and it is incorporated.[121] We can connect this enjoyment with Eros. Indeed, this drive aims at fusion, which leads to symbiosis and the disappearance of the Self. As such, Eros is the terrain of the woman, where there is an 'other' *jouissance* that inspires fear.

There is an Apollonian pleasure on the other side. It is tension-relieving. It also stops somewhere. It is limited. It is the phallic *jouissance*, the phallic pleasure Freud talks about. Lacan also calls it *'la jouissance de l'idiot'*.[122] It is a tiny but safe pleasure in which the subject persists. It is partial, leads to separation and to tension reduction through the orgasm that brings an 'unwanted and abrupt end to the ecstatic being outside itself of enjoyment'.[123] We can connect this pleasure to Thanatos. It causes the disintegration of the twosome, where the fusion stops, and the lovers can say, 'I *come*, I *come*', but also, as Verhaeghe notes, '*I* come, *I* come'. For what comes is indeed their (subjective) I that frees itself from ecstasy; before, their I was far from it.[124] It is the human territory, of pleasure and sadness after the loss of symbiosis: *omne animal post coitum triste* or, as Paul Moyaert says: 'We all share the same fate: we cannot share each other's fate'.[125]

10 Desire

Finally, a term that constantly recurs with Lacan and is absent (except as '*Wunsch*') from Freud is, of course, '*désir*'. You can desire to become famous, long for a handsome man, for a fast car, for a romantic date, a lovely house, a nice holiday, an exciting exhibition, or a gourmet dinner. All these provide pleasure, but you can hardly call them needs. Nor can you ask for help or call 911 for them. What would one answer to the question, 'I desperately need good sex!' Unconscious desire must be distinguished from drive. Even in the womb, the baby sucks its thumb. This is not out of oral need or desire but oral drive. An *enfant sauvage* may satisfy its sexual drive by masturbating, but this has nothing to do with desire. The drive can be satisfied auto-erotically (as opposed to need), but appetite should not be confused with hunger. You can fulfil your needs with a Baxter or tube feeding, but this feeding is neither delicious nor pleasant. Who would crave it, let alone consider it a proof of love? Sex can be asked for, but it does not satisfy a physical nor a psychological need, so why else do we ask for sex other than as proof of love? The erogenous pleasure it provides does not reduce tension but maintains it. It gives enjoyment only due to proper 'use' of the body parts and activities that serve it (cf. *jouissance* as usufruct).

In Lacanian terms, desire appears in the interval between need and demand. Or it appears at the edge where demand is subtracted from need. In need (Fr: '*besoin*') we appeal to (Fr: '*demande*') the big Other. Their answer always falls short or beyond what we ask for, creating an 'extra' constitutive of desire. We can still articulate our needs as much as we want. Our demand has to slip through the language bottleneck, and the latter thereby gives rise to our (so typically human) desire. Earlier came the question of whether animals could lie. Should we still ask whether they can desire? To ask the question is to answer it![126]

The objects that we, humans, long for are finally also imaginary: the Thing, object small a, phallus. The Thing is the object of loss; it haunts our lives in the guise of object small a, and we are in pursuit of possessing or embodying the phallus through which we could, in turn, fulfil the desire of the big Other. The demand is spoken, but what you ask can never fully express what you want. Especially since '*cet obscur objet du désir*' is hidden from your consciousness. First, the baby cries. It asks something, but it doesn't know what. By acquiring language, the child chooses words from the mother tongue by which it is surrounded: bottle, tut, mama, bear. But what it desires may be something completely different. It may be something that doesn't even exist! Even if the child gets what it has asked for, it may be sad, angry, disappointed or disillusioned. It is clear by now: not in its need, but in its desire. Where the child's demands and desires are still simple, they increase in precision and complexity throughout our lives. Not that chocolate, but that one. Not this rug, but that. Not the North Sea, but the Mediterranean and so on.

11 Love

With all the data from attachment theory, ethology and infant research, it has now been conclusively proven that we do not only demand or desire material objects. Something as immaterial as love is also vital to the human child; in this sense, it contains a component of need. Desire grows and flourishes on this soil of a need for love. Love is giving what you don't have, and the effort you make for the other is a measure of the love you express. Our most complicated demands and desires, therefore, revolve around love and sexuality. First, they are neither visible, tangible, nor (unlike hunger or thirst) satisfiable. Moreover, they are not directed at objects but at subjects whose desire may or may not and more or less can or will answer ours.

Probably one of Lacan's most famous slogans is '*Le désir, c'est le désir de l'Autre*'. Desire is the desire of the Other. This is both a subjective and objective genitive. We desire what the big Other desires; on the other hand, we also desire to capture the big Other's desire. Desire desires desire, but the desire of the big Other is and always remains inscrutable and enigmatic. When can we ever feel one hundred per cent certain and/or secure about this? The fact that this is never the case makes us long for such certainty. Desire, in turn, gives – fortunately! – also a particular *drive* and hence *jouissance*.[127] In that sense, it is desirable to (be able to) experience desire, and the lack of desire is probably one of the main components of depressive feelings of all kinds.

Love and desire are at odds. In his *Three Essays*[128] and his contribution on the most widespread humiliation in love life,[129] Freud had already discussed the tension between tenderness and sensuality, between love and (sexual) desire. He argued that people often fail to integrate these two strivings and considered this phenomenon an outgrowth of the incest prohibition. He compared it to digging a tunnel, detailing the difficulty of matching both sides.[130] I paraphrase Lacan with an even more strident statement in one of his most famous Seminars: 'I love you, but because something in you (the object small a) makes me incomprehensibly covet you, I also *mutilate* you'.[131] Indeed, this desire does not care about the Other in its subjective alterity but sees this other merely as an object of pleasure and enjoyment. In other words, desire and love are also in a tense relationship with Lacan.[132] Desire is part of love, but desire is aimed at partial objects[133] that attract or excite us, while love is aimed at the being and/of the whole person.

Not only (infantile) sexuality but also self-love can be a difficulty for our love life. To what extent is the other loved in his alterity? Or does the other serve mainly as a narcissistic extension or a (small) other-equal? Feeling God in the depths of our thoughts is all good, but are we also God in the thoughts of our beloved? And what about the ambivalence that characterises any long-term object relationship?

One last complication in love emerged after Freud's publication on the life and death drive. There is a discord in the life of the drive itself, which Lacan links to the two different kinds of enjoyment just described.[134] It is a duality that, according to Verhaeghe, makes human sexuality by definition '*fascinans et tremendum*': we long for what at the same time also frightens us the most: a fusion with the big Other[135] The total discharge and the dreamed unity is impossible for the subject[136] There is only partial satisfaction, even (or perhaps especially) when the Masters and Johnson couple frantically try to 'come' simultaneously.[137] According to Lacan '*Il n'y a pas de rapport sexuel*'.[138] The partners never achieve a (fully) compatible Yin and Yang-like relationship. In this sense, the encounter between man and woman is fatally a 'failed' encounter.[139] It inevitably collides with the rock of castration.[140] The only thing that provides a mutual coupling is the crazy little Thing called love.

12 What Finality?

Jacques Lacan is very influential today in human and cultural sciences. Within mental health care, however, he enjoys a dubious reputation. His theory there is often perceived as too intellectualistic. It is considered too far removed from (psychiatric and psychotherapeutic) practice, it underestimates the importance of (the imaginary of) emotions and affects and its practice is characterised by (ultra-) short sessions and an ultra-silent attitude of its practitioners.[141] Unlike Freud, Lacan did not discuss his dreams nor utter a word about his analysis. In his teaching, he drew only on others' clinics and did not add new domains or formations to psychoanalysis. However, his thinking is manifestly distinct from that of the other post-Freudians. He restores Oedipus and the castration complex and lifts them to a higher level of abstraction. As a result, they shed more light on their ever-changing manifestations in time, space and culture. He reinforces the state of the father and installs the primacy of the phallus and the signifier, placing humanity in a radically different because denatured light. For him, the human condition is inevitably marked by faltering, misunderstanding and lack, and *the* mental health does not exist.[142] For Lacan, the psychoanalytic process revolves around the pot unceasingly.[143] After all, the heart of the matter remains as opaque as the navel or mycelium from Freud's dream theory. In an allusion to Donald Winnicott, the essence of the so-called true self is *incommunicado*. The essence is that there is no essence. We merely incessantly produce words/signifiers through which, like Baron Von Munchhausen, we pull ourselves by the hair out of the swamp (of the Real).[144] Except for rare neologisms, they always come from the big Other. Only their selection and combination make up our individuality.

We can resist like the proverbial devil in a holy water barrel, but the symbolic castration is inescapable. There is a gap between man and Thing, and 'never the twain shall meet'.[145] In more contemporary terms, there is only the LGBTQ++++ of countless stories and varieties as we relate to the small other and the big Other, the law, the Thing, object little a and phallus.[146] It is sufficiently clear: for Lacan, psychoanalysis is not a cure-all, although, of course, 'cure' is excellent.[147] Hidden in our symptom is the core of our truth, and it is (like every person and process) radically singular. We gain more insight into our affairs through psychoanalysis, but a complete understanding (and even less: a firm grip) is unattainable. When we seek help, we want to find out more about ourselves and go to someone we think knows (it) and with whom we can find out more.[148] It is a journey into the insides of our nature where the landscape of our mind passes by the window, and we dwell at length on milestones or other landmarks. Meanwhile, we drain the breeding ground of our symptoms. These are just surface symptoms of an iceberg that is mainly underwater. We examine and experience what damage it does and whether and how we can bring it to melt.

13 Seduction

After this long Lacanian excursion, I will end with another (in some ways 'crazy') approach to eros and eroticism. It can be found with Jean Laplanche, a compatriot and former adept of Lacan. He is now widely known for his classic *Vocabulaire de la Psychanalyse* but also his theory of original seduction.[149] We saw that Freud first assigned a crucial causal role to adult 'seduction'. Within his *Neurotica*, a traumatic aetiology (invariably of a sexual nature) was at the root of hysteria.[150] But soon, he would downplay the causality of this 'trauma'. It is (only) a trigger of or affecting the child's polymorphic perverse disposition. Perversion was first located primarily in adults, later primarily in the child. Jean Laplanche tied back into Freud's *Neurotica* with his general seduction theory.[151] His concern was with seduction as structural/universal rather than accidental trauma.[152] Already, according to Sandor Ferenczi, a 'confusion of speech' inevitably arises between the childlike, playful language of tenderness and the adult language of sexual passion. Thinking of Winnicott's holding, the clay of infantile sexuality is moulded by the caretaker (usually the mother). The adult cannot help but unconsciously respond sexually to initial interactions with the infant. Willingly or not (s)he communicates fantasies and effects in these intimate contacts.

Laplanche's theory connects two mutual concepts: the fundamental anthropological situation and repression as a faulty translation. The asymmetry characterising the early childhood relationship is that of the 'innocent' child still stripped of a sexual unconscious in the presence of an adult who is scarred/divided by this sexual unconscious.[153] This asymmetry is not thought of in the relational or intersubjective current. It repeats itself in part within the therapeutic relationship where the 'treatment of the enigma' can be resumed.[154] Indeed, in Laplanche's view, the unconscious results from a kind of translation error.[155] For example, the mother, while breastfeeding her baby and pampering him, will respond sensually and sexually. Her bosom is imbued with sexual meaning and sensations, her body responds to touch, and she has all kinds of fantasies. This 'communication' is unconscious, non-verbal and continuous. The child encounters confusing, puzzling messages that it cannot understand nor integrate but which leave their mark on its innate sensitivity and sensuality. What the child absorbs in terms of sexuality is mysterious, overwrought, unexpressed and also unworded. It is passed on from generation to generation. Laplanche postulates that in this asymmetrical process, instinct is transformed into human sexuality and the subject forms.[156] According to him, the child is affected, as it were, by more or less enigmatic adult sexuality. It organises its sexuality around these (micro-) traumatic events from its life history. This leads to a private psychosexual trajectory that acts as an implicit template for later desires and arousals.

Laplanche makes a sharp epistemological distinction between psychoanalysis and psychology. To him, it is the boundary between self-preservation and sexuality. Instincts (attachment included) are evolutionary and innate. They belong to the Ego- or self-preservation drives. They are not part of infantile sexuality, which, after all, is not innate. The latter is the derivative of the adult's sexual fantasy that gives compromising messages under the guise of care and safety.[157] Another noteworthy addition by Laplanche[158] is that gender identity results more from parental identification *by* than from identification *with* parents.

Not so different from Lacan, for Laplanche, human sexuality develops based on symbolic-imaginary structures that precede the child. The pleasure principle governs them, but unlike need and demand (*besoin* and *demande*), desire (*désir*) depends entirely on fantasised conditions imposed on objects and activities. Laplanche has argued how fantasy forms the crucial link between the external sexuality of maternal enigmatic messages and the internal of the so-called 'object-source'.[159] This source object is Laplanche's word for the repressed source of drives: the untranslated part of maternal seduction. There must be a pre-existing somatic reactivity, but it takes a seduction by the archaic mother to turn it into a drive.[160] At that infantile moment, the child tries to decipher the sexual (and therefore arousing) message, and autoerotic prurience arises. What is not contained sinks into the unconscious. It persists there as a hard and real core of unconscious fantasies. It is as opaque and non-symbolisable as Freud's navel of the dream, the drive-root of the symptom, or Lacan's non-symbolisable Real.[161]

14 Landing

This book part has dwelt on two pillars or poles within psychoanalytic work. We can summarise them as mentalising developmental aid versus interpretive cutting-edge technology. They define the nonspecific agenda of the therapeutic relationship and the specifics of psychoanalytic work in a narrower sense. Classically Freudian, the patient becomes *sadder but wiser* in the process. After all, the psychoanalyst is not an illusionist but a disillusionist,[162] and the clinical psychotherapy discussed in the next part is not a *wellness* clinic. In his famous one-liner: where the Id was, (the) Ego must become. It is a process that Freud compared to draining the Zuyderzee. In the process, the pleasure principle gives way to the reality principle. The intention is that the patient can face true reality and his true self. Ideally, ego functions such as impulse control, frustration and anxiety tolerance increase. Both the Ego- or self-preservation drives and the sexual drive should be able to be used better and more flexibly, and preferably in as pro-social a direction as possible. Meanwhile, our Ego must learn to ride the horse of its Id and to free itself sufficiently from the excessive yoke of its Superego. Psychoanalysis helps us to get adequately over ourselves to increase our capacity for object love. Although the analyst cloaks themself in ignorance and neutrality, they value life over death, Eros over Thanatos, and truth over lies.

Depending on the current, different aspects are focused on each time. The Kleinians mainly emphasise integrating good and evil, love and hate, and increased symbolising capacity. With his container-contained model, Bion and his followers elaborate on this. They also draw a trail to the relational movement by emphasising and exploiting the communicative value of projective identification. Winnicott is at the root of both *two-person* and self-psychology. Thanks to him, the transitional space (of play) is now considered a matrix of creativity. The capacity for un-integration manifests phenomenologically in being able to be *alone* and being able to *be* alone. Finally, according to Kohut, we need figures who fulfil a self-object function throughout our lives. Various psychopathology and acting-out behaviour are understood by him as degradation products when they fail and consequently fragment the self.

As an intermediate conclusion, we can say that in dialogue and contradiction, Freud and his psychoanalytic progeny set the beacons within which an integration between psychiatry and psychoanalysis can be achieved. In all psychopathology, three factors in varying alloys play a role in the pathogenesis. First is the biological factor: predisposition and drives ('*l(a) cause*'). The attachment factor is the relationship to the first significant others (the small other and the big Other). Thirdly, there is the subject's (S) ever-private life history in which specific patterns are automatised/repeat themselves. Answering this complex pathogenesis in an integrated way often starts best within the framework of clinical psychotherapy. For a lot of patients, it announces itself as a last resort. They have usually gone through an entire Calvary and, in the process, have often swum many waters within mental health care. In the best case, they can land sufficiently well to lead their lives differently. Even among mental health professionals, clinical psychotherapy is unfortunately largely unknown and/or unloved. In the meantime, however, clinical psychotherapeutic treatment for people with severe and/or 'early' disorders appears to open new perspectives effectively.[163] In recent years, it has also ensured that psychoanalysis, somewhat tarnished by the scientific world, has been 'reintroduced' by psychiatry.

Notes

1 Sigmund Freud (1912–1913 p 211).
2 Goethe (1790) *Faust* I, 3.
3 'In the beginning was the Word, and the Word was with God, and the Word was God'. From a Lacanian perspective, it is all about the (function of the) Father and the primacy of the signifier.
4 Jacques Lacan distinguished logical and chronological time to consider the specific temporal aspect of deferred action or *Nachträglichkeit*. See Eric Porge (1989).
5 There are no written sources for prehistory, and its deposit is implicit.
6 Julia Kristeva (1984).
7 For Lacan motherese becomes *lalangue* (1971–72 p 14b). Llanguage has become its standard translation (Nobus & Quinn, 2005). See Malloch & Trevarthen (2009) for 'communicative musicality'.
8 Paul Verhaeghe (2002a p 148ff) attributes four functions to language: mastery, identity acquisition, communication and awareness.
9 Rudi Vermote (1994).
10 Julia Kristeva (1984).
11 Walter Schönau (2002).
12 Digital or binary: 1/0, present/absent. Lacan refers to a sequence of heads and tails that produces an ordering absent in the Imaginary (Lacan, 1957 p 48).
13 The primary process is the unconscious's mode of functioning. Connections are not logical but associative, and the pleasure principle rules. The secondary process characterises conscious thinking, where rationality and reality principle prevail.
14 It is the refusal of (symbolic) castration. Sigmund Freud (1905c p 142): 'At the time when the child learns to handle the vocabulary of his mother tongue, he takes evident pleasure in experimenting playfully with this material and, without committing himself to the requirement of meaning, joins the words together to sort out the loop effect of rhythm or rhyme. This pleasure is gradually prohibited to him, until only the meaningful word compounds remain permissible to him.' Lacanian neuropsychoanalyst Ariane Bazan (2011) calls this 'disambiguisation'.
15 Jacques Lacan (1955b) in (1966).
16 Frédéric Declercq criticises the idea of a 'gradual' transition from onomatopoeia to symbolic language in (2000 p 85ff).
17 With his Neuropsychoanalysis Mark Solms taps into the *earliest* Freud (Kinet, 2023a).
18 The imaginary order links the (specular) Ego with the small (mirror) other, whereas the symbolic order links the subject (S, Freud's Es/Id) with the big Other of law and language. The big Other *makes* the subject outside the subject's awareness.
19 The Id and the Real (as the energetic-material), the Ego and the Imaginary (which we share with mammals) and the Superego and the Symbolic (as the typically human set of laws, norms, prohibitions, etc.).
20 According to Lacan, the drive is situated in the Id. The unconscious is the realm of desire: a defence against the drive.
21 For Lacan, the infant is immersed in *jouissance:* it is not about satisfaction of the need, but of the drive (1986).
22 Lacan (1973) draws inspiration from Aristotle in the distinction he makes between different causalities: the necessary, the accidental/contingent and the impossible. The necessary is the *automaton* as what does not cease to write itself

(*ce qui ne cesse pas de s'écrire*). It is repetition at the level of signifiers. It is *lawful*. The accidental/contingent is what ceases not to write itself (ce qui cesse de ne pas s'écrire). It is the tuchè or chance: unpredictable. The third category is the impossible as the Real that (by definition) is not symbolisable. It is what does not cease *not to* write itself (*ce qui ne cesse pas de ne pas s'écrire*).

23 *Jouissance* is a key concept with Lacan. Phenomenologically, it implies a combination of pain and pleasure. It is considered crucial by Lacan in the compulsion to repeat. Drive and *jouissance* always say: More! More! Hence the title of his XX Seminar (1975b): *Encore!* It is why Lacan calls every drive a death drive. As such Lacan's death drive must be distinguished from the biological drive to return to the inanimate/inorganic. Lacan's concept of the drives is altogether removed from the realm of biology. Drives differ from biological needs in that they can never be satisfied. The purpose of the drive is not to reach a final destination but to follow its aim (Lacan, 1981b p 168). *Jouissance*/enjoyment resides in the repetitive movement of this closed circuit. Desire is a defence against a limitless losing oneself in *jouissance* (Lacan, 1966a p 699).

24 Self-psychology focuses mainly on our sense of self or self-image, respectively as proprioception or, in its specular guise, the looking-glass self. Often, Ego and self are confused with each other. The former is a supposed mental apparatus, while the self relates more to our imaginary and symbolic identity. Regulating a sense of self and self-esteem is one of the functions of the Ego. The subject the Lacanians talk about is a *res cogitans*/thinking thing that is hidden under both and is never (completely) covered by the Ego or the self.

25 Van Haute (2000). Lacan opposes every attempt to explain human phenomena *solely* in terms of adaptation (Lacan, 1966a p 158, 171–172). Reality is not a simple objective given to which the Ego must adapt, but it is precisely a product of the Ego's fictional misrepresentations. There is an illusory sense of adaptation that blocks access to the unconscious. The analyst is not the arbiter of the patient's adaptation (nor his own), nor do they impose its power (Lacan, 1991b p 323).

26 '*Le symbole est le meurtre de la Chose*' in (1953) in (1966 p 319).

27 Hunger, thirst and sleep are in se *satisfiable needs*.

28 Jacques Lacan, '*l'objet de la psychanalyse et le manque d'un objet*' (1953 ibidem) in (1966a p 268)

29 Jacques Lacan (1953 ibidem in 1966a p 272).

30 Jacques Lacan poses the question of truth not from an I that thinks, but an I that *speaks*. The word is both instrument of falsehood and receptacle of ambiguity, and it underlies the domain of truth (Fromentin, 2021 p 234).

31 The clearest example is toilet training but also what and how we eat, dress, enjoy ourselves etc is determined by (the desire of) the big Other.

32 This is also a concise definition of repression: that which is conspicuous by its absence.

33 In the English translation of the collected work edited by James Strachey (the so-called Standard Edition), '*Trieb*' is incorrectly translated as instinct and not drive. The calf knows what to do when it becomes a bull. There is no (crisis of) adolescence in the animal because everything is fixed in the Real of the chromosomes. Not only does drive differ from instinct, but also the colloquial and personal German *Ich* is lost in translation to the Ego.

34 Moustapha Safouan (2005 p 57–59).

35 Regarded as the apotheosis of 'development', while Lacanians view it as a concoction (Van Haute, 2000 p 140)

36 Vincent Hanna/Al Pacino in Michael Mann's *Heat* (1996): 'All I am is what I'm going after'.

37 'The mind is inflicted upon mammals who are not adapted to it' (Bion, 1975 p 161).
38 Philippe Van Haute, (ibidem p 25–26).
39 Lacan even refers to algorithms (1957 p 515).
40 Term coined by Gilles Deleuze (1992).
41 This fundamental difference between '*le sujet de l'énoncé*' (the subject of the spoken) and '*le sujet de l'énonciation*' (the speaking subject) comes up repeatedly with Lacan (Lacan, 1958–1959 lesson 3/12; 1967–1968 lesson 6/03). The unconscious subject is situated at the level of speaking, and the imaginary subject at the level of the spoken. The first subject is continually vanishing under the signifying chain (Lacan, 1970 p 194). That is why, in a Lacanian view, the dimension of the subject exists only as a *hypokeimenon* or as an assumption (Lacan, 1968–1969 p 90).
42 '*L'inconscient est structuré comme un language*' (Lacan, 1953).
43 The stone is a dark granite stone that was discovered in Egypt in July 1799. It contains a bilingual text written in three different writings, and it played a crucial role in deciphering hieroglyphics.
44 Ferdinand De Saussure (1916).
45 Ariane Bazan (2011) would even say motoric because the signifier is uttered (even in silence) by the appropriate (and I phrase it deliberately broadly) body parts.
46 Lacan (1966a p 502).
47 Paul Verhaeghe (2002a p 55) explains how this conjugation is only possible because the symbolic lacks a signifier: a sliding puzzle can only shift if one box remains empty.
48 Following Aristotle, the animal has *nous* (intellect) and *technè* (ability) but no *epistemonikon* (knowledge). Beavers build a dam, spiders weave a web, and birds fly in circles, but they do not know the ordering principles.
49 For example, it smiles when a balloon rises, thus defying gravity.
50 A nice analogy is the Id as a force field that arranges the molecules in the liquid crystal display in such a way as to promote them into readable letters or characters (see Kinet, 2023). It is a variant of Freud's Mystical Wonder Block (1925c) as a metaphor for unconscious, conscious and perception. You write with a stylus on the celluloid protective layer (perception). You can read what appears on the underlying wax paper (conscious). Still, even after you have erased/pushed away, the signifier is immortalised in the lower wax layer (the unconscious) and, given the proper technique, can be found there.
51 De Saussure (1916 p 124). Lacan calls these axes, respectively, those of *la langue* and *la parole*. The first is paradigmatic and metaphorical, as in, for example, the eye of the needle or a star is born. The words eye and star derive their meaning not from the dictionary but from the context and subtext in which they appear. When the metaphorical dimension of language is disrupted (as in psychosis), the formulation of 'the eye of the needle' or 'a star is born' can acquire terrifying connotations. *La parole* is syntagmatic and metonymic, e.g., High Street says, a sail appears on the horizon, I take the salmon.
52 Nobus (1997), Lacan (1949). There is a gap between *le Moi (m'aître/m'être)* and *être*. This gap is closed by the symbolic-imaginary. Intimate connections emerge that last throughout our lives between body and world. On the one hand, a child sees nothing but images of its corporeality; on the other, it learns to represent and animate the outside world through its body. All of (post-) Kleinian thought, for Lacanians, revolves around the imaginary colonisation of that first outside world: the maternal body. Lacan reads their transference-

countertransference continuum as a dual (imaginary) relation, which he believes the analyst must renounce. For Lacan, the analyst has primarily a symbolic function.

53 For the connection with self-awareness, see, for example, Heyes (1998). According to primatologist Frans de Waal (2005), the chimpanzee also has self-awareness. Aggression, competition and concern for conspecifics are part of its mindset.

54 Lacan (1949). Lacan's conclusion from ethological findings by Konrad Lorenz and Nikolaas Tinbergen is that images also spur animal development. The unity or wholeness anticipated in the mirror stage masks natural imperfection and thus has an orthopaedic function.

55 I would like to refer to the famous words of the French poet Arthur Rimbaud (1871): 'C'est fou de dire: je pense. On devrait dire: on me pense... Je est un autre.'

56 There is a distinction between the 'felt self' and the 'seen self'. The former refers to our inner body and skin; the latter is an image of ourselves from which we are separated and alienated.

57 The healing and wholeness of the whole versus the crumbled body 'le corps morcelé'.

58 The impact of a depressed mother (Green) or the absence of a mother in institutional children (Spitz) in terms of failure to thrive has been described many times. In a good-enough situation, the child is treated with attunement and delight, support and expectation, knowledge of history and context and, more generally, the complexity of another's complex subjectivity.

59 Paul Verhaeghe (2009a)

60 'L'inconscient, c'est le discours de l'Autre' (Lacan, 1959 p 549).

61 Lacan (1960a p 677). Peter Fonagy and other voices from attachment theory zoom in on the formative function of mirroring, but Lacan equally emphasises the distortion or repulsion it can cause.

62 Lacan (1949 p 96; 1960 p 675).

63 Lacan (1960a p 655).

64 Language allows us to name all kinds of fragmentary affects or sensations. They become feelings that we can place in a story, relate to events and characters. They not only textualise but also contextualise the affect.

65 Nor is the aggressive tension inherent in the attachment/mirror stage conceived in attachment theory. Lacan speaks (about the Imaginary) in a neologism of (difficult to translate) 'hainamoration': a mixture of love, hate and admiration (Lacan, 1973).

66 Paul Verhaeghe (1994 p 58).

67 Verhaeghe repeatedly quotes Spinoza (XI 48–51): 'cogitatio adaequata semper vitat eamdem rem'. An adequate thought always avoids the same thing (in this case: Thing).

68 the law is intrinsically part of the Other and the symbolic order: if I call someone father or mother I implicitly invoke the incest prohibition see Schokker & Schokker (2000 p 28).

69 Jacques Lacan (1986 p 101).

70 Schokker & Schokker (ibidem p 81 and 135).

71 We never really possessed the object small a. It paradoxically appears only as a lost object. There was no original state of complete jouissance. The law makes object small a arise only in retrospect as the location of a mythical pleasure. Initially, we are only a disparate bundle of unmediated jouissance. Only with the 'isolation' of an object small a does a desire caused by it come into being. This

object small a remains out of (empirical/phenomenological) view. It is like the vanishing point in a painting: invisible but at the same time constitutive of the representation.

72 Hans Andreus (1975 p 101).
73 Bruce Fink (1997 p 51) When it falls away, the Coke of the amorous relationship turns into a *flat* Coke.
74 Paul Moyaert (1994 p 21).
75 Slavoj Žižek (1992 p 8).
76 Paul Moyaert (ibidem p 154ff). It is an intersubjectivity that, *nota bene,* also characterises Winnicott's transitional object see Moustafa Safouan (2005 p 174).
77 Slavoj Žižek (1996 p 222ff).
78 Ethel Person (1989 p 13–14).
79 Jacques Lacan (1975 p 132).
80 Ethel Person (ibidem). We constantly meet people we already knew in our unconscious. We say: it feels as if we have known each other for a long time (if not: all our lives). I briefly continue on Freud's mystical wonder block from note 62. Memory traces/signifiers derived from sensual impressions are stored forever in our unconscious. The *jouissance* associated with them becomes associated with certain empirical traits, and it sets the beacons of our libidinal life. A glance, a voice, a gesture becomes involuntarily intertwined with it and becomes a component of our most basic fantasies. More than their meaning, the materiality of such signifiers is operative. They have something analogous/semiotic because they are indexical or iconic rather than symbolic. They refer like a trail or a broken branch to a passerby (in the case of the index) or they refer like a tall tower to the phallus or like gently rolling hills to the breast (in the case of the icon). Our unconscious is constantly hunting for libidinally invested traits associated with a fantasised completion: the mirage of the lost but regained paradise.
81 Paul Moyaert (ibidem).
82 Jacques Lacan: '*le phallus est* raison *du désir de l'Autre*' in (1958) in '*Ecrits*' (1966 p 693).
83 Slavoj Žižek (1997b p 204).
84 To be clear: the simplest and most mundane objects or projects can act as object small a and take the place of this Thing. The sublime object is '*Un objet élevé à la dignité de la Chose*', an object elevated to the level of the Thing: Lacan's famous definition of sublimation. Something then comes to occupy a certain structural place: a simultaneously sacred and forbidden place of supposedly boundless *jouissance* (Žižek, 2019 p. 221).
85 Many psychiatric problems are characterised by questions related to sexual identity and orientation, especially those that occur during adolescence, which, incidentally, drags on longer and longer over time...
86 Sigmund Freud (1924b).
87 Sigmund Freud, (ibidem p 85).
88 Sigmund Freud, (ibidem p 90).
89 Leaving aside the (in)accuracy of Freuds descriptions: Lacan produces a much more abstract/metaphorical view on the Oedipus and castration complexes and he thus elevates them to more universal, timeless proportions.
90 Sigmund Freud (1905a).
91 In the anal-sadistic phase.
92 Also called the infantile genital organisation.
93 Sigmund Freud (1923b p 79–80).
94 Chronologically first cognitively: object-permanence and only a lot later affectively: object-constancy.

95   For this universal (ontogenetic instead of phylogenetic) root of the Oedipus complex, see Claude Le Guen (1974).

96   It plays no role in this matter whether it is the father as a figure or someone/something else performing the function of 'third party'.

97   About Freud's alleged phallocentrism: according to Alenka Zupančič (2017), Lacan uses the signifier 'phallus' not because men have a penis. Indeed, he does not mean to idealise an accidental characteristic of men. It would be a mistake to replace phallus with a more neutral term (and *a fortiori* with the uterus). Although it can appear erect and symbolise power undefinedly, we receive it as a signifier offered by nature mainly because half the world's population does not have this visible (!) body part. This 'cut' of the organic makes the phallus the signifier par excellence. The phallus is a heterogeneous element, yet it determines Symbolic's grammar.

98   The child is at the mercy of '*une loi de caprice*' of the (maternal) Thing (Lacan, 1994 p 69, 187).

99   For example, to her partner, her work, and some pleasure or recreation.

100   Jacques Lacan (1958b in 1966 p 693).

101   Jacques Lacan repeatedly calls the penis a signifier that is 'given' to us by nature.

102   Jacques Lacan (1973 p 95).

103   Capitalised Law because it refers to the Name/No of the Father that separates us from the maternal Thing.

104   Jacques Lacan distinguishes between the ymbolic, the imaginary and the real father and links this to three logical stages of the Oedipus complex. The symbolic father (-function, because also incarnated by (m)Other) is representative of the (law of) language: the No and the Name of the father which guarantees the symbolic castration. It installs an early-oedipal triangle: mother–child–phallus. The mother supposedly desires the (imaginary) phallus. The child is frustrated by this and tries to identify with it. In a second (logical) time, there is the imaginary father. It is the all-powerful (God the) father who castrates the mother denying her a *jouissance* (literal translation: use of her fruit/usu-fruct) of the child. Finally, it is the *real* father (as the man who *actually* enjoys the mother) who castrates the child so that it can no longer be all or mother's phallus.

105   Paul Moyaert (2004 p 43–48).

106   Jacques Lacan, '*le désir est l'envers de la loi*' (1962) in '*Ecrits*' (1966 p 787). Desire is the flipside of the law.

107   In an allusion to Charles Baudelaire's '*les Fleurs du Mal*'.

108   In an episode of *Inspector Morse* set in the milieu of drug addicts, a mantelpiece read: 'Protect me from what I want'.

109   Jacques Lacan (1994 p 69).

110   For Freud, the mother was the lost paradise with which the child wanted to reunite; for Lacan, the mother is (also) a creature of enjoyment by which we are in danger of being devoured. Recalling *Le crocodile croque Odile*, he wields the infamous image of the mother's desire as the maw of a crocodile that would devour the child, should the father not stop it (the phallus). Or the image of the mother as a praying mantis of whom (because masked myself) I do not know how she sees me and whether or not she will devour me after coitus. The protective role of the phallus is also evident in the *Odyssey* where the sailors tie themselves to the mast (!) to resist the Sirens' lure.

111   Jacques Lacan (1991b p 17). That *jouissance* leads to death is evident, for example, in the clinic of anorexia nervosa or toxicomania, where the patient draws a direct line to the Thing. See the film *Trainspotting*: 'I chose not to choose life. I chose some Thing else'.

112 In contrast to the grubby and traumatic reality faced by, say, centers addressing child (sexual and other) abuse.
113 Philippe Van Haute (2000 p 191, 233).
114 Paul Moyaert (1994 p 94).
115 Paul Moyaert (1998 p 237).
116 Jacques Lacan (1975b p 109ff).
117 Paul Moyaert, (ibidem 1994 p 96–99).
118 Slavoj Žižek (1997b p 49).
119 Camille Paglia (1992).
120 Jacques Lacan, (ibidem p 68–70). Paul Verhaeghe relates it to '*das Primäre Befriedigungserlebnis*' (the experience of satisfaction) of Freud (1995 p 2).
121 Paul Verhaeghe (1994a p 166).
122 Jacques Lacan, (ibidem p 75) or in other places '*jouissance de l'organe*' or '*jouissance de masturbation*'.
123 Paul Moyaert (1991 p 40).
124 Paul Verhaeghe (1998 p. 168).
125 Paul Moyaert (ibidem 1998 p 80).
126 Two witty statements by Wittgenstein. A dog is afraid his master will beat him, but not that his master will beat him tomorrow. Or: when I got home, I expected to be surprised, but there was no surprise, so I was surprised.
127 In this Lacanian chapter, there are some more words on *jouissance*. In a notary context, it means usufruct. Only after 1960 did it evolve into a concept of its own, distinct from pleasure. The pleasure principle limits jouissance and paradoxically commands the subject to enjoy as little as possible. Jouissance, conversely, involves a constant tendency to exceed this law or limit and go beyond the pleasure principle. The prohibition of jouissance is inherent in the symbolic structure of language and in the context of the castration complex. In it, the subject gives up the attempt to have/be the imaginary phallus of the mother. They withdraw from and protect themself from enjoyment of the (first) big Other who uses them (incestuously) as a fruit. Jouissance, according to Lacan, lays the path to death (Lacan, 1991b p 17). Its enjoyment is more impossible than forbidden. Towards the end of his teaching, Lacan (1975b) distinguishes between phallic jouissance and feminine jouissance, which he also calls the enjoyment of the big Other. The former bears a resemblance to Freud's libido (regarded as masculine). The last is supplementary, unbound and lies beyond the phallus (ibid. p 69) in unmentionable and unspeakable ways. Obeying Shakespeare's dictum (brevity is the soul of wit): *Jouissance + Nom du Père = Principe de Plaisir.*
128 Sigmund Freud (1905a).
129 Sigmund Freud (1912a p 186).
130 When it does succeed, it gives a *Lucky Strike*: the cigarette brand of the gold-diggers who rarely *found* gold.
131 Jacques Lacan (1973).
132 Paul Verhaeghe (2022 p 31): 'Those who want ultimate pleasure end up in perversion and those who want ultimate love end up in madness'.
133 Desire is in a sense fetishistic: focused on breasts and buttocks, penis and (muscle) balls.
134 In the Oedipus complex revised by Mark Solms there is conflict inside the Id between seven drives. For example, CARE and ATTACHMENT conflict with SEEKING, PLAY, FEAR, RAGE or PLEASURE.
135 Paul Verhaeghe (1996 p 199).
136 The entanglement of two bodies is never unifying because the body of one enjoys a part of the body of the other, see Moustafa Safouan (2005 p 301).

137 It is an image frequently used by Paul Verhaeghe (1998).

138 Slavoj Žižek (1997a p 112) In the first part of a commercial, a girl walks along a stream, sees a frog, kisses it, and the frog turns into a handsome young man. The man casts an eager glance at the girl, kisses her, and she turns into a beer bottle. The woman sees in Him a full phallic presence, while the man reduces Her to a partial object/consumption product.

139 Jacques Lacan (1973 p 53–55, 66–67): *'une rencontre toujours manquée'*.

140 Sigmund Freud (1937a p 262). It is about the rejection of femininity with its being at the mercy of the enjoyment of the Other.

141 See earlier note on the inspection of two IPA committees and his dismissal. Personally, I maintain a classical/fixed duration of sessions both individually and in groups. In a (semi-)residential setting, however, I adopt an elastic rather than inflexible approach. You have to (dare to) tread uncharted paths to arrive at a psychoanalytic event in the encounter with the psychiatric patient. This is also evident in my forthcoming *Psychoanalytic Psychotherapy in Psychiatric Practice. Clinical Portraits* (Routledge).

142 Jacques Lacan (1991b p 374–375).

143 *'Fragments are the only forms I trust'* says the narrator in a short story by Donal Barthelme (1981).

144 Marc De Kesel on this 'Münchhausen paradigm' (2019).

145 A famous verse by Rudyard Kipling from *The Ballad of East and West* in T.S. Eliot (1941).

146 In Freud's time, sexuality and gender were closely related. His psychology involved the oppositions active–passive, phallic–castrated, male–female within which we try to determine our 'position'. Today, we have evolved away from these fixed frameworks, and our (gender) identity is more fluid: a search for one's own identity amidst the 1001 faces of Eros (McDougall, 1996). Nowadays, a puzzled and puzzling neo-sexuality becomes paramount. It has to be understood in its particularity. LGTBQ++++ refers to a plurality that should be analysed (sufficiently) instead of banalised.

147 Jacques Lacan (1953 p 305–314).

148 Jacques Lacan (1973).

149 Jean Laplanche was in Lacan's analysis until 1963. Still, he and some of Lacan's other seminarians (among others: Daniel Lagache and Daniel Widlöcher) broke away to found the *Association Psychoanalytique de France* (part of the IPA) (Roudinesco, 1993). This IPA barred Lacan as a training analyst, while several of his disciples became prominent members. Besides Laplanche: Jean-Baptiste Pontalis, Didier Anzieu and Daniel Widlöcher, who even became president! (Bailly, 2012).

150 Sigmund Freud (1896).

151 Jean Laplanche (1987).

152 For this distinction, see Verhaeghe (1997).

153 Hélène Tessier (2014 p 171).

154 Jean Laplanche (2011 p 280).

155 Ibid. p 115.

156 Kulish (2019).

157 Hélène Tessier (ibid. p 179).

158 Ibid. p 181.

159 Jean Laplanche (1999).

160 Jean Laplanche (2002 p 52).

161 Zeuthen & Gammelgaard (2010 p 11).

162 Antonie Ladan (2007).

163　General studies that demonstrated effectiveness, without comparing them with other forms of treatment, e.g. Tucker et al. (1987), Stone (1990) and in recent years studies with more *'strength of evidence'* e.g. Doidge (1997), Chiesa et al. (2003) Bateman & Fonagy (1999, 2000, 2001, 2004). Corveleyn et al. (2005) Leuzinger-Bohleber (2002). Vermote (2005). Leichsenring & Rabung (2011), Leichsenring et al. (2019), Leichsenring et al. (2022).

Part III

Psychiatric Practice

Chapter 9

Freud & Co in Psychiatry

Cutting-edge Technology and Development Aid

I Current Psychoanalytics[1]

As recently as 1983, Bruno Bettelheim stated that psychoanalysis was the treatment of choice for mental illness in the United States, as medicine was for physical illness.[2] However, with the rise of biological psychiatry and pharmacotherapy, with the triumph[3] of symptom-focused and short-term behavioural therapies, and as a result of *ad hominem* criticism of Freud's person, psychoanalysis has in recent decades been losing this undisputed leading role in psychiatric treatment. For the managed care industry today, most disorders within the DSM should be treated through a judicious pre-scription of medication and a predetermined number of (reimbursable) ses-sions, and this is based on 'scientifically' accepted criteria. Yet a turnaround has been occurring again for a few decades. Existing psychoanalytic forms of therapy are becoming more systematised and protocolled. In terms of symptomatic improvement, they can demonstrate comparable and even longer-lasting efficacy than, for instance, (cognitive) behavioural therapy.[4] Numerous studies have been done on the effectiveness of longer-term treat-ments,[5] and the basic concepts of psychoanalysis have been scientifically tested.[6]

Because of their only temporary and transient effect, short-term and (superficial) symptom-oriented treatments (as opposed to psychoanalytically inspired ones) are increasingly coming under threat.[7] There is also a new profiling going on within psychoanalysis where, in addition to the role of interpretation, the importance of the therapeutic relationship[8] is emphasised. More attention is paid to mental processes than to mental content,[9] and cognitive and neuroscientific research findings are increasingly being inte-grated into psychoanalytic theorisation and practice.[10] Finally, research around attachment[11] and mentalisation, secure or otherwise, shows undis-putedly that the quality of both is (interconnectedly) protective against the occurrence of psychopathology. On the one hand, both are also transmitted trans-generationally: parents with insecure attachment and/or limited men-talising ability have corresponding children. On the other hand, increasing

DOI: 10.4324/9781032698052-12

mentalising capacity in parents has positive effects towards 'mental health' not only for themselves but also for their children.[12]

Such findings have greatly served the prestige and importance of a psychoanalytic approach to psychiatry. Consequently, thanks in part to the mentalisation-based semi-residential treatment of severe personality disorders (which has proved superior to drug, social-psychiatric and behavioural therapeutic approaches),[13] psychoanalysis has made its re-entry into the treatment guidelines of the American Psychiatric Association. In my country, a large-scale process-outcome study by colleague Rudi Vermote[14] on 78 patients has confirmed the compelling (and also lasting in *follow-up* research) therapy results in severely personality-disturbed patients.

2 Sophisms

However, by most 'lay people' (including within the mental health community), psychoanalysis today is still identified with and reduced to one well-defined form of treatment, namely the typical couch cure. They perceive this as an outdated and ultra-long-lasting undertaking for a select group of intelligent, affluent and, in many ways, hyper-complicated patients who, in their eyes, find a peculiar 'pleasure' in squeezing (or having squeezed) the depths of their souls. Moreover, the world of psychoanalysts seems to them a closed (if not incestuous) universe of professional navel-gazers meeting in hermetic cenacles. When they 'come out', they speak a barely comprehensible jargon, in which *sex* plays an all too obvious central role. After all, this psychoanalytic world seems to be made up of the most diverse, conflicting and sectarian circles. A certain dogmatism sometimes makes them seem far removed from the open mind they are supposed to have.

If psychoanalysis reaches out, it will have to admit that even in matters such as these, there is no smoke without fire. We will deal *à décharge* more extensively with the divisions within the psychoanalytic world and its use of language. In the section that follows, we will discuss the typical cure. The division within the psychoanalytic world understandably raises a lot of eyebrows. What would science still mean if the difference between geocentrism and heliocentrism were a matter of opinion? However, we can compare post-Freudian psychoanalysis to post-Newtonian physics. His theories remain valid (except for the ultra-small and the ultra-large). Opinions differ only on what took place several billion years ago or beyond the view of the electron microscope. Moreover, theoretical differences often involve a different research object, field of study, practice, or foreign language and culture.[15] Divisions remain perhaps most significant between the (Lacanian) *Association Mondiale de Psychanalyse* and the *International Psychoanalytical Association.* Community aside, this mainly concerns the importance they give to language and biology, humanities and natural sciences, respectively. Even during a congress of the IPA dedicated to this, it was admittedly revealed that within its fold, there are very different views on the (nature of the) scientific status of psychoanalysis.[16] Discussions on this, however, proceed through rational argumentation and in all intellectual serenity.

Some, following the model of the natural sciences, strive for a theory of everything.[17] They see it as a scientific task to find an all-encompassing and as 'conclusive' as possible system underlying the psychological and psychopathological. They often come from academic circles. In contrast, others (who usually start mainly or exclusively from clinical practice) uphold and defend the value of theoretical pluralism. After all, all phenomena can be approached from several '*vertices*'.[18] For them, each theory must remain (in Bionian terms) unsaturated[19] for truth to slip into it.[20] Does not the particularity of any psychoanalytic encounter presuppose a maximum openness and receptivity perhaps best served by a broad theoretical bandwidth?

3 Faith

It is yet another variation on the difference between psychoanalysis as a science, as a (form of) psychotherapeutic art and skill and as a movement of faith, in which, as it turns out, these registers are not mutually exclusive. Jacques Lacan (who may nonetheless be regarded as the great system-builder par excellence): '*Ce que le psychanalyste* doit *savoir: ignorer ce qu'il sait*'.[21] And furthermore: '*Il n'y a pas d'Autre de l'Autre*'.[22] There is no guaranteeing master. Every symbolic system is based on nothing more than convention, that is, in a sense, on nothing. Unless, of course, one believes in a (God-the-) Father, for instance, in Freud as the Godfather of psychoanalysis or in one of his disciples who is considered the ultimate guarantor figure.[23] All this is inevitable for any symbolic enterprise around which people group, including the psychoanalytic one. Indeed, the lack of an object (Lacan's object small a) is the cause of desire. So, it also causes the desire of any symbolic system to recover this lost object (or rather, this lost Thing).[24] But whether it is faith, science or art, every symbolic system, by definition, falls short of eliminating the lack by which it is caused. There is an ever-impossible encounter. At the horizon of the big Other, only the 'structural muteness of the Real' and of the *Thing in itself* remains.[25]

It is also integral to psychoanalysis's scientific aspirations that it develops its language. Indeed, many of its terms appear in common parlance. Moreover, they refer to matters of paramount importance in everyone's life: love and relationships, desire and death, happiness and suffering. But in a psychoanalytic context, these terms often have well-defined meanings. Psychoanalytic publications are teeming with technical terms and jargon to counter such confusion. Lacan and Bion[26] even pursue an algebraic formulation that deliberately moves away from intuition, imagination, and common sense. Such technicity has no place in the language used during the psychoanalytic encounter. To a broader audience, it also often needlessly damages the reputation of psychoanalysis. Nevertheless, a critical note may perhaps also resonate with the latter. Is it not surprising that it commands reverence and awe when Einstein uses mathematical formulas? And at the same time, that adverse reactions (ranging from anger to hilarity) can be observed when scientists attempt to capture the complexity of human and/or subjective phenomena in formulas? On pain of nullity, should such subjects then all be offered as sweet cake or fast food? Why is an instant understanding of these issues imperative?

Both Freud, Winnicott, Bion and Lacan[27] also make 'a drawing' occasionally. Freud talks about the topics of unconscious, preconscious and conscious, and later in his work, he divides the psyche into three agencies: Id, Ego and Superego. Lacan develops his topology with his registers of the Real, the Symbolic and the Imaginary, his ring of Möbius,[28] his bottle of Klein, his Borromean knot and so on. In short, instead of words, psychoanalysts sometimes use images to describe the psychoanalytic field. In both cases, the conceptual frame of reference determines whether, how and with what precision the territory can be studied. In the meantime, we should not forget that the word can never (fully) capture the Thing,[29] and the map never (fully) 'covers' the territory.[30]

As we will see below, several psychoanalytic authors after Freud designed their own (more or less sophisticated) language and their own (more or less sophisticated or comprehensive) maps. They then focused mainly on an area that remained virtually unexplored by Freud: the (early) mother–child relationship[31] and that of woman.[32] What will follow in this chapter is, to a large extent, a stimulus to identify ourselves with the Inuit. Because they (according to legend) have as many as a hundred words to name snow, they view their seemingly monotonous, white world with much more shading and nuance than we would suspect as outsiders.[33] At the same time, a warning must be issued against snow blindness. Indeed, we will find that all sex seems to have vanished from the theories of Melanie Klein, Donald Winnicott and Wilfred Bion.[34]

From classical Freudian and Lacanian quarters, this is considered the result of a blind spot. Had Freud not considered the primordial role of sexuality as one of his most important discoveries? Isn't psychoanalysis, in a sense, a theory of infantile sexuality? But first, psychoanalysis has extended its scope of action to problems where man's identity, integrity or survival as a subject is threatened. Moreover, it is not so much concerned with sex in its ordinary sense of genital activity but also with the pleasurable/enjoyable experience of oral and anal, of sucking and biting, of pissing and pooping, of voyeurism, exhibitionism and sadism. It is the universe Melanie Klein discovered and described in real-time from psychoanalytic play therapy with children affected by severe psychopathology. It is a Hieronymus Boschian world of good and bad breasts, penises and toxic bowel movements that shows that in the little child, besides a divine,[35] there can also be a sinister side of, for instance, murderous cannibalism. And as for sex anyway, it is only Jacques Lacan who has added to the enigma of our erotic life several new ideas and theorisations, thinking primarily of object little a, phallus and *jouissance*. Therefore, the always problematic nature of their mutual relationship gives Eros (in Joyce McDougall's words) a thousand and one faces.[36]

4 Neurosis and the Typical Cure[37]

The neurotic, and *mutatis mutandis*, the analysant, is sometimes regarded as a *'malade imaginaire'*:[38] someone who imagines his illness. 'It's all just in the mind' is then said, which, as will be shown, is in a certain sense true. Conversely, it often happens that the analysant themself starts looking for trauma, a 'real' reason on which they can hang the cause (*'causa'*) of their suffering. Or that they no longer believe in health at all. According to Jules Romains, every healthy person is – in a way – ignorant of their illness: '*Tout homme bien portant est un malade qui s'ignore*'.[39] It is a poor consolation that everyone would be sick in the same bed.

What is addressed in the psychoanalytic treatment is not the visible but the largely hidden psychological suffering that is not understood by the person concerned (and *a fortiori* by those around them). It is more potent than themself and forces itself upon us repeatedly, no matter how hard we try to push it *away* in all possible and impossible ways. These are, for instance, fears, insecurity, feelings of inferiority, shyness, compulsions, doubts and/or inhibitions related to all kinds of difficulties in love, play and work. Usually, these problems do not show on a person's face, especially since the person in question tries to present themself as well as possible and function according to wishes or expectations. Who hasn't experienced feeling like a rock without showing it to the outside world? How many crises play out unseen in and/or around us, and how many dramas appear *ex nihilo*, like a bolt from the blue? This concerns the 'classical' conflict and psychoneurosis with its hypertrophy of the symbolic-imaginary, in which repetitive patterns of thought, feeling or behaviour can be related to (early) childhood history and our then, always more or less phantasmatically distorted relations with significant others through interpretation and (re-)construction. They are mental representational disorders, where the psyche and the mental have developed sufficiently. The only way out is to arrive at a lived understanding of the psychogenesis and psychodynamics of the problems. It presupposes a return to how and when things went wrong in life history. Which forces or elements in the person conflict with each other, and which unsuccessful attempts at self-healing has the patient cobbled together at that time as a sometimes elegant, sometimes forced 'solution'?

The Oedipus complex often plays a crucial role in these neuroses. This complex is defined as the set of romantic desires and hostile feelings the child experiences towards its parents and continues to operate in the unconscious (towards other parental figures). They will then lead to all sorts of intrusive feelings of rivalry, jealousy, competition and/or sexual desires for 'forbidden' or 'impossible' partners.[40] They also trigger all kinds of neurotic psycho-pathology, with sexual and narcissistic pleasure being hampered by inhibitions, symptoms and all sorts of fears. In its 'positive' form, the Oedipus complex is characterised by death wishes for the same-sex parent and erotic desire for that of the opposite sex. In its 'negative' form, just the opposite occurs. However, elements of both forms are mostly present in intertwined ways. The complex peaks between three and five during the phallic phase. During this period, the child 'knows' only the phallus, which, by its presence or absence, is considered characteristic of the gender difference. With the formation of a (predominantly paternal) Superego, the Oedipus complex is repressed during the latency years. It has a revival during puberty and then culminates more or less satisfactorily in a well-defined object choice.

All psychoanalysts regard the Oedipus complex as structuring both personality and later psychopathology, both of which are, after all, understood in their relation to this complex.[41] Classically, the treatment for this (largely Oedipal) conflict- and psychoneurosis is couch-based psychoanalysis. Technically, within the cure, a return ('regression') occurs to the point where and when the neurosis was born (the point of fixation). In this way, a lived insight can be gained about how it worked (or didn't). Indeed, this insight must arise *in vivo* within the living reality of the therapeutic relationship. As a result of the transference, this can more or less be seen as a new edition of the past. However, the analyst does not play the game. Indeed, as a participating observer, they will consistently remember the total transference situation as an expression of the analysant's unconscious and/or inner world. The reality of the unconscious that thus appears will have to be translated in due course. Everything is (re-) experienced in the here and now of the encounter. Moreover, all this is accompanied by an analytic labour that is the opposite of dream work.

5 Cutting-Edge Technology

It is a complicated and cutting-edge undertaking that invariably takes time.[42] That neurosis is a mild form of psychopathology, therefore, deserves to be refuted. Recurring difficulties in love, play and work can indeed drive one to despair, especially if the person in question realises that all this mischief (in a way that is unfortunately difficult to grasp) has to do with *themself*. Invisibly, the neurosis gobbles up energy that does not remain indefinitely available for the chores of real life. The neurotic's environment also suffers to a greater or lesser extent from their psychopathology. The patience and understanding of significant others are either limited or may be tested excessively and intolerably. Treatment of this psychopathology is also no *sinecure*. Among other things, it requires perseverance on the part of the patient, the utmost tact, expertise, and diligence on the part of the analyst, and sufficient love of truth on both.

From the 'classical' Freudian analysis perspective, the analyst is a surgeon, detective and archaeologist. They engage in cautious yet incisive dissection[43] of resistance and defence mechanisms. Like a detective,[44] they search logically for truth and meaning. Like the famous Peter Falk/Columbo, they often play dumb. They go against the 'culprit' and their relentless flow of deception, lies and deceit,[45] but without damaging the relationship of trust required. Finally, the analyst's method is similar to that of the archaeologist who tries to (re-)construct from non-verbal sources the (pre-)history of the analysant.[46] The discovery of the unconscious can then be equated with the writing and rewriting of one's own (infantile) history.

Lacanian-understood psychoanalysis adds some accents of its own here. Here, it is not so much about liberating the patient's Ego as it is about releasing the patient *from* their (specular) Ego.[47] Here, the way to achieve this is to promote free association per se. This free association is nothing more or less than the constant sliding of the narrative/signifier chain (the Symbolic), the only remedy against the pseudo-mastery of the Ego and the Imaginary. In this way, the true subject or the subject of the unconscious[48] can rise, namely the subject as desiring. Also, the Lacanian approach is very text-oriented. Words are highlighted, and punctuation in the sentence is emphasised or changed. The signifier chain is like a laundry line on which an affective charge is hung with clothes pegs (the signifiers). The wind that the analyst blows through the process both tilts the clothes pegs and shifts the load so that, surprisingly, an altogether different laundry wash hangs on the thread over time!

On the one hand, there is free association as surrendering to something in us that thinks and something in us that speaks: the *'ça parle'*. This *res cogitans*, [49] this Thing in us that thinks, is something very intimate and alien at once. It is, according to a neologism by Lacan, *'extimate'*.[50] It resides at the core of our being, and simultaneously, it escapes us in unrecoverable ways. It is something that ultimately springs from our *soma*, from our body as a disjointed conglomeration of organs. It also receives words that seem to come from elsewhere, from the big Other. Yet the neurotic should not be decapitated. They are not meant to become completely I-less. At times, there must be a *'prise de conscience'*,[51] an awareness where they must also precisely realise what they are saying. In this sense, there is a constant back and forth within the psychoanalytic process. The patient oscillates between un-integration[52] and integration. Sometimes, they let go and let things come as they come; other times, they try to reconcile things. For the therapist, too, there is a pendulum swing between an analytical position or discourse and a master position or discourse,[53] depending on whether they suspend their knowledge or provide help. Thus, psychoanalytic and psychotherapeutic moments characterise every psychoanalytically understood therapeutic process.

Either way, the protective blanket of imagination and symbolisation[54] comes off bit by bit, allowing the neurotic to get (back) in touch with the Real of Thing, drive and trauma. By definition, it makes the typical cure a complex and terrifying undertaking that can sometimes be disruptive. As such, it is suitable only for certain patients. Those most eligible for analysis in the typical cure are people who (despite their psychological suffering) have sufficient basic trust, stability and resilience. Their problems are mainly related to the housekeeping of pleasure and enjoyment, and their anxieties are not of a psychotic order: they are not so much related to maintaining identity or integrity. More generally, they can call on the necessary 'resources' to get through such an undertaking without too much adversity (i.e. needless mess and misery). As such, the cure allows them to move from neurotic, frozen choices to more conscious and personal ethical decisions. What interpretation do I give to love and sexuality, to work and relationships? How do I relate to loss, mortality and the many lacks and losses that characterise life anyway? In short, how do I relate to the Things of Life?[55]

6 Leaving the Couch

However, apart from those with some form of prior knowledge, few people ask for psychoanalysis themselves. Most people who suffer psychologically try to help themselves. When they ask for help (often after a long time), they initially turn to a GP, a psychologist or a psychiatrist. Many difficulties are then 'met' by the prescription of psychopharmaceuticals and/or a supportive attitude of empathetic listening. Witness the number of intoxications that wash up in emergency departments. Many also 'accidentally' end up in mental health care, where they usually receive fast-forward solution- and symptom-focused assistance. It is only when such cases drag on, worsen or keep recurring that the question arises among themselves or those around them whether there is a need for a more 'thorough' approach.[56]

However, another problem immediately arises: do they have sufficient capacity to qualify for a psychoanalytic cure? Almost all patients who end up in hospital services (psychiatric or otherwise) for reasons of psychological suffering or disorder are unwilling or unable to undertake this time- and money-consuming undertaking for various reasons. The nature and severity of their psychopathology will also often make a conventional cure impossible. For instance, their condition or level of functioning does not allow it. Prior interviews (which are always face-to-face) almost invariably reveal a history of broken trust, loss and abandonment, traumatic events, substance abuse and interpersonal problems. It also makes them feel they would struggle to stick to the 'framework' of the cure. For instance, they feel unsafe, threatened or abandoned and need tangible support and/or grip. Psychoanalysis is, therefore, most commonly applied in the form of psychoanalytic therapies. According to Otto Kernberg,[57] they are even beginning to play the de facto leading role in the psychoanalytic treatment of neuroses.

As will be shown below, the patients who are (have to be) admitted to the psychiatric hospital are even worse off. Their condition has the proportions of a major psychiatric disorder requiring professional care; they are caught up to their ears in substance abuse and dependence and/ or without understanding how or why; in several areas of their lives, they often make irreparable messes. As a result of all this, they are increasingly and in multiple ways at risk of ending up on the margins of society, where it is not pleasant to dwell (except, perhaps, temporarily and for the affluent or spoilt).

Psychoanalytic treatment can often only start within a sophisticated clinical psychotherapeutic milieu, as is offered in some specialised psychiatric settings. There is a significant need to draw on post-Freudian developments for such 'early' disorders. According to Freud and the poet William Wordsworth, 'the child is father to man'. However, it has since become clear that for the more severe than neurotic disorders, it is not the child but the infant that plays the leading role. Melanie Klein invented play therapy for the psychoanalytic treatment of children. Her experiences also have many implications for the technique in adults. Moreover, through her work with severely disturbed patients, she identified many phenomena and mechanisms from early (pre- or infra-verbal) childhood that are also relevant to 'early' disorders in adult psychiatry. Wilfred Bion extended psychoanalytic activity to psychotics and worked with and in the group in which, incidentally, he also discovered many psychotic fears and phenomena. From these experiences, he developed a theory of technique and a theory of thinking. Donald Winnicott was not just an analyst but worked for 40 years as a paediatrician with mothers and their babies. After 20 000 consultations with these 'couples', it is doubtful if there is an analyst who has more to say about their misadventures.[58] From the direct child observations of René Spitz, Henri Wallon, Margaret Mahler and Daniel Stern, much could be deduced about the first years of life. For the infants, both dietary and emotional and mental nutrition proved *vital*.

With John Bowlby, a whole series of large-scale research on attachment was started, which has been pursued in recent years by Fonagy and his collaborators in reciprocal intertwining with reflective functioning and mentalisation. The result is that no one in the world of psychiatry and psychotherapy can now deny that the emotional and psychological quality of our initial relationships plays a decisive role in the occurrence of or protection against psychopathology. If necessary, we must 'feed' or 'arm' the subject (with basic trust and safety, mentalisation capacity, containment). Ultimately, we try to get 'in touch' more profoundly to determine the subject's most proper and personal relationship with the Real.[59] How all this is realised in group psychotherapy and/or within clinical psychotherapy ('multiple-treater setting')[60] is elaborated in the next section, but I will end this chapter with some thoughts on the need for (this time) positive (instead of negative) capability.

7 Positive capability

In an editorial in Dutch *Tijdschrift voor Psychiatrie,* Joris Vandenberghe discussed the tension between clinical and managerial thinking.[61] At the basis of clinical thinking lies the therapeutic relationship with the patient. Establishing and maintaining this relationship on good and bad days is an art and a skill. It requires commitment and attachment, bearing and tolerating, boundaries and understanding. The counsellor is not a technologist under whose prescription the patient is treated but explores with, around and within each unique patient the always shadowy and complex roots of evil. This involves Evil as *'le Mal'* (Charles Baudelaire), which simultaneously implies the dimension of pain. Diagnosis is a tentative process that leads only to preliminary working hypotheses that never fully cover the truth. Therapy is a shared responsibility and enterprise in which the patient does much themself (but not alone) and whose outcome cannot be precisely guaranteed.

Management logic is primarily opposed to this clinical logic because it constantly aims to align resources and goals judiciously. Terms like Human Relations Management, project operation, audit, result-oriented strategy, personal development plan, efficiency and quality review are in the zenith here. The basis for this is planning and steering by measurement, analysis and control. The approach is rational and goal-oriented based on figures and tables. The world of acronyms like PDCA, SWOT, SMART, the Bradford factor, balanced scorecard and other paraphernalia seek to make the cogs of the modern organisation run smoothly. To illustrate this tension between clinical and management thinking, I would like to refer to the following witticism: for management, the ideal hospital is one without doctors and without patients! However, anyone responsible for (semi-)residential (e.g. clinical psychotherapy) psychoanalytic work must manage and lead. A lot of *positive capability* is needed to sail against the wind/resistance from patients, family, referrers, health authorities and the treatment team and stay psycho-analytically 'on course'. It is a matter of pertinent Real politics combined with the ethical 'economics' of *Saving Private Ryan.*[62]

In these economics, neither people nor resources are spared to save some-thing private. We know the heroic form of this 'something' from Antigone and Socrates, Galileo and Luther, Mahatma Gandhi and Martin Luther King: people willing to die for their cause. Or through the works of great artists such as Caravaggio, Goya, Van Gogh and Bacon. But in the broad (and less sensational) sense, many people dedicate their lives to a cause. They try to make 'something' of it and ignore the utility or other benefits it would bring them. According to Belgian *peintre maudit* Philippe Vandenberg, every oeuvre costs a human life.[63] Psychoanalytically, *something* (Thing) *private* is about a highly personal cause for each patient. To rescue it, we would give our lives...

Notes

1 The title of the Dutch language book series I started in 2005. It produces an average of two books a year.
2 Bruno Bettelheim (1983 p 40).
3 Various forms of psychotherapy score similarly: the 'dodo bird verdict' after an episode from Lewis Caroll's *Alice in Wonderland*: 'everyone has won so all must have prizes' see Fisher & Greenberg (1996 p 207). Explanations: the multi-dimensional clinical reality and 'non-specific' factors such as support, empathy and a therapeutic relationship with a reliable other. See Wampold et al. (1997) and Luborsky et al. (2002).
4 Considered are 'transference focused psychotherapy' (TFP, Kernberg et al., 2002), 'mentalisation based treatment' (MBT, Bateman & Fonagy, 2004) and dynamic interpersonal therapy (DIT) as highly protocolised, on which extensive scientific effect research has been conducted. In an earlier meta-analysis by Leichsenring and Leibing (2003) psychodynamic therapy has a large overall effect size of 1.46 (1.08 self-report measures, 1.79 observer-report measures) while cognitive behavioural therapy has (only) 1.00, 1.20 0.87, respectively. Moreover, the longer the psychodynamic treatment, the greater the effect. See most recent Leichsenring et al. (2011, 2022).
5 See Doidge (1997 p 102–150), Leuzinger-Bohleber (2002), Leichsenring, (2005), Johansson et al. (2010).
6 Patrick Luyten (2001).
7 Joseph Corveleyn et al. (2005).
8 This is much more important than the specific therapeutic factors see Miller et al. (1997) and Hubble et al. (1999 p 1–19), which is why the way of handling the (transference) relationship is promoted to the *essence* of psychotherapy by Paul Verhaeghe (2005b).
9 Antonino Ferro (2015 p 132): 'The purpose of the analysis is to work not so much on insight, the overcoming of splits, repression, or historical reconstruction, as on the development of the instruments for thinking'. Question mark!
10 Willem Van Tilburg (2000 p 119).
11 Attachment is a specific affective bond with someone from whom security is expected and which is internalised as 'felt security' an 'inner working model'. It can be tested in children using the Strange Situation Test (Ainsworth et al., 1978) and in adults by an attachment interview (Main & Goldwyn, 1995).
12 Main and Goldwyn (ibid.). Peter Fonagy (2001), and Fonagy et al. (2002).
13 See various effectiveness studies Bateman and Fonagy (1999, 2000, 2001 cfr supra), Perry et al. (1999), Gabbard (2000a, 2001).
14 Rudi Vermote (2005b).
15 As can be shown, for example, about 'theoretical' differences regarding primary narcissism (Kinet, 2005).
16 Recently in a couple of pages: Mark Solms (2018a).
17 Robert Wallerstein (2002 p 1253).
18 A term Bion prefers to that of viewpoint. Like Lacan, he prefers mathematical abstraction (Bion 1974 p 88–89).
19 Martin Charcot: '*la théorie c'est bon mais ça n'empêche pas les faits d'exister*' in: Peter Gay (1989 p 57).
20 The poet Dylan Thomas, in his *Poetic Manifesto,* says that the best craftsman always carves out holes and chinks in the interior of the poem so that something not in the poem can slip, crawl, flash or thunder into it, see Wasch (1998).
21 Jacques Lacan (1955 in 1966 p 349). What the analyst should know: ignore his knowledge. There is no big Other of the Other.

22 Jacques Lacan (1991b p 393–394).
23 Donald Winnicott has been careful not to form a 'school' around him. Of course, a whole range of psychoanalysts are working in his 'line': Charles Rycroft, Marion Milner, Masud Khan, Christopher Bollas, et al. Jacques Lacan wanted to dissolve his school with his *'Je ne suis pas Lacanien, je suis Freudien'* (in his Séminaire de Caracas, 1981) or (in his *'Lettre de dissolution de l'école Freudienne de Paris'* of 5 January 1980): *'Ce problème se démontre tel, d'avoir une solution: c'est la dis – la dissolution'*. The post-Lacanian era is characterised by a kind of 'bible study' of his texts.
24 Finding an object is a re-finding (Freud 1905a p 155). This involves a sublimation, elevating the object to the dignity of the Thing see Jacques Lacan (1986 p 133).
25 Frédéric Declercq (2000 p 70).
26 Lacan's and Bion's thinking count about 35 and 50 algebraic symbols, respectively. According to Bion's *Grid*, the 'algebraic calculus' and the scientific deductive system are the highest in his Theory of Thinking. However, its use during the session implies a minus K. There, all -isms are sophisms.
27 Jacques Lacan with his ingenious *'graphe du désir'* in (1960 in 1966 p 817).
28 Möbius' ring, in particular, clarifies a lot of things. If we turn an elongated and narrow strip of paper lengthwise over 180°, glue the ends together, and run our finger along one side, we gradually end up from the inside to the outside or vice versa. It makes inside and outside and psychoanalytic change 'tangible'.
29 Jacques Lacan, *'le symbole est le meurtre de la Chose'* in (1953 in 1966 p 319).
30 Schaeffer (1989 p 781–794).
31 Didier Anzieu (1975).
32 Sigmund Freud (1926) where he calls woman a 'dark continent'. The riddle for him is: *'Was will das Weib?'* Serge André (1986).
33 According to the famous philosophical 'Sapir-Whorf hypothesis' or 'linguistic determinism' (see Benjamin Whorf, 1940 p 212–214), our conceptual system directly influences how we think about and experience the world. According to Whorf, the Inuit would also literally 'see' the snow differently; the veracity of his claim is in doubt, given the peculiarity of the Inuit language, but the *principle* of linguistic determinism seems to stand.
34 With them, too, virtually no word on perversion as a structurally distinct psychopathology.
35 The primary narcissism of 'His Majesty the Baby' (Freud, 1914c).
36 Joyce McDougall (1996).
37 The typical cure is (as Anna O. noted) essentially a 'talking cure' see Peter Gay (ibid. p 70).
38 See Molière's comedy (1673).
39 Jules Romains (1924).
40 Respectively as variations on the parricidal (parental murder) and incestuous theme, see the 'rat man' who is so wildly sexual that he says you'd kill your father for it see Peter Gay (ibidem p 247).
41 Laplanche & Pontalis (1967).
42 Michel Quinodoz (2013).
43 A surgical term for clearing the area to be operated on using a scalpel (and other surgical instruments).
44 The Wolf Man (one of Freud's most famous patients) writes in his memoirs that Freud regularly read Sir Arthur Conan Doyle's Sherlock Holmes stories (Obholzer & Pankejevv, 1982).
45 Slavoj Žižek (1996 p 71–93) contrasting the cool of Sherlock Holmes with the 'hardboiled private eye' descending in some quest into some *Heart of Darknes*, in

my view a nice metaphor for the less classical/orthodox forms of psychoanalytic work.

46 Sigmund Freud (1937b p 217).

47 Andreas De Block (2003 p 124). This does refer to the Ego as Lacan conceives it: imaginary/specular.

48 Lacanian, this subject is *between* the Es and the (imaginary) I. It is like Baron Munchhausen pulling himself out of the swamp by his own wig or like Felix the Cat jumping in the animated films from a fictional point above the abyss see Marc De Kesel (2002 p 35).

49 An allusion to the Cartesian dualism between the *res cogitans* and the *res extensa*, a thinking thing and a thing extended in space, between spirit and matter, see René Descartes in his *Meditations* (1989 p 47).

50 A term by Jacques Lacan as a mixture of intimate and external. This *hybrid* status characterises both the Real of Thing and object a and the Symbolic of language and big Other within and around us. See the Schokker brothers (2000 p 62).

51 Difficult to translate: how the conscious *grabs* the unconscious.

52 Winnicott distinguished unintegration from disintegration. It is about the capacity to be alone in the presence of someone else (1958). Blaise Pascal (1669 p 136 my transl.): 'All the miseries of men have but one cause, namely that they are incapable of remaining quietly in a room'.

53 For a clear description of the discourses, see Paul Verhaeghe (1994a).

54 Ludi Van Bouwel (1998 p 38).

55 Lacan repeatedly talks about the Thing or '*la Chose*'. But also about '*la Cause*' or '*l'a cause*'. He also called his school '*école de la cause freudienne*' which is at once '*une cause perdue*' and '*une chose perdue*': a lost Thing and a lost cause.

56 A large-scale US study showed that most patients entering analysis had tried shorter forms of psychotherapy and medication before resorting to analysis, see Doidge et al. (1994).

57 Otto Kernberg (1999).

58 Neville Symington (1986 p 315).

59 '*Savoir y faire avec son symptome/sinthome*' as an absurd and Real enjoyment see Jacques Lacan (2005b).

60 In the UK one speaks of *Clinical Psychotherapy* see for example https://www.kcl. ac.uk/study/postgraduate-taught/courses/clinical-psychotherapy and in the US of multiple-treater settings (Gabbard, 2014 p 164).

61 Joris Vandenberghe (2007).

62 For an essay dedicated to *Saving Private Ryan*, see Mark Kinet (2023d).

63 Philippe Vandenberg '*Tout oeuvre coûte une vie humaine*' (2006).

Chapter 10

Group Psychotherapy
The Unconscious Live on Stage

1 The Group[1]

We are thrown into the world naked and needy at birth because we are physiologically immature. We do not choose where our cradle stands. Not the astrological, but the psychosocial constellation is decisive from the start.[2] Most of us have known some kind of primaeval honeymoon, but some were in a way already lost before birth. It is a statement that is often echoed by psychiatric patients: very early in my life, it was too late. They must learn by trial and error from mistakes often made *before* them. Moreover, we are born into the dreams of others, but some of us remain trapped in them. Even when the dream becomes a nightmare. This is all analogous to what happens when we suddenly find ourselves in a 'random' treatment group.

Sociologists speak of the primary group.[3] It is a group within which personal and enduring relationships are created and maintained. With family and village as its prototype, the primary group has its values, norms and behaviour patterns and thus forms an implicit micro-culture. In a supposedly natural way, it is in all our fibres. Sociologist Pierre Bourdieu calls this a *habitus*.[4] It results from primary socialisation and ensures, for instance, that children of artists move through the art world with great ease and naturalness. In contrast, others fatally retain something artificial about it. The secondary group should be explicitly distinguished from the primary. Here, we have the choice of joining it or not. This choice is determined by whether this or that group *tells* us something. To find any object is to see some*thing* in it or to find something in it. You join a group because of shared characteristics, desires, dreams, problems or defences. In secondary groups, such as teams of all kinds, members maintain formal, instrumental relationships with each other. This is to achieve specific shared goals. *The raison d'être* of this secondary group is rational rather than emotional. It is also variable in composition: changing members does not mean this secondary group ceases to exist.

Even for Aristotle, household members and family were not to be reduced to biological relationships. Instead, it is essentially a configuration, varying in

DOI: 10.4324/9781032698052-13

time and culture, of interrelationships, commandments and prohibitions, rights and duties, not least in who, how and what can be 'enjoyed'. In Lacanian terms, the big Other enters our psyche and makes us a *zoon politikon* or political animal.[5] Therefore, Freud's Oedipus complex should be understood as an initial symbolic structure: a social order *inside* the family. The Oedipus complex and mirroring contribute to our drive or affect regulation and identity formation. For example, for the optimal psychological development of the child, the parent's love for each other is more important than the parent's love for the child. If the parents have an unsatisfactory relationship, a skewed triangle may develop, with one or both parents seeking satisfaction from the child. Thus, the child is not sufficiently confronted with loving parents in an erotic couple. It seems more in tune with the mother and/or father than their partner, and it thinks it can or should satisfy their desires. The boundaries between the sexes, between generations and those related to incest become unclear. What falls short is the paternal function (not to be confused with the father as a traditional figure), which by law must prohibit and protect. Thus, boundless love is curbed, where parent and child merge in a pathological (or even lethal) manner.[6]

Most (semi-)residential psychotherapeutic programmes and environments are teeming with group work.[7] It, therefore, seems appropriate first to put group functioning in psychiatry under the psychoanalytic microscope. In inpatient care, several small treatment groups (8–12 people) usually follow the work types[8] of their therapy programme. On the other hand, large-group meetings (sometimes up to 40–60 people) also often occur, such as ward– and patient–staff meetings.[9] There is also a lot of group work within the team. Indeed, various team meetings sometimes focus on direct patient care and other times on departmental operations or treatment culture. Particular group dynamics can occur in these groups that need to be recognised and remedied. After all, they hinder the work of the group and the work of the individual members who are part of it. Apart from the broader psychoanalytic thinking already referred to, it is Freud and Bion, in particular, who can be inspiring in understanding such group dynamics.

2 Freud's Group

Freud himself wrote extensively about groups twice. With his 'scientific myth' from *Totem and Taboo,* Freud latched on to evolutionary-biological findings to expose the phylogenetic antecedents of the Oedipus complex.[10] In it, Freud speaks of a kind of primordial group. Drawing on a variety of archaeological and anthropological sources,[11] Freud constructs in this treatise a mythical primordial horde led by a jealous and violent, polygamous and monopolising father[12] who kept all the females to himself and chased away the sons. Eventually, the rebellious brothers united, and they killed this primordial father. His body was then eaten in an attempt to adopt his feared and envied traits and powers. Tormented by remorse and guilt because of this useless murder, a common totem was chosen, usually an animal that symbolised the father and around which a cult began to develop. Killing this animal became taboo. Only sporadically (e.g. annually) this animal was ritually killed and eaten. A taboo also came to be placed on women, namely an incest prohibition or an exogamy prohibition. The place of the primordial father must not be taken. To Freud, this is the foundation of civilisation, exposing a phylogenetic original sin and exhibiting a structure reflected in many revolutions. Also, we have probably all witnessed it already: not only Pope ('Papa') John Paul II was canonised with skilful haste immediately after his death ('*Santo Subito!*'). Of course, in all this, we recognise some ingredients of the Oedipus complex (ambivalence of the sons towards the father, taboo on parricide and incest). Still, some of this is also recognisable in group dynamics. In particular, large unstructured groups can regress as a result of internal or external stress to the extent that a *revival* of the primal horde occurs.[13]

Another critical text by Freud related to (large) groups is *Mass Psychology and Ego-analysis.* [14] In this writing, he gives the phenomenological description of masses a psychoanalytic underpinning and, *en passant*, takes a run-up to his later structural Id/Ego/Superego model.[15] First, Freud describes the mass and its influence on the individual. The mass is more unstable, irrational, immoral, unloving and unrestrained than the individual. Individual achievements fade, and particularity diminishes. Conflicting conceptions coexist without conflict. The impossible does not exist. A collective soul comes alive in the masses, and the individual acquires a sense of invincibility. Action is predominant over reflection. Thoughts and feelings are oriented in one direction. The civilised individual becomes a barbarian and impulsive creature in the crowd. There is a desire for illusion, not truth. There is impressionability and credulity. There is a tendency towards extremism and a need for a strong leader. The reader no doubt recognises fascism at the macro level and the unconscious at the micro level in these descriptions. However, according to Freud, there are potent remedies against these destructive processes of the masses: continuity, tradition, institutions and structures, in other words, law and order or, more topically, 'checks and balances' of a symbolic framework.

Freud wonders what holds a crowd together, even against common, objective interests. His answer: love, to be understood as a libidinal investment between group members. In English, you have *a* mob and *the* mob. The authors Freud consulted talked mainly about spontaneous crowds (a mob) that are volatile, like a lynch mob. He delves into artificial masses such as the church and army (the mob). These have an elaborate structure headed by a leader believed to love all members, making them equals. Bonding with the ruling opinion or the opinion of those who rule is a prerequisite for bonding among themselves. Love focuses inward, lovelessness (to even hatred) outward.[16] The danger of a Holy War is evident here.

Freud tried to understand the state of mind of the masses psycho-analytically. He points to the much-described phenomenon of 'contagion' in groups. He relates this to suggestion, and through analogies with infatuation and hypnosis, he concludes that a primitive mass can be defined as a collection of individuals who choose the same object (a person or idea) as their Ego-ideal and identify with each other in their Ego. Through this double bond consisting of a horizontal identification with each other and a vertical identification with the leader (as the incarnate ideal), he believes the mass phenomena, as mentioned above, can then be explained. They are processes that threaten the independent and mature functioning of the participants in every group to a greater or lesser extent.

3 Bion's Group

Bion also devoted many psychoanalytic reflections to group dynamics and, together with Wolf, Salvson and Foulkes, may be considered one of the pioneers of psychoanalytic group therapy. Unlike Freud, he indeed *worked* in and with groups.[17] Therefore, he could write a book entitled *Experiences in Groups*.[18] He described the group from the inside and argued that the emotional storm that can sometimes arise between analysant and analyst becomes an emotional whirlwind in groups. Bion dealt with the group like an analyst deals with his analysant and, in other words, left the leader's place *vacant*. Such unstructured groups were found to be hardly capable of achieving their goals because of intense emotions that determined the group's functioning but were not recognised as such by the members. He observed that the group developed group transferences characterised by unspoken and unconscious assumptions. In doing so, he distinguished three variants of assumption regarding the nature of the group, its leader and its task: the dependent, the fight-flight and the pairing group. He considered these basic assumptions (BA) as regressive transference resistances of the group with the typical characteristics of splitting and projective identification,[19] loss of individual distinction, diminished reality testing and reduced belief in possible progress through work and suffering.

A balance between the working group and basic assumption culture characterises every concrete group. The more predominant the former, the more rationally and maturely the group strives to fulfil its task as effectively as possible. It then consists of mutually separated, unique individuals, each working together from their own personality and/or discipline and/or expertise and contributing to the conscious, rational task of the group. They do not let their positive or negative emotions interfere with this. The leader is also chosen not for their charisma but for their competence. For example, the task may be insight-giving treatment of patients (for the team as a group) or free association to gain insight into their problems (for the patients as a group). Members tackle this conscious task, considering their abilities and limitations and mutual differences of opinion and others. They explore internal and external realities as realistically and truthfully as possible. This workgroup culture is never a permanently acquired fact. It is always compromised by disruptive factors inside and outside the group.[20] The danger of emotional regression to basic assumptions is always lurking around the corner, with the group more concerned with itself (namely, defending itself against its anxieties) than with its task in external reality.

Bion distilled three unconscious and regressive basic assumptions that undermine rational group functioning. In the absence of a father, the group *dreams* of a leader. Either to go to war against a common enemy, or to be led to some Promised Land, or in the form of a couple expected to bring some Messiah into the world. Especially in the most primitive schizoid-paranoid or *fight-flight* group, a leader is often 'chosen' who conforms to the *dark triad* that characterises so-called 'strong men'.[21] Like (for example) Putin, Erdogan, Bolsonaro, Duterte or Trump, they embody a cocktail of narcissism, psychopathy and Machiavellianism and sooner or later, the group becomes the victim of their character pathology.[22] It is essential in clinical psychotherapy to (be able to) recognise these phenomena. It comes down to problematising this regression and especially to getting the various members of the group to (re)adopt their separate positions. After all, a working group culture is characterised by no more or less than members doing their (in this case, psychoanalytic) work.

4 Psychoanalysis in the Group

What this work implies touches on the ideological debate[23] within psychoanalytic group psychotherapy. There is a camp of those who do psychoanalysis *in* the group.[24] As in the cure, this involves the particularity of the subject and their life history being analysed. The group setting only leads to other emphases, such as a more prominent role of (multilateral) transference and enactment at the expense of the dream as the royal road to the unconscious. Additional assets are therapeutic factors specific to (almost any) group work. The other camp focuses instead on the communication matrix of the group, adopting a particular group-analytic frame of reference.[25] Our clinical psychotherapy explicitly situates itself in the first 'camp'. Speaking about or addressing *the* group, we regard it as merely imaginary.[26] With a nod to a well-known Lacan slogan: THE group does not exist.

Working in/with groups, on the other hand, implies many specific therapeutic factors.[27] The early pioneers of group psychotherapy already mentioned them. In a military hospital in New York, Wolf observed that patients identified with each other in groups. A mutual sympathy and understanding spontaneously developed.[28] In 1938, he began working psychoanalytically with groups, and he is the founder of group psychoanalysis. The primary objective is becoming a subject, (re)constructing one's life history and detecting repetitive patterns. The English pioneer Foulkes started group psy-chotherapy in 1940, and he, too, retained several specific therapeutic fac-tors.[29] The patient comes out of isolation and enters a situation where he feels adequate. He can express himself freely and is on an equal footing with the other group members. The group provides an opportunity for mirror reactions,[30] where people can recognise morbid thoughts, feelings or impulses in each other, mitigating feelings of shame and guilt. Repression is more easily noticed in the other person, and projective mechanisms open up the possibi-lity of recognising the repressed in oneself. What is discussed in the group is also not without therapeutic effect on the other group members, even if they only (seem to) listen.[31]

Following a visit to England and his introduction to the group experiences of (then unknown) Bion and Rickman, Lacan[32] stressed the importance of horizontal identifications and the relevance of transference phenomena within the group. The group provides an opportunity to develop relation-ships with peers and parent/authority figures. At the same time, both brother–sister and mother–father transferences can be established and ana-lysed, and these multiple transferences are the main asset of psychoanalysis in the group.[33] More generally, patients who have benefited from group therapy themselves report some things as therapeutically effective. For instance, insight, learning from each other and a feeling of belonging are experienced as critical healing factors. In the group, catharsis occurs, group work provides an opportunity to mean something to others, the loneliness of psychological suffering is alleviated, and the dimension of hope takes root. All this occurs in and is peculiar to each form of group work.[34]

While many patients initially shy away from group psychotherapy because of all kinds of anxieties, resistances and prejudices, inpatients are *forced* to come into contact with various forms of group work and experience its advantages first-hand. In group psychoanalysis, all topics (including the most shameful and guilt-ridden) can be discussed, and here, too (as in the cure), the only resistance is ultimately that of the therapist! Finally, working with groups allows for homogeneous and/or specialised help. It can lead to a specific treatment program, e.g. for young drug users, trauma patients, bor-derline patients, adolescent problems, etc. Group work installs a therapeutic environment and can also fit better (than individual forms of treatment) in a broader milieu therapy setting. Finally, given the scarcity of human resources and specialised *know-how,* group treatment is also an economic advantage. In this way, a structured therapy program can be provided for many more patients within the same time frame.

Besides the already mentioned authors, our group psychotherapy model is most inspired by more recent analysts like René Kaës, Claudio Neri, Robert Hinshelwood, Didier Anzieu and, in the Dutch language area, Tom Berk.[35] Kaës and Neri[36] hail the thinking-together and the field that emerges as a kind of analytical third within the group. This thinking-together ('*co-pensée*')[37] can be an intense and satisfying experience, with a playful alternation of giving to each other and receiving from each other. When group members are thus involved in each other's inner world and can contribute to each other's evolution, a sense of being capable of good things grows, which benefits self-esteem. Hinshelwood describes how the group can be a fragile, rigid or flexible container.[38] The former involves a group that cannot bear the tensions, fears, overwhelming emotions, and fragments. In a rigid group, no emotional resonance occurs, group members remain isolated with their preoccupations, and no links are established. For a group to be therapeutic, it must function as a flexible container. This means there is an emotional commitment of group members to each other and a culture to reflect on these relationships.

As a psychoanalyst, I agree best with French psychoanalyst Didier Anzieu, who talks about the group illusion or the group as a fantasy of its members. This also concurs with Michel Thys.[39] He talks about the *group as a hole* (without w): a hole through which we fear being sucked in, but also an emptiness that yearns to be filled by us or, perhaps better: plugged. It ties in with the group as *Gestalt* of the archaic mother from whom we expect understanding and assistance on the one hand but by whom we are in danger of being eaten up. Unless the father stops this with his phallus because the laws and limits he imposes are prohibitive and protective.

I can also broadly identify with Tom Berk's work on psychoanalytic group therapy. Still, I propagate some fundamentally different accents, which differ according to the principles and finality of our practice.[40] For instance, it is primarily about psychoanalysis *in* and not *of* the group.[41] For the group, I do not pursue a good rapport between patients. Negative feelings should be analysed and not avoided. Nor do I let genetic factors rest at all. I would say on the contrary. It is always the same song with everyone; what is repeated must be remembered and worked through.[42] Above all, the basic rule remains. Free association and free discussion are different. The former is a *special*, the latter a *social* rule. After all, the analyst's desire involves a psychoanalytic process in each individual's mind. What I have in mind here is not so much the interpersonal as the intrapsychic, and not the similarity or mirroring, but what makes a difference.

5 Live on Stage

I need to talk about transference and countertransference to recognise how much content comes alive on stage in group therapy. Broadly understood, it is about the emotional reactions the patient triggers. Heinrich Racker distinguishes a concordant from a complementary countertransference.[43] In concordant countertransference, there is empathy or identification with the patient's subjective self-experience of that moment. For example, the therapist goes out of their way to help and understand the patient, but is destroyed each time, just as the patient used to be knocked down again and again by a parent despite great efforts. Here, the therapist feels what the patient themself is experiencing (consciously or unconsciously). In complementary countertransference, the therapist is forced to identify not with a self-representation but with an internal object in the patient. The therapist is soloed with that internal object because the patient cannot bear it themself and so 'evacuates' the object. For instance, the therapist catches themself reacting coolly and detachedly to the patient's emotional expressions. They recognise themself as a narcissistic mother who does not take her child's needs seriously or even ridicules them. Or they aggressively reprimand patient A, to the visible delight of patient B, who had outsourced their homicidal *sibling* rivalry to the therapist through projective identification.

For Freud, countertransference was an adverse phenomenon. He understood it simply as the counterpart of the patient's transference. After all, the therapist, too, has transference reactions of which they can be or become more or less aware.[44] Lacan, too, finds countertransference a difficulty.[44] For him, counter-transference is a form of resistance from the therapist. He defines counter-transference as the totality of prejudices, passions, inhibitions and limited knowledge or information due to the analyst at a given point in the therapeutic process. Post-Kleinians, in particular, came to regard countertransference as an essential tool. It comes to be closely related to projective identification. It is a difficult concept that has undergone quite some evolution. For instance, projec-tive identification evolved from a pathological defence mechanism in Melanie Klein to a regular form of non-verbal communication. From an attempt to rid oneself of unbearable content to a way of making emotional contact and, finally, from an intrapsychic to an interpersonal phenomenon.[45]

The starting point for this evolution was Wilfred Bion, who explicitly dis-tinguished between normal and pathological projective identification.[46] According to him, an average degree of projective identification forms a foundation for mental development. It is the earliest form of empathy; it lays the foundation for symbol formation and the development of the self and object relations.[47] Thomas Ogden even promotes projective identification *via regia* to psychological change.[48] From nothing is sicker to nothing is heal-thier than projective identification![49] A great confusion between subject and object usually accompanies projective identification. Hence, there is a dis-tinction between projection and projective identification. In projection, the subject feels alienated from and out of touch with the object; thus, there is a psychological distance between the two. In projective identification, on the other hand, the subject feels closely connected to the object and wants to maintain a link with it through omnipotent control.[50]

6 Via Regia

Projection is pure evacuation. Projective identification is also communication instead of a temporary deposit or delegation. Projecting on someone remains superficial; on the outside, the object can easily brush it off, and it doesn't *enter*; projective identification as projecting *into* someone goes deeper, really settles in the other person who can't just shake it off.[51] The patient wants a specific object relationship confirmed or actualised in the therapeutic interaction.[52] They exert emotional pressure on the therapist to play the corresponding role. Each group member who appears on the group stage carries their script, their unconscious scenario, formed throughout their life history. It consists of fantasies about themselves, the others and all their interrelationships. Everyone experiences the group situation from their inner world and will also behave accordingly. Unconsciously, the patient sometimes also tries to seduce or manipulate others to play specific roles. Thus, in group therapy, the inner group comes *live on stage*.

It is very original that Joseph Say[53] introduces an alternative term for a dilated form of projective identification. He calls it 'projective recruitment', which is especially common in group psychotherapy. It retains the idea of an active process of denial, dispossession and externalisation in the social environment. The mechanism originates in the subject, but they recruit the other to embody and interpret this split-off piece. This is not done haphazardly, but the other is, as it were, typecast. They possess pre-existing attributes that are not created but *accentuated* by projective identification.

With the life history and resulting object relations in mind, I am relentlessly alert to detect repetitions in the group. Transference reactions towards the therapist, fellow group members and the group as a whole allow a vivisection of feelings and sensitivities or – in the case of trauma – of triggers and hypersensitivities and their defence against them. In a constant back and forth, current experiences are interpreted and related to older and/or deeper patterns. Former president of the *International Psychoanalytical Association* Horacio Etchegoyen, in his standard work on the foundations of psychoanalytic technique, defines the psychoanalytic method in one sentence: psychoanalysis is a method that recognises the past in the present and distinguishes them through interpretation.[54] This psychoanalytic work is possible in group and individual psychotherapy. However, the Via Regia to the unconscious in the group is not the dream. The royal road is that of transference and countertransference. It is always to be interpreted only within the context of the therapy and the history of those participating in it.

Notes

1 Group psychology is primarily studied by social psychology and contains a veritable library of publications from that angle alone. The approach adopted here is psychoanalytic and psychotherapeutic, which does not prevent a lot of common ground with now almost classical findings on the often problematic impact of the group. Think of the banality of evil (Arendt, 1963), the so-called *groupthink* (Janis, 1972), the *bystander effect* (Latané & Darley, 1970) or the experiments that have also become so well-known on the broader population, such as Stanley

Milgram's *Obedience to authority* experiment (1974) or Philip Zimbardo's *Stanford Prison Experiment* (1971/2007).

2 See also the voiceover accompanying the opening images of the feature film *Mystic River* (2003): 'I always think that things you don't choose make you who you are. Your city, your neighbourhood, your family…'

3 Daniel Farberman (1985).

4 Pierre Bourdieu (1989).

5 John Ackrill (1994).

6 Mark Kinet (2019).

7 For an overview of the therapeutic factors specific to group work, see Bloch & Crouch (1985).

8 Types of work include group psychotherapy, occupational therapy, creative workshops, movement therapy, etc.

9 Patient–staff or community meetings where treatment culture is discussed with all patients and all team members present (1–2x/w).

10 Sigmund Freud (1912–1913).

11 Which were disputed by later authors without necessarily detracting from the psychic reality of the myth.

12 In current (biological-ethological) terminology, this involves the so-called alpha male.

13 According to Jongerius and Eyckman (1993), the large group exerts a strong regressive suction and participating in it isn't very comforting because it cannot be grasped. If in the small group, it is sometimes difficult to *feel*; in such large groups, it is rather challenging to *think*, cf. Hartman (1982) and cf. Bion's schizoid-paranoid *fight-flight* group further.

14 Sigmund Freud (1921).

15 Sigmund Freud (1923a).

16 Sigmund Freud (1921 p 252).

17 Along with John Rickman and others at Northfield military hospital (GB).

18 Wilfred Bion (1961).

19 It also confirms the almost systematic occurrence of primitive defence mechanisms such as splitting and projective identification, especially in large groups; for example, Winner & Ornstein (1994) and Robert H. Klein & Serena Lynn-Brown (1987).

20 The individual may also regress to being preoccupied with and defending themself against inner fears and/or conflicts due to a disturbing factor and thus start functioning less well in external reality.

21 Nai & Toros (2020).

22 *Groupthink* (Janis, 1972) reduces judgement. In the company of idiots, we become idiots along with them. Freud's urban and contemporary Karl Kraus: 'The secret of the demagogue is to make himself as stupid as his audience, so they believe they are as clever as he.' in Manfred Kets de Vries (2021).

23 A quote from Durkin (1964).

24 As the founders, we refer to Wolf & Schwartz (1962).

25 Sigmund Foulkes (1964), Foulkes & Anthony (1983).

26 To be compared with the '*alters*' of multiple personalities, i.e. dissociative and thus imaginary as well as defensive formations against the real of drive and trauma and (symbolic) historiography. The more the therapist goes along with this imaginary formation the more it multiplies. Analysis of its defensive function is, therefore, the message.

27 They have already been extensively documented and objectified; see, for example, Bloch & Crouch (1985).

28 Wolf & Schwartz (1962 p 2).
29 Sigmund Foulkes (1964 p 33–34).
30 Malcolm Pines (1984). The group member relates to the group as the baby relates to the (archaic) mother. It is the register of the imaginary with its illusions of equality, (h)recognition and understanding: a source of protection and resistance.
31 Given the importance currently attached to reflective functioning (Fonagy) and mentalisation (Bion), the added value of group psychotherapy is also evident here: the patient can, as it were, look into the heads of their fellow group members and is also 'fed' by their mentalisation.
32 Jacques Lacan (1947).
33 Wolf et al. (1993 p 4).
34 Irwin Yalom (1970), Jongerius and Eyckman (1993) and Sigrell (1992).
35 Berk is not the only one, but it is the most important for me. Wilfred Bion (1961), Sigmund Foulkes (1964, 1967), Didier Anzieu (1975), René Kaës (1994, 2000, 2004), Claudio Neri (1997), Robert Hinshelwood (1987) Tom Berk (2005).
36 Claudio Neri (2009).
37 René Kaës (1994).
38 Robert Hinshelwood (2005).
39 Michel Thys (2009).
40 Tom Berk 2005 p 185ff, Kinet (2009, 2011).
41 See also Wolf et al. (1993).
42 Sigmund Freud (1914c).
43 Heinz Racker (1957).
44 Jacques Lacan (1952).
45 In this discussion, I follow the line of thinking of Thys (2015).
46 Wilfred Bion (1959 p. 103).
47 Malin & Grotstein (1966).
48 Thomas Ogden (2002).
49 Quoting Michel Thys (ibid.).
50 Thomas Ogden (2012 p 278, 296).
51 Brown (2011 p 50–52).
52 Joseph Sandler (1987 p 43).
53 Joseph Say (2011).
54 Horacio Etchegoyen (1999 p 112).

Chapter 11

Clinical Psychotherapy

An Attempt at Integration

1 Complexity Trumps

We can distinguish several major 'classes' within adult psychiatry. There are the (classical and major) psychotic disorders and mood disorders, the disorders related to substance abuse or dependence, the (neurotic) depressive and anxiety disorders and personality disorders. The 'distinction' between these disorders is highly relative.[1] First and foremost, this has to do with the already denounced overvaluation of the DSM classification, in which diagnoses are reified as if they were referring directly to a natural order.[2] However, thirty-eight per cent of people who have a 'mental disorder' at some point in their lives have so-called co-morbidity.[3] In patients requiring residential treatment, psychopathology rarely even occurs in a 'pure' form. The orthogonal distinction between syndromal and personality diagnoses does not exist in practice. About sixty per cent of psychiatric and addiction problems involve at least one full-blooded personality disorder.[4] The prevalence of personality disorders in the general population is 15–20 per cent. This makes them (along with anxiety and depression) among the most common mental disorders. Considering the subclinical severity of many syndromal and personality pathologies, we can say that diagnostic alloys are ubiquitous.

The previous chapters discussed the always complex and multifactorial pathogenesis[5] that characterises psychiatric disorders. In the genesis of all psychopathology, there is always an intertwining of predisposition and drive, attachment to and relationship with first meaningful others, and ever private and subjective life history. The conclusion is simple: complex causation = complex treatment. The fundamental inadequacy of a unilateral therapeutic approach in psychiatric disorders may by now have been sufficiently demonstrated. The consistently severe and/or recurrent problems that lead to residential treatment require, *a fortiori*, psychiatric and psychotherapeutic treatment that acts either simultaneously or consecutively on these divergent points of intervention. We particularly want to emphasise this because the bio-psycho-social model (which has also been making its presence felt in medicine for a few decades now), while receiving much lip service, has not

DOI: 10.4324/9781032698052-14

yet penetrated the mental health system nearly enough. Moreover, since the unconscious only exists for those who listen to it,[6] many do not consider its peculiar laws. When asked where much psychopathology comes from and even more so what it means, the answer – paraphrasing President Bill Clinton – should be: 'It is the unconscious, stupid!'

2 Risks

Indeed, often, the response to psychological suffering is far too short-sighted. An overly symptom-oriented treatment risks covering up the importance of the subject and their life history. Such an approach also neglects the decisive role of attachment (which is recorded in implicit memory and, as a primary transference, determines our relationship with others). The possibility of discovering the deeper determinants of psychological and interpersonal problems and working with increased awareness is lost in the process. As a result, relapse often occurs after temporary improvement, with all its discouraging or actual implications, both for the person concerned and for their environment. Every crisis or problem carries the seeds of growth and insight within it. However, medical/psychological knowledge under which the subject disappears makes harnessing this progressive potential difficult or impossible. 'I have endogenous depression', 'I have chronic fatigue syndrome' or 'I am a borderline' too often means the end of the story.

However, an overly one-sided psychoanalytic approach also has its pitfalls. It can, for instance, misunderstand or deny the causality of the Real (disposition and drive) and neglect the role that a medical-psychiatric intervention has to play in this matter. For a long time, the prescription of psychopharmaceuticals was considered incompatible with a psychoanalytic process.[7] However, a major mood disorder may be denied in its constitutional determination, depriving the patient needlessly of effective help (e.g. antidepressants, mood stabilisers) with more or less catastrophic consequences. A person can lose themselves in substance abuse or addiction without a necessary directive intervention, breaking the cycle that is evolving into a vortex. A more contemporary example is autism spectrum disorder. At the neurocognitive level, these patients' brains ('the computer') work in atypical ways. Like a grain of sand from the Real, it ensures that their mental engine runs square 24/7. Especially when this difficulty is not, or only belatedly, recognised, they have often silently put up with simultaneously invisible and misunderstood suffering for many years so that sooner or later, they become exhausted, if not develop burnout.[8]

3 Indications?

From too classical psychoanalytic views on indication, many patients also remain deprived of appropriate psychoanalytic treatment. The question is whether this or that patient is 'eligible' for a 'psychoanalytic' way of working. By 'psychoanalytic' is meant only that method which is characterised by a neutral and abstinent attitude on the part of the therapist,[9] who supports as little as possible and interprets as much as possible. For people with limited mentalising or introspective abilities (who therefore somatise and act out) or, more generally, the more severe personality disorders, a psychoanalytic approach understood in this way is not suitable. The result may be that treatment gives way to some 'counselling'. Helping patients in a supportive manner to function at an acceptable level and/or keeping them 'out of psychiatry' becomes objective number one. This type of patient does not achieve a more psychotherapeutically ambitious undertaking, which can only be provided within the caring and structuring holding and facilitating environment of the (semi-)residential setting. It is often necessary to put errant patients on a track that more fundamentally offers new perspectives. This is particularly the case with much more 'severe' psychiatric disorders and with patients with structural (as opposed to neurotic) psychopathology.[10]

It would lead us too far from the present scope to discuss individual psychoanalytic therapy's developments in detail. From the beginning of the psychoanalytic movement, there was a search for how to activate and/or shorten the analytic process. Indeed, Franz Alexander[11] pioneered this matter. From him also came the term 'corrective emotional experience'.[12] Peter Sifneos,[13] David Malan,[14] Habib Davanloo[15] and Edmond Gilliéron[16] developed their psychoanalytic forms of therapy theoretically and technically at the end of the last century. They all proceed face to face, continue at a lower frequency (once to twice a week) and are basically of shorter duration than the classical cure.[17] Sometimes, a particular focus, objective or deadline is set. We have already pointed out that the difference in the psychoanalytic process realised by such therapies can often only be determined afterwards. According to Kernberg,[18] psychoanalytic therapy is gradually evolving into the preferred treatment, even for neuroses, which were traditionally considered the indication for the typical cure. At the beginning of this century, more protocolised psychodynamic treatments also appeared, such as inter-personal dynamic therapy, transference-focused psychotherapy or mentalisation-based treatment.[19] Each manages to achieve demonstrably similar results to other forms of psychotherapy.[20]

While the psychoanalytic community sometimes maligns these therapy forms,[21] they have undoubtedly contributed to the survival and perceived relevance of psychoanalytic thought in psychiatry. More supportive but psychoanalytically understood forms of therapy have also significantly broadened their clinical applicability to less classical areas of indication.[22] That clinical psychotherapy as a form of applied psychoanalysis within the psychiatric hospital can offer a particularly effective treatment for a lot of 'troublesome folks'[23] with largely untreatable psychopathology seems to be a well-kept secret (known only to its practitioners)!

4 Sociotherapy and Milieu Therapy

In the early 1980s, there were already calls for promoting sociotherapy as *the* pre-eminent speciality of clinical psychiatry.[24] Sociotherapy was understood as providing a temporary, unnatural, artificial and, above all, sophisticated treatment environment for the patient. Sociotherapy is the methodical handling of the living environment within a functional unit for (semi-)residential treatment. In recent years, the term milieu therapy has mainly been used as a more modern, somewhat extended, and broader variant of the earlier term.[25] Janzing and Lansen[26] define milieu therapy as the methodical establishment of a stable, well-organised and well-connected social organisation. This organisation is characterised by an overall vision and integration of methods, techniques, means and attitudes which are interrelated to a particular therapeutic goal. For his part, Jongerius[27] defines environmental therapy as using all aspects of being hospitalised (living, working, leisure) in the context of the individual patient's treatment goal. It is the continuous attempt to arrange the three constituent elements of the environment (staff, buildings, organisational structure and living rules) so that the patient can benefit from them to achieve the goal he has set for themself.

What is stressed by all[28] is the importance of inner consistency and cohesion in the therapeutic environment that lends a frame of reference and structure to the interpersonal relationships offered to the patient. Developing an overall vision that acts as a guideline and consistently has its actual realisation in all concrete provisions is essential. In terms of objectives, two things recur time and again. The first objective is to control and limit pathological behaviour, and the second is the development of personality and/or skills.

Janzing and Lansen distinguish three types of milieu therapy. In supportive milieu therapy, a society is established within the department characterised by structure, flexibility and simple rules. Reconstructive milieu therapy is exploratory and often takes shape within a psychotherapeutic community. It is a treatment community where patients and staff work on severe psychopathology understood as an expression of (early childhood) life history. Psychopathology and symptomatology are considered to be rooted in the earliest stages of life (attachment, oral phase, separation-individuation phase and so on). In the social therapeutic milieu, the pathology is assumed to be situated in the social role and interaction. A strongly democratically structured micro-society is set up where there is room for 'normal' social intercourse and where social rules apply. It is assumed that personal growth and change come about through social learning.

5 Clinical Psychotherapy

Clinical psychotherapy is a well-defined form of 'milieu' therapy. It does not involve psychotherapy in the hospital ward (which could also be done on an outpatient basis or in the psychiatric ward of a general hospital) but psychotherapy *via* the hospital ward. The inpatient situation itself is structured psychotherapeutically. As such, it is offered only in certain psychiatric hospitals. Clinical psychotherapy must be distinguished from institutional psychotherapy ('*psychothérapie institutionelle*'), which is characterised by the installation of a psychoanalytic ethic in a psychiatric institution primarily concerned with treating psychosis.[29] The clinical psychotherapeutic milieu is characterised by clear boundary demarcations within treatment teams and between team and patients, steadfast working arrangements and the discovery of (transference) relationships between patients and caregivers and between patients. Psychotherapy is present in two guises: as a guiding principle for environmental structuring on the one hand and as a working type (alongside, for example, psychomotor therapy, creative therapy and so on) of the therapeutic programme on the other hand.

We can think of this environment as a place where, in an atmosphere of care, protection and 'shelter', people can work on their problems. A transitional space is created, which must be warm and safe enough for patients to expose themselves. After all, they must be able to loosen or remove their 'clothing' of usual defence mechanisms and play the therapeutic game in this (semi-)unclothed state.[30] This presupposes clear rules and chalk lines. Observing and monitoring this symbolic structure of laws, rules, norms and boundaries gives the interactions a meaning-giving frame of reference. It makes it possible to notice acting out/boundary violations in time and problematise them by discussing them individually, in a group and with the entire department. All this contributes to the 'holding/facilitating environment' and gives the patient (external) structure and grip. By analogy with the team members, the patient is an expertly unequal but ethically equivalent co-player in this therapeutic event. Participation and empowerment for all (patients and team) is the message.

The entire treatment milieu is teeming with rules, boundaries and laws. Acting out and transgressions (given the nature and severity of psychopathology) are central. Initially, they are listened to as a treasure trove of information from the unconscious. Only in case of insufficient results are limit-setting measures taken in this regard. The therapeutic programme is offered as (almost full-time) work and is intrinsically anti-regressive. We assume that the transferences and resistances occurring during this work will illuminate the subject's particularity and psychopathology. Again and again, we pose as employers and reflect on the difficulties, anxieties or resistance patients experience. Patients are asked to constantly mobilise the executive functions of their Ego (to expand or conserve their skills following the motto 'use it or lose it'). This has a very anti-regressive, supportive and structuring effect and provides the opportunity for reality confrontation.

The therapeutic programme is also composed of a balanced and varied menu. It consists of activities or therapies, which proceed methodically and with appropriate techniques within a framework (consisting of duration, frequency and working arrangements) monitored by the therapist's continuous and reliable presence. The care and diligence with which the therapeutic process and the framework are handled are essential to both the safety or holding provided and the opportunity for experimentation and change. There must be room for verbal and non-verbal activities (expressive and result-oriented, experience- and process-oriented). Both methods that use materials (e.g. art workshop) and those that use one's body/person (e.g. dance therapy) will find a place in the programme. Numerous moments are provided to open one's 'book', but equally to learn to close it again. Of further importance is a rhythmic, alternating programming of these various forms of activities and therapies. Depending on the specificity of the treatment group, the ratio of complementary components of the menu may be different. Also, what falls outside the therapeutic programme in the narrower sense (night duty, leisure time and so on) should, as far as possible, be able to occupy its own specific and thought-through place within the environment, striving for consistency, both towards the team and towards the patients.[31]

Psychoanalytically inspired clinical psychotherapy is almost extinct in the Netherlands but is still represented in about twenty places in Belgium. It is an intensive treatment in which the therapy programme is offered as a kind of work. People are thus confronted with difficulties or limitations. They are stumbling blocks to self-knowledge and a source of resistance of all kinds. However, unlike the therapist's resistance, their analysis contributes substantially to awareness. It can also increase the patient's reach or range in several areas of life.

6 The Team as Environment Mother

While 'classical' psychoanalytic work is mainly about free association, interpretation and working through patterns of repetition, more basic work must be done in clinical psychotherapy. This broadly involves establishing basic safety and trust, developing reflective functioning and mentalisation, and elaborating and integrating (inner) object relations. The psychiatric nurse plays a central role. Several dimensions can be discerned in it. They are the primary contact person, lay the foundation for (psycho)therapy, are a culture carrier and organisational pivot figure and (depending on the type of milieu therapy) set this or that 'technical' act.[32] They and the physical nurse have several functions in common. They are continuously present, approachable and have the polyvalence of a front-line worker. Nurturing and nursing refer to watching over and caring for vital functions such as eating, drinking, sleeping, etc. The patient should and can turn to the nurse with all their needs and demands. The nurse is the first intermediate station that decodes and filters the distress signals, tries to remedy the distress themself, and organises referrals in a focused and dosed manner if necessary. All this represents the dimension of primary care and contact. The nurse tries to provide this in a way that Bruno Bettelheim describes as 'not perfect but good enough'.[33]

The psychiatric nurse also contributes to the (psycho-) therapeutic basis.[34] In this context, we return to the concept of containment introduced by Bion. We proposed it as an ingredient of good mothering. The mother tries to recognise and respond to her child's needs and fears. She gives meaning to fears, limits them, and tries to contain, keep and tolerate destructive contents in particular. She may also be called a 'translation device'. While accommodating negative feelings, she remains 'good' and can endure and survive this attack. Through her understanding capacity, she is constitutive in constructing meaningful psychic content, and by tolerating unbearable feelings, she gives them communicative value and existence. Transposed to the therapeutic situation, containment means that all psychic contents are bearable, not destructive. Everything the patient says can be integrated, and what initially seemed indigestible can be made digestible with the help of a tolerant and understanding (m)other. We can also imagine the psychiatric nurse forming an envelope[35] around the patient and guarding them from (traumatic) overstimulation both inside and outside.

Translated concretely into clinical practice, the nurse must be able to handle the patient's anxiety and distress, to limit them and not be overwhelmed by them. The nurce can think about them in an attempt to 'mentalise' them. All this must allow the destructive spiral of acting out and re-acting-out to be avoided and help keep problems negotiable and workable. The psychiatric nurse is the therapeutic milieu's pivotal figure and culture carrier. They thus play a crucial role in the organisation, which they embody to a large extent. Depending on the type of therapeutic milieu, additional, more technically coloured interventions will graft themselves onto these basic functions. These are the socio-therapeutic interventions appropriate within one's treatment philosophy. These can occur within an individual contact, during a group or ward meeting, and be reconstructive, supportive or socio-therapeutic.

Clinical psychotherapy requires a closely-knit, well-integrated, multi-disciplinary team within which sustained reflection and open communication are possible. Within this team, there is a culture of participatory reflection characterised by expertise inequality (the occupational therapist has different expertise from the psychiatric nurse) and ethical equivalence (everyone has the same right to speak). Besides being prepared and able to think together and feel together, it is also necessary to be together and do together. This requires the necessary guidance and authority at several levels and areas. After all, psychoanalytic work and clinical psychotherapy is not a *laisser faire, laisser aller*. It touches on persistent misunderstandings related to a misunderstood non-directive attitude and neutrality attributed to psychoanalysis.

7 The Paternal Authority[36]

First of all, guidance is indeed needed in the psychoanalytic process. Not everything can or should be analysed. The focus should be on the unconscious formations: the symptom, the parapraxis, the dream (in group psychotherapy and clinical psychotherapy especially), the transference, and the patient's acting out or enactment. All kinds of things (e.g. affects and all kinds of 'hassles'/acting out) should ultimately be put into words as much as possible. Even the analyst's silence is not a sign of passivity but is (however paradoxically) of the order of the *act*. The only motive for silence is the analyst's desire that the 'truing' would occur.

In direct patient care in clinical psychotherapy, there is also a need for guidance, limit setting and support. The need for care and the ability to take up one's responsibility must constantly be assessed stage-specifically. The understanding we try to bring to this work's difficulties does not stand in the way of the imposition of rules (e.g., the ground rule of free association).[37] Technical neutrality is characterised by a most objective, committed attitude to the patient and their problems, a steadfast effort to help the patient clarify the nature of those problems and a position that maintains equal distance from the opposing forces at work in the patient's psyche. The analyst's frantic efforts to prevent the patient from knowing anything about their own personal life imply a striving towards misunderstood (and counterproductive) anonymity, leading to contrived, unnatural behaviour. In contrast, the analyst is supposed to behave as naturally as possible within the boundaries of their specific professional role. The position of a blank screen does not mean that the analyst's personality should remain invisible but, above all, implies a natural and authentic respect for the patient's freedom to come to their own decisions and choices.[38]

Furthermore, there is a strong need for milieu therapy leadership in clinical psychotherapy. On average, team members working in clinical psychotherapy settings are highly skilled and qualified. Moreover, the dimension of vocation comes into play. After all, their choice of profession and commitment is often based on personal motives rooted in their history and development. They put their heart and soul into their work. Kernberg[39] puts the following (ideal) requirements on this authority: high intelligence for strategic and conceptual thinking, personal and non-corrupt sincerity, capacity for deep object relations for realistic evaluation of employees, healthy narcissism (i.e. self-affirming rather than self-defeating) and lastly, prudence and responsible anticipatory paranoia. The willingness and ability to take maximum account of one's share adds to this. This willingness and ability are (evidently) essential for all mental health professionals.

Unceasingly, the manager(s) should monitor and facilitate the working group culture. Ditto for necessary basic capabilities that must be sufficiently present within the entire team, such as holding, containment and affect attunement.[40] They are overlapping ingredients of good-enough mothering,[41] besieged daily by destructive forces in the patients and the team. Important values within the environment are neutrality and abstinence on the one hand and tolerance, empathy and compassion on the other. Neutrality, as mentioned, is not absolute: we are on the side of life, not death, of construction and not destruction, of truth and not lies. On the other hand, we will suspend our personal opinions and views as much as possible to allow patients to make their own ethical choices. Abstinence is also not constipation. It is not depriving the patient of any expression of commitment but rather a sustained respect for the limits inherent in our professional role. Tolerance is needed to bear and endure. It should not be confused with the permissiveness of 'anything goes'. After all, understanding does not imply permitting. While boundaries are constantly set, boundary violations are treated primarily therapeutically and not repressively. Empathy is a necessary condition for the proper recognition of psychological suffering and is the nonspecific psychotherapeutic factor par excellence. Compassion implies a willingness to undertake the inevitably long, arduous and painful (transference-countertransference) labour of the psychotherapeutic process.

8 Psychoanalytic?

In clinical psychotherapy, transference,[42] enactment and acting out are the gateways of choice for analysing what is going on in the unconscious. Patients tend to repeat what they have made of their first relationships with significant others. A typical question asked within a psychoanalytic treatment philosophy is what the patient does to us and induces in us. Here, we make interpretive and mentalising use of our feelings, thoughts and behaviour generated by the encounter with the patient. The question is how the inner state of the patient and therapist can explain the event or hassle in the here and now.[43] Clinical psychotherapy is a highly effective form of psychotherapy for classic non-analysable psychopathology. Patients who tend to evacuate intolerable contents through substance abuse or acting-out behaviour, who need additional help and support due to the severity of their psychiatric symptomatology or whose problems must be understood as a deep-seated developmental disorder need a temporary 'holding environment' that can provide them with the necessary care in a dosed manner. Clinical psychotherapy is also particularly effective for complex neurotic problems. In outpatient psychotherapy, the patient is never so intensely engaged with themselves and with their inner world. They are too distracted by the external reality of everyday life for that. Moreover, getting to the point after the latest news is not always easy. Full-time engagement in clinical psychotherapy offers a much more intense immersion in one's inner world. Ego-syntonic[44] personality elements can more easily be 'promoted' to symptom status and thus made accessible for analysis.

The entire inner and psychic reality gradually unfolds within the clinical psychotherapeutic milieu. This psychic reality becomes almost omnipresent in clinical psychotherapy, with the various team members within their therapy or activity as its privileged witnesses. The (early) childhood constantly reproduces itself in the living reality of clinical ward life. Pathogenetic constellations from the past come alive on stage. The clinical psychotherapeutic environment becomes a theatre of inner objects. Using this as a treasure trove of information from the unconscious is the unsurpassed power of (semi)residential psychoanalytic work. It often opens a unique avenue of access to the realm of the unconscious and the primal repression from the first years of life. Indeed, it provides us with circumstantial evidence based on which we can (re)construct prehistory and patients' first relationship to the big Other. Various traumatic constellations can also come on stage and become available for psychoanalytic research.

Given the above, clinical psychotherapy can be understood as the (re-) construction of transferential experiences congruent with the inner patterns/ scenarios of object relations.[45] We refer to Klein's concept of 'memories in feeling'. Provided with the necessary mentalisation, change occurs through implicit/procedural rather than explicit/autobiographical memory.[46] Not so much what the patient *declares,* but how they *are* in the transference provides information about their psychic reality. Only in this way can we access the very earliest childhood. It was a (primal) time when we were (protected to a greater or lesser extent by a stimulus barrier, a container, a skin ego or *arrière-mère*) at the mercy of structural (the drive) and/or accidental (e.g. sexual abuse) trauma.

In a broad definition, clinical psychotherapy can be designed to treat a whole range of psychiatric problems.[47] However, the perspective used here is that of clinical psychotherapy as a form of (semi-)residential psychoanalytic programme for an intertwined set of anxiety, mood and personality disorders.[48] In developing this clinical psychotherapeutic milieu, the starting point was not which patients qualified for our way of working. Instead, the question was and is how we should set up our clinical psychotherapy to get patients with such a wide variety of psychopathology to work psychotherapeutically and psychoanalytically.

The binding and guiding principles are not only the clinical psychotherapy methods and techniques described so far.[49] The integrating principle was foremost a psychoanalytic ethic.[50] Our aim is not merely symptomatic improvement or syndromic clearance. We also, and above all, wish to offer developmental help employing constructive psychotherapy in cases of actual pathology and the defect model (e.g. in borderline and trauma patients). In the psychopathology that corresponds to the conflict model, we aim to offer a lived insight into the psychogenesis and psychodynamics of psychological suffering/dysfunction through reconstructive psychotherapy. Ultimately, we want to bring patients to the point where they can make conscious and personal ethical choices. For example, what does being a husband, wife, father, or mother mean to me? We try to bring these patients to the position of absolute difference. Concerning love and sexuality, law and authority, lack and death, some are on the lookout for a conventional answer; others succeed in creating some invention.[51]

9 Psychotherapy and Pharmacotherapy

A psychoanalytic process is initiated in various patients beyond psychiatric and psychotherapeutic care, often well beyond the (semi-)residential treatment episode(s). This psychoanalytic treatment philosophy does not prevent the most judicious use of the entire arsenal of psychiatry and psychotherapy. The combination of psychotherapy and pharmacotherapy is the rule. Exceptionally, on the indication, behavioural therapy,[52] relationship or family counselling or therapy[53] are added to the psychoanalytic approach. However, this is done so that means and methods remain coherent and convergent to the abovementioned psychoanalytic goal. Pharmacotherapy, in particular, can be seen in this perspective as framing a broader psychotherapeutic event. The word 'framing' should be understood as 'establishing the conditions within which psychotherapy can be possible and effective'.[54] This is very different from pharmacotherapy, seen as a *passe-partout*: a key that fits all the locks.

Pharmacotherapy primarily focuses on the syndromic disorder. In this case, efforts are made to keep prescribing simply and unambiguously, whereby the pharmacy can come to serve the word and not the word to serve the pharmacy. This medication policy generally remains maximally constant, except in cases requiring adjustments. As a matter of principle, this is done as much as possible within the team consultation to minimise the (counter-transference) reaction requiring a change in prescribing behaviour. We can call this classic psychiatric pharmacotherapy, and in major psychiatric disorders, it is always a *sine qua non* for further inpatient or outpatient psychotherapy.

For dysthymic, anxiety or other neurotic symptomatology, the disabling nature and/or the burden of suffering will determine the drug recipe. Indeed, when these symptoms have too high a volume, they can no longer be considered significant by the patient and lose their indicative value in the psychotherapeutic process.[55] In this view, pharmacotherapy is sometimes a necessary and temporary adjuvant to psychotherapy. Especially in the case of personality disorders, the psychopathology may be so disruptive (we think of fugues, (auto)destructive acting out and so on) that the establishment or maintenance of a therapeutic alliance is threatened. In that case, pharmacotherapy can be part of attempts at limit-setting. In both the latter cases, we could speak of psychodynamic pharmacotherapy. Psychopharmaceuticals do not focus on pathology but are used to respond to discordant psychological functions or forces. This is in line with the views of Hungarian analyst

Leopold Szondi,[56] in which psychopathology is seen to be related to a conglomerate of 'vectors' and drives. For instance, contact, paroxysmal phenomena, mood, drive, reality testing, etc., can be modulated by psychopharmaceuticals in their various sub-profiles.

This psychodynamic pharmacotherapy can ideally be realised in a measured way within a (semi-)residential psychoanalytic psychotherapeutic treatment. The pervasiveness of complex psychopathology, in which there is a coexistence of major psychiatric disorders and more neurotic or personality disorders, requires rational pharmacotherapy.[57] It should be based on current biological psychiatric insights in the case of psychiatric pharmacotherapy and a thoughtful and deliberate psychotherapeutic strategy in the case of psychodynamic pharmacotherapy.[58] For instance, it should not be prompted by the urge to immediately evacuate the patient's or therapist's unbearable feelings.

10 Psychopathology

Regarding pathogenesis, we have repeatedly referred to the two poles of the defect model and the conflict model, between which there is a continuum. To what extent has the alignment and mirroring of the first significant others (the Other) been able to provide an answer to the Real ('*l(a) cause*') of disposition and drive? To what extent have an Ego, a self, secure attachment and a mentalising capacity developed in the process? Diagnostically, this corresponds to the contrast between mental process disorders and mental representational disorders,[59] as well as between actual pathology and psychopathology.[60]

At the psychotherapeutic level, the corresponding poles for 'treatment needs' in the first category are support, construction/subject amplification, holding and containment. Insight, reconstruction/interpretation, and frustration are critical in the second category. The unconscious manifests itself, on the one hand, mainly under the form of transference and *enactment* and on the other via free association and dream production. The attitude of the psychoanalytic psychotherapist should be sufficiently elastic in the first regard and inflexible in the second. The setting will (have to) be (semi)residential rather than ambulatory to enable the analytic process in some and bring it to fruition in others. We refer in this context to a statement by Hinshelwood, who pertinently and succinctly summarises the indications for the various forms of inpatient psychotherapy as follows: 'Mental health institutes exist for people who cannot contain themselves'.[61]

To make the whole of this situating of psychopathology and psychotherapy clear and understandable, we place it all in Table 11.1.

The psychopathology we treat within our clinical psychotherapeutic milieu mainly responds to the characteristics described in the central column. Syndromally, it primarily consists of dysthymic disorders and anxiety disorders

Table 11.1 Situating of psychopathology and psychotherapy

	Actual Pathology	*Psychopathology*
Pathogenesis	Defect model Real Symbolic hypotrophy	Conflict model Symbolic-Imaginary Symbolic hypertrophy
Diagnosis	Mental process disorders Actual pathology Structural pathology	Mental representational disorders Psychopathology Neurotic pathology
Psychotherapy	Support Construction & subject-amplification Holding and containment	Insight Reconstruction and interpretation Frustration
Psychoanalysis	Transference and enactment Elasticity (Semi-)residential	Free association and dream Inflexibility Ambulatory

(especially free-floating anxiety and post-traumatic stress disorders). However, this symptomatology is primarily considered an epiphenomenon of the more severe and complex personality disorders, which we, therefore, prioritise as the principal diagnosis.[62] Dysthymic disorders involve (possibly worsening episodically to major depressive proportions) chronically depressive symptoms.[63] Usually, they have already led to various stages of mental health care, which, however, have remained without lasting results or in which the condition has progressed from bad to worse and is accompanied by increasing psychosocial deterioration and/or suicidal tendencies. Such depressions are, of course, treated *lege artis* with pharmacotherapy but are mainly the focus of a broader clinical psychotherapeutic project.

First of all, all intrapsychic and interpersonal difficulties invisibly drain much energy from psychism and, to a greater or lesser extent, lead to 'depressive' symptoms such as apathy, lethargy and loss of interest. Lingering unconscious feelings of guilt related to forbidden aggressive and/or sexual impulses are almost always present. The depressive mood is often also the result of (narcissistic) disorders in the regulation of self-esteem. Finally, often at play is a misunderstood early childhood depression that remained hidden for a long time under the hypomanic and/or hyperactive character defence of a False Self. Sooner or later, it led to a massive and therapy-resistant depressive decompensation that struck like a bolt in the blue to the person and/or his environment. Short-term and/or symptom-oriented treatments were invariably perceived by these patients as lacking holding and containment and thus as disastrous repetition of past rejection and/or misunderstanding and/or abandonment. The ultimate reason and existence of this type of depression must first and foremost be recognised because it is usually rooted in (early) childhood development marked by severe deficits and/or trauma. It can often only be remedied through (deep enough) regression within a caring mother environment. Unbound ('diabolic') death drive can result in stubborn (auto-) destructiveness that needs to be borne, contained and countered by a lot of life drive due to the team.[64] Anxiety disorders are also prominent in most patients, pointing to the disruptive influence that non-mentalised contents exert on psychism. Diagnostically, the vast majority of these anxiety disorders correspond to free-floating anxiety disorder and/or panic disorder, which can be considered actual pathology. If phobic and/or obsessive-compulsive psychopathology has developed out of this actual pathology, this sometimes requires additional symptom-oriented help following a behavioural therapeutic signature. After all, this symptomatology can make more or less 'normal' functioning completely impossible.

In terms of personality disorders,[65] we can add to the distinction between actual and psychopathology that between structural and neurotic pathology. In the former, the other is used as an auxiliary Ego, a self-object, or a narcissistic extension. The other continues to play a vital, indispensable and, precisely for that reason, frightening role in maintaining psychic equilibrium.[66] From an Ego-psychological and object-relational angle, we saw that Otto Kernberg[67] describes all this in terms of 'levels' of borderline and neurotic personality organisation. Sidney Blatt[68] has been engaged in clinical and scientific work on personality disorders and depression for 30 years. We saw that he distinguishes between anaclitic and introjective psychopathology. It is a dichotomy that can be added to the previous one and may partly parallel it. In anaclitic psychopathology, interpersonal issues of caring and connectedness are paramount. Separation and abandonment anxiety predominate, helplessness trumps, and there is a considerable need for supportive and nurturing contacts. Introjective psychopathology centres on issues of self-image, separateness and independence, often accompanied by a compelling perfectionism. The main concerns are self-esteem and self-doubt. Feelings of guilt and shame predominate. There is more hopelessness than helplessness. The distinction between these two poles of psychopathology described by Blatt[69] also guides the type of psychotherapy help by which they are best helped. Anaclitic psychopathology (at least initially) needs more care and support, while the introjective one has to be addressed through a more 'classical' insight-giving/interpretive approach.

11 Drive and Trauma

Post-traumatic stress disorder is by far the most common among anxiety disorders, as about half of our inpatients have experienced cumulative or complex trauma. Before dwelling on this trauma longer, we would like to point out that there is an essential overlap between traumatic neurosis and severe personality disorders.[70] Qua differential diagnosis, however, traumatic neurosis is more likely to involve splitting the self and consciousness ('dissociation').[71] Indeed, the danger is primarily external and invokes defence mechanisms with which a defenceless prey protects itself from the predator, such as *freezing* and *defeat*. Respectively, the subject defensively reduces itself to dead matter or (acts as if) it surrenders since it considers itself incapable of *fight* or *flight*. In severe personality disorders, the danger is more internal (predisposition and drive as 'structural trauma'). Then, splitting (all-good/all-bad) of the object and the relationship to this object is more likely to prevail…

Accidental trauma can be descriptively defined as an intense event to which the subject cannot react adequately, which causes distress and which can produce more or less long-lasting pathogenic effects. Clinically, it is always about something unspeakable, and economically, it is about an increase in stimuli that cannot be handled, to which the subject is passively and defencelessly exposed, distorting the inner homeostasis dramatically and unexpectedly. The impact of trauma is always definite because it will graft itself onto the patient's personal history and phantasm. *Grosso modo* its pathogenic impact is all the greater when a secure attachment is lacking.

In Freud's first theory, he attributed to trauma a central role in the pathogenesis of neuroses. The treatment consisted of recollecting specific (early) childhood traumas and the psychic elaboration and release of the corresponding blocked affects through catharsis. In the terminology we used, the Real was bound to the symbolic-imaginary by processes of mentalisation and symbolisation. On completing his *Neurotica,* Freud's conception of trauma shifts sharply. The incident becomes traumatic only because of the drive and phantasm activated by it. The aetiology of neurosis[72] is conceived more as a complementary series. The predisposition and primordial time plus infantile event(s) cause a libido fixation on which an incident can graft itself with pathogenic consequences. In this new view, trauma becomes pathogenic only at two moments in time. First, the child undergoes sexual 'seduction' passively and unpreparedly. Only in the second instance (mainly at the time of puberty) does this infantile event become traumatic. It does so '*nachträglich*', by deferred action, via afterwardsness.

Indeed, the child becomes 'aware' of the sexual/incestuous/violent character of the trauma only in a delayed relay. In this line of thought, the trauma becomes *a* rather than *the* decisive element in the pathogenesis. Indeed, Freud starts to pay more attention to the phantasmatic organisation around infantile sexual experiences. There are two possible evolutions. Either trauma 'triggers' the decompensation of a pre-existing neurotic structure, or the trauma triggers a traumatic neurosis in which this trauma plays a decisive role in symptomatology (dissociation, amnesia, alienation, avoidance, re-experiencing, nightmares and so on).[73] This symptomatology is interpreted as an attempt to process and bind unprocessed traumatic content psychologically. A characteristic is the sometimes traumatophilic-seeming repetition compulsion as an attempt at mastering. This can lead to an astonishing passive–active[74] reversal, which is incomprehensible for the person involved and those around him, whereby the 'victim' becomes a 'perpetrator', laden with violent feelings of shame and guilt.

Psychodynamic research on trauma and its treatment remains very scarce to date.[75] Co-morbidity with other problems is the rule. A shift from a dis-order-centred to a person-centred approach is also needed in this field.[76] Increasing convergence between psychodynamic and cognitive-behavioural approaches is taking place.[77] Both attribute a traumatic impact to the massive feelings of abandonment (anxiety, sadness and anger) in an unbearable situation because the mentalising ability is lacking. *Mutatis mutandis* psychotherapy focuses mainly on building/restoring secure attachment and mentalisation.[78] Judith Herman and Bessel van der Kolk are two international trauma authorities who have put complex PTSD and developmental traumatic disorders on the map, respectively.[79] They result from exposure to severe stressors of a repetitive or long-term nature that caused harm and/or were added to abandonment by caregivers or other (presumed) responsible adults, particularly during critical periods of development such as early childhood and adolescence.[80]

The psychoanalytic therapy of trauma has nothing to do with the kind of retrospective compassion that characterises quite a lot of trauma help.[81] Some psychoanalytic focal points in trauma treatment are, first and foremost, the restoration of basic safety and trust. The clinical psychotherapeutic milieu's warm, safe and protective holding environment is ideally suited for this. Restoration of symbolisation and mentalisation (defensively switched off to parry degrading de-subjectification) is also the order of the day in clinical psychotherapy. Replacing dissociation with integration and working through guilt associated with fears, passive–active reversal and/or involuntary sexual response are things that can be brought about within (preferably individual) psychotherapeutic sessions. There is always great anger towards the perpetrator and the environment that was inevitably perceived as negligent. The issue is to bring it to its full potential in the most constructive way possible.

The libidinal re-investment of the erogenous and relational body is a delicate and long-term task which can be experimented with within the protected ward life. To this end, the trauma victim will have to reappropriate sexual, affective and dependent tendencies to develop and/or restore the capacity to love. Last but not least, there is invariably the difficult-to-handle negative transference in which the therapist may be perceived as a perpetrator or perverse abuser. The positive transference of fellow patients can be the touchstone through which such transference distortions can be noticed and analysed. Given the betrayal and abandonment that are inextricably linked to trauma, a supportive, caring and restorative approach aimed at a corrective emotional experience in the relationship with the therapist is needed above all. It can be fuelled by psycho-educational ingredients whose sole purpose is to facilitate discussion of the most shameful and guilt-laden contents.[82] It is one of the countless 'unorthodox' turns into which the psychoanalytic therapist must wriggle to bring patients who have often been touched or disturbed to the depths of their souls 'closer to the truth'.[83]

12 The Tiger Whisperer

In classical psychoanalytic work, an almost scientific attitude prevails with the analyst. The patient has sufficient resources to carry out the psycho-analytic process themself (but not alone). They have enough basic security, a sufficiently differentiated image of themself and meaningful others. The Ego and self are sufficiently stable and developed, with sufficient mentalising capacity. The main issue is to gain insight into the psychogenesis and psychodynamics of phenomena repeating themselves throughout the life story and help the patient draw the necessary lessons from them. A state of reverie and negative capability does help the analyst engage their twilight sense, read between the lines and look at things obliquely[84] to let something of the underlying essence come to them.[85] This undoubtedly contributes to good timing and a tactful, digestible paraphrasing of the analyst's interjections.[86] Sometimes, they will try to facilitate a halting free association; they will let silence 'work' or provide punctuation. When interpreting they will follow the motto '*la matière ne suffit pas, il faut aussi la manière*'.[87] Matter and manner are both essential.

In most patients in need of residential treatment, the psychotherapist needs to support mental processes on top of this 'classical' work and provide the necessary holding and containment to that end. Bion and Winnicott's thinking is an indispensable inspiration in clinical psychotherapy. Technically, there is a much greater need for support in these patients, to be understood as the externalisation of an inner attitude of attention, empathy and commitment. In his interventions, the psychotherapist emphasises mentalisation, subject amplification and construction. They adopt a user-friendly attitude and offer to be 'used' as a development object. All this presupposes a more pronounced activity on the part of the psychotherapist. Tuning into and resonating with the affects, the mirroring and ongoing symbolisation are of the utmost importance to form a bond and create a psychic space and envelope. On the one hand, the psychotherapist must have the necessary elasticity and flexibility to venture more interactively into the encounter. Indeed, an overly defensive rigidity prevents the chance of 'moments of meeting', which are necessary to make *It* happen. On the other hand, they must have sufficient solidity to withstand and/or limit destructive attacks[88] on their thinking and professional activity.

Patients will often benefit from the psychotherapist's occasionally poetic use of language (or even some mystical disposition). Poetry means (apart from any artistic appreciation) the combination of a compression of language and an expansion of meaning.[89] The most diverse psychoanalysts emphasise the importance of words that touch the patient,[90] of 'weak', unsaturated interpretations[91] that act as a kind of container/recipient into which the patient can release their own unbearable and/or unthinkable contents or into which something of their truth or meaning can slip. In this way, an intersubjective world is also born from the encounters between patient and analyst, which becomes a tangible hold for the patient and a unique and enduring product of a shared experience and history.[92]

It introduces into the difficult psychoanalytic work of and with these patients something of the order of the aesthetic. For Immanuel Kant, beauty is '*was ohne Begriff allgemein gefällt*'.[93] It is an understanding-without-understanding that is also peculiar to poetry.[94] Through its form, every work of art contains a promise of inwardness. The aesthetic object is (like the transitional object) a subjective object or quasi-subject.[95] Jacques Lacan speaks of '*la fonction du beau*' in connection with this aesthetic.[96] According to him, only the distance congealed in the aesthetic image allows one to enter the dimension of the Real.[97]

Furthermore, as for mysticism, for Lacan, mysticism is an imaginary way of feeling more whole while evading the destructive impact of a real *jouissance*. In his view, only the psychotic is in immediate contact with the Real. He is even 'insanely' at its mercy. Bion has a different opinion on this.[98] He advocates a mystical attitude of 'being in O' for the analyst.[99] For him, this mystical attitude can open up access to a 'mystic/genius/messiah idea', and only this kind of idea can bring about what he calls 'catastrophic change',[100] in which the (also internal) Establishment with its 'classical' thinking patterns ('rigid motion transformations')[101] is broken.

In an autobiographical essay at the end of his life, Bion says the following: '...All my life I have been imprisoned, frustrated, dogged by common sense, reason, memories, desires and –greatest bug bear of all – understanding and being understood'.[102] We can compare this to what the French artist Yves Klein said following the introduction of his monochrome paintings: 'In front of any painting, figurative or non-figurative, I felt more and more that the lines and all their consequences, the contours, the forms, the perspective, the composition became exactly like the bars on the window of a prison'.[103] Psychoanalysis can bear a resemblance to a whodunnit with the therapist as the detective. Still, it can also have something of a shared adventure in which both participants turn into escape artists like Houdini.

In most 'early' and severe psychiatric disorders, however, the patient is at the mercy of unbound and, therefore, dangerous to destructive forces. They feel as if they were haunted by a tiger that has become increasingly wild due to misunderstanding or poor care. Inside and/or outside, they feel cornered by a raw world of drive and trauma, exposed to which they feel naked and defenceless, helpless and abandoned. They need protection, warmth and care from people who use all their physical, emotional and mental abilities to help them out of this often life-threatening distress. In the Oscar-winning feature film *The Horse Whisperer*, Robert Redford/Tom Booker says at one point to Kristin Scott Thomas/Annie MacLean (who has fallen in love with him as a married woman): 'Knowing is the easy part; saying it out loud is the hard part'.[104] It is recognisable for what goes on in a classical psychoanalytic process among neuroses. We might call the clinical psychotherapist more of a tiger whisperer. They often have other cats to flog, namely those without easy parts. After all, knowing more about tigers does not make them any less dangerous.

Language fails. All its arrows fatally miss their target. The scourge of language has left us all with the same disease. Jacques Lacan calls it the unconscious: an ailment no one cures.[105] For Wilfred Bion, the conscious is finite and the unconscious infinite.[106] In his words: 'Psychoanalysis itself is just a stripe on the coat of the tiger. Ultimately, it may meet the Tiger – The Thing Itself – O.'[107]

Notes

1 Van Os et al. (2019): 'A growing body of knowledge indicates that mental illnesses are seldom "cured" and are better framed as vulnerabilities. Important gains in well-being can be achieved when individuals learn to live with mental vulnerabilities through a slow process of strengthening resilience in the social and existential domains.'

2 For example, Erik Nieweg (2005b) differentiates between varying epistemological premises (nominalism, realism, pragmatism) and argues about this overvaluation of the DSM (p 693–694). On the risk of reification, see Vanheule (2015).

3 Bruffaerts et al. (2004 p 75–85). There is 45% 'co-morbidity' in the Netherlands and 56% in the United States.

4 Verheul & van den Brink (1999). More precisely the prevalence of borderline personality disorder is 12% in an outpatient and 22 % in an inpatient population (Leichsenring et al., 2024).

5 See, for example, for depression Corveleyn et al. (2005) and for borderline personality disorder Bateman and Fonagy (2004 p 1–38).

6 Juan-David Nasio (1988, 1992).

7 On the added value of pharmacotherapy in combination with psychotherapy, see, e.g. Thase & Jindal (2004) and Bateman & Fonagy (2004 p 195).

8 Hull et al. (2017); Grant et al. (2022).

9 Sigmund Freud advised that the analyst would lend themself as an opaque projection screen for (transference) fantasies (1912b p 97). In his actual practice, however, he was present in the consulting room as a warm, amiable and real figure. See Harry Stroeken (1987).

10 De Wolf (2002). *Grossly,* this involves the neurotic vs borderline register, actual pathology vs psychopathology (Verhaeghe), the defect model vs conflict model, and mental process vs mental representational disorders (Fonagy).

11 E.g. Alexander & French (1946).

12 From contemporary outcome research, support, empathy and relationship seem to be as important vehicles for transformation and 'structural' change as

interpretation; see, for example, Wallerstein (1986), Sandell et al. (2000), Leuzinger-Bohleber (2002).

13 Peter Sifneos, (1979).

14 David Malan (1979).

15 Habib Davanloo (1990).

16 Edmond Gilliéron (1983, 1997).

17 Just as Freud is said to have discovered the unconscious, Davanloo is claimed to have discovered how to work with it! His technique anticipates contemporary TFP (Clarkin et al., 1999, 2007; Kernberg et al., 2002). For other solid and more recent publications, cf. e.g. Gilliéron (1983), Crits-Cristoph and Barber (1991) and in Dutch Pierloot and Thiel (1986) and Tom Berk (2001).

18 Otto Kernberg (1999).

19 DIT, MBT and TFP join earlier protocolised three-letter therapies such as CBT and DGT. See also Doering et al. (2010) and Gabbard (2014).

20 Leichsenring et al. (2004), Leichsenring et al. (2005), Leichsenring et al. (2022).

21 Sigmund Freud (1919) contrasted psychoanalytic gold with the copper of suggestion. See instead: 'that a considerable range of changes in symptoms, character traits, personality functioning and lifestyle rooted in lifelong and repressed inner conflicts were brought about through more supportive psychotherapeutic modalities and techniques' and these changes are 'indistinguishable from those brought about by typically expressive-analytic means' (own translation, Robert Wallerstein, 1988b p 146).

22 Lester Luborsky devised a protocolised yet high-quality psychoanalytic psychotherapy centred around the 'core conflictual relationship theme' (CCRT) (1984). See also Rockland (1989) or, in Dutch, the article series (1987, 1988) by De Jonghe et al. or Derksen & Markx (2003).

23 As our northern neighbours sometimes call severe personality disorders.

24 Dutch language *Journal of Psychiatry* (1981) 5: theme issue sociotherapy.

25 Sociotherapy is understood more in opposition to psychotherapy. It involves interactional learning within the here-and-now of life on the treatment ward. Question: what is repeated, while memory is the field of psychotherapy; see, for example, Linden (1984).

26 Janzing and Lansen (1985).

27 Jongerius and Rylant (1989).

28 Also by foreign authors, see Almond (1974) and Heim (1985).

29 The Mecca of institutional psychotherapy is *La Borde* (France). It has left-political, anti-psychiatric, Lacanian roots, and its leading figures are Tosquelles and Oury. See Marc Ledoux (2004).

30 On top of the mentioned specific factors of group therapy, clinical psychotherapy offers a caring mother who *picks up* (absorbs) and *touches* the baby (in the patient). See Bolten et al (1988 p 34).

31 The most recent publications also include structure, consistency, coherence, flexibility and dosed care intensity (Bateman and Fonagy, 2004 p 183).

32 This technical act depends on the kind of milieu, the kind of patient, the kind of problem that manifests itself.

33 Bruno Bettelheim (1990). I like the saying: 'Perfect parents exist, but they don't have kids'. 'Perfect' parents blame and burden their children.

34 In Bateman and Fonagy's MBT, the nurses realise treatment almost entirely under the supervision of an analyst. See Bateman and Fonagy (2004 p 205). Interpreting and helping to integrate the inner object relations externalised in transference is the psychoanalytic psychotherapists' job (Verheugt-Pleiter and Deben-Mager, 2005).

35 See the concept of Didier Anzieu (1994) and previous chapters.

36 Maternal and paternal refer to traditional 'role behaviour' and have nothing to do with anatomy.

37 Step-down treatment with a decrease of care and increase of task effort and responsibility is of prime importance, which manifests itself, among other things, in adapting the setting (24-hour treatment, day treatment, outpatient) in function of the psychoanalytic process and the evolving 'treatment needs', see Marco Chiesa et al. (2003), Ogrodniczuk et al. (2001).

38 In doing so, we fully endorse the views of Kennedy (1993) and of Kernberg (1996).

39 Otto Kernberg (1984a).

40 Daniel Stern (1985).

41 For a comprehensive discussion of all this, Vliegen & Cluckers (2001a).

42 Ralph Greenson (1967) distinguishes three components in the relationship with the therapist: the real relationship, the therapeutic alliance and the transference relationship. Horacio Etchegoyen limits them to the real and transference relationship (1999), and Jacqueline Godfrind (1993) distinguishes two parallel streams *within* transference: the narcissistic/primary and the Oedipal transference.

43 Bateman & Fonagy (2004 p 203). Indeed, a huge gap often exists between affective experience and its symbolic representation (ibidem p 205).

44 Character traits are Ego-syntonic. In group and clinical psychotherapy, they create dissonance and are 'promoted' to symptoms.

45 Peter Fonagy (1999).

46 It is a plausible explanation for why psychoanalysis has two mutative factors: interpretation and the 'moment of meeting'; see Stern et al. (1998 p 903–904).

47 For a recent compilation of psychoanalytically based psychosis treatment, see Smet et al. (2003).

48 For a more detailed description of a concrete operation (Kinet, 2003).

49 Vermote et al. (1998).

50 Paul Moyaert (1994) and Marc De Kesel (2002) on Lacan's Seminar (1986).

51 The Queen of England asked Prime Minister Disraeli what his gospel was. His reply: 'Majesty, it is the blank page between the Old Testament and the New Testament'. In Marc Philonenko (2004 p 16).

52 For example, for symptomatic neuroses *par excellence,* such as phobia and obsessive-compulsive disorder, which can be highly disabling and sometimes require an additional, more symptom-focused approach.

53 For example, when the patient is part of a 'system' that hinders or makes any change impossible due to its symptomatic pseudo-equilibrium and morphostasis. Or when the patient is caught up in a 'collusion' with their partner, as described by Jurg Willi (1983 p 43–54): 'We can live neither with nor without each other'.

54 Pierloot & Thiel (1986 p 4).

55 When children hide something, they say 'hot' and 'cold' according to whether we approach the hidden or move away from it. Increase and decrease in symptoms have similar indicative values, cf. the signal function of anxiety, Sigmund Freud (1923a).

56 Jacques Schotte (1990, 1994) and Fons Van Coillie (2000).

57 'not whether but how the combination of psychotherapy and medication is beneficial' (Gabbard, 2014 p. 157).

58 Marcia Kaplan, who devotes nuanced reflections to this challenge (1997).

59 Fonagy et al. (2002).

60 Paul Verhaeghe (2002a).
61 Robert Hinshelwood (1987 p 232).
62 Theo Ingenhoven et al. (2000) and Kinet (2003).
63 For psychoanalytic reflections on depression e.g. Myer Mendelson (1993), Sidney Blatt (2004) or Jos Corveleyn et al. (2005).
64 In physical medicine, the temporary taking-over of essential/vital functions is customary.
65 See Rudi Vermote (2000).
66 Gerald Adler, concerning the borderline, speaks of the 'need/fear dilemma' (1979). Gabbard (2014) speaks of a bi-dimensional transference: on the one hand, the transference of past experiences and, on the other, a self-object transference in which there is a need for repair because of the therapist.
67 Otto Kernberg (1984b).
68 Sidney Blatt (2004) and Corveleyn et al. (2005).
69 He also reaches these conclusions through meta-analysis of other studies such as Wallerstein's Menninger Psychotherapy Research Project (1986). We recall that this showed that support and interpretation equally produced 'structural' personality change, which, on closer inspection, is related to the mentioned 'division' into types of psychopathology. It is a different process and outcome, also confirmed by the recent large-scale study by Rudi Vermote (2005b).
70 There is 70% overlap between borderline and trauma. Besides predisposition and dysfunctional attachment, trauma plays an important role in the patho-genesis of borderline personality disorder, see Fonagy et al. (2002) or recently Leichsenring et al. (2024): 'There is convincing evidence to suggest that the interaction between genetic factors and adverse childhood experience plays a central role in the etiology of BPD'.
71 While repression prevails in inner conflict, dissociation prevails in trauma (Spiegel, 1991). The trauma can neither be thought nor articulated. The Ego splits off and dissociates the unsymbolised experience to avoid destruction. See also Kluft (2000).
72 Sigmund Freud (1916–1917).
73 The trauma remains *real.* Somatic and sensory sensations (e.g. a smell, pain in the underbelly) underlie dissociative defences.
74 Anna Freud attributes this to identification with the aggressor (1936).
75 Roth & Fonagy (2004).
76 Luyten et al. (2008 p 41).
77 Joe Allen (2013) and Kudler et al. (2009).
78 In multiple studies, RCTs showed that MBT is more efficacious here than TAU even after an 8-year follow-up (Bateman & Fonagy, 2008). Group psychother-apy also contributes to better efficacy (Ford et al., 2009; Fallot & Harris, 2009; Shea et al., 2009). See also Glen Gabbard (2014 p 299): 'Recovery of traumatic memories is not the goal of psychotherapy'. It is mainly about restoring trust and mental processes.
79 Judith Herman (1992, 1993); Bessel Van der Kolk (2005).
80 Ford & Courtois (2009 p 13).
81 Following his dispute with Otto Rank, Freud denounced an overly simplistic therapeutic approach to trauma. He compared it to a fire brigade that removed a fallen oil lamp that caused the fire. Of course, all damage must be inventoried and repaired as much as possible. (1937a). In psychic causation, cause and effect are disproportionate.
82 On trauma and psychotherapy, see Kinet (2016, 2023d) or Franckx & Hebbrecht (2023).

83 Gert Peelen (2001).
84 Slavoj Žižek (1996). The skull at the bottom of Hans Holbein's painting *The Ambassadors* is an anamorphosis seen only through a fleeting side-glance when leaving the exhibition room (Lacan, 1973 front cover and p 75–109).
85 Thomas Ogden (1999).
86 '*Le lion ne saute qu'une fois*' (The lion jumps only once) in Sigmund Freud (1937a).
87 Serge André (2003).
88 Destructive attacks may come from the narcissistic, omnipotent, and envious part of the patient or from a terrorist part that is split off (borderline) or dissociated (trauma) doing its destructive work.
89 Thomas Ogden (2002 p 206).
90 Danielle Quinodoz (2003).
91 Antonino Ferro (1996, 2015).
92 Thomas Ogden (1994). There is a *colloque singulier* between mother and child, between poet and muse, between lovers (Victor Hugo: '*Qu'est-ce que des amants? Ce sont des nouveaux-nés*') and between patient and therapist.
93 Immanuel Kant (1790/1987).
94 For a more detailed elaboration (Kinet, 2005c p 118–121).
95 See reflections on this quasi-subject Mikel Dufrenne (1967 p 196–197).
96 Jacques Lacan (1986 p 271).
97 Marc De Kesel (2002 p 220–221).
98 Lacan distinguishes three structures: psychosis, neurosis and perversion.
99 One of the ardent contemporary proponents of this mystical attitude is Michael Eigen (1998) and (2004)
100 For a brief and clear description of the '*genius*' and '*catastrophic change*': disruptive change with emotional upheaval (Bion, 1965, 1966, 1970) see Grinberg et al, (1971 p 17–21). He also talks about the poetic language of achievement that departs from O. The analyst waits for the moment when O finds a form or a thought finds a thinker. This happens in his terms thanks to (an act of) faith (Bion, 1970 p 30). Cf Pablo Picasso: '*Je ne cherche pas, je trouve*'.
101 Wilfred Bion (1965 p 15–16).
102 Wilfred Bion (1997 p 578).
103 Yves Klein (1959) in Harrison & Wood (p 804) With his *Yves Klein Blue* he really went '*ins blaue hinein*'.
104 Robert Redford (1998). From a psychoanalytic view, this film is about an oedipal/triangulated configuration and the transference of love towards a therapist.
105 Moustapha Safouan (2005 p 396): '*L'inconscient est une maladie mentale dont on ne se réveille pas*'.
106 Riccardo Lombardi (2015).
107 Wilfred Bion (1975b). It touches on Imanuel Kant's sublime: point of fear and of awe (see Civitarese (2014); Doran, 2015).

Chapter 12

Epilogue
A Remedy by Truth

After the psychodynamic psychiatry described, I will again end on a psychoanalytic note. No history of philosophy lacks Freud (or, more generally, a psychoanalytic input). That psychoanalysis and philosophy have common ground is obvious. First, the patient is more or less out of their wits and seeks help to become wiser about their problems. The desire for wisdom is an obvious motive for psychoanalysis, just as sufficient love of truth underlies it. According to Paul Ricoeur, Freud, like Schopenhauer, Nietzsche or Marx, belongs to the '*philosophes du soupçon*'.[1] Together with Heidegger, they can be considered the first deconstructivists. In plain language, they all want to eliminate illusions and appearances. Psychoanalysis also implies a peculiar philosophical anthropology. It dethrones the sovereignty of the Cartesian *cogito*. Given the predominance of the Id and unconscious, humans are not our own masters. Language is our home, but it is also a prison from which we want to escape. It creates a lack of being that makes us long for a surplus of enjoyment that we assume beyond language. This, however, is unjustified because such enjoyment is paradoxically destructive and unenjoyable. We must make do with the pleasure principle (or its upgrade: the reality principle) and life's *small* things. We must stay at a respectful distance from the Thing with a capital letter and not want to go *beyond* the pleasure principle.

Perhaps psychopathology, furthermore, has not so much to do with genes or the brain but simply with issues we do not want to know about. They relate to love and sexuality, destruction and aggression, selfishness and narcissism.[2] But equally to spiritual matters. Even in a world from which evil, violence and injustice had been banished, human beings would struggle with parting and loss, with illness and mortality, with differences between people, generations or genders. In his *Ethica Nicomachea*, Aristotle talks about three different forms of knowledge: *epistemè, technè* and *phronesis*. The first contains knowledge that is context-independent, universal and immutable and based on an analytical rationality. Examples are physics and mathematics. Then you have *technè*, which is pragmatic, context-dependent and production-oriented. It uses instrumental rationality and determines, for example, architecture or other applied sciences. Finally, there is the *phronesis*, which is

DOI: 10.4324/9781032698052-15

also pragmatic and context-dependent but uses a value-based rationality.[3] According to Paul Verhaeghe, it is essential for regulating interpersonal relations and characterises the psychoanalytic enterprise par excellence.

One of its objectives is for the patient to be able to make more conscious choices in these matters. For this, they must first be able to develop mentally.[4] After all, sufficient maturity is needed to participate fully in adult life (including ethically and legally). Furthermore, they must be able to detach or distance themself sufficiently from their determinedness to set (*'auto-nomos'*) their own law. Towards the end of the psychoanalytic process, the patient can sometimes come close to the opaque kernel of their being. This refers to their symptom's (drive-) root or the basic phantasm as an unconscious cognitive and affective script that structures their relationship with the world. They can align with convention but also arrive at some more creative discovery. Both may involve, à la Nietzsche, a kind of *amor fati*, embracing one's fate. This is expressed in formulations such as the invention of a sinthome[5] or 'Enjoy your symptom!'[6] Paraphrasing JFK: 'Do not ask what you can do for your symptom, but what your symptom can do for you!' Psychoanalysis, thus pursued, leads to making an absolute difference.[7] This has nothing to do with a willed eccentricity, extravagance, or the narcissism of small differences.[8] After all, the latter is a purely imaginary affair in which differences are cultivated to distinguish one's image. Instead, it has to do with a relationship to the Real that is authentic and unique.[9] Indeed, one of our most private elements is the highly particular ways we avoid pain or unpleasure and the possible or impossible ways we try to enjoy ourselves.

From an adaptive perspective, truth is evolutionarily significant. It pays off in the struggle for life. That is why, according to the philosopher of science Maarten Boudry, truth is always better than lies.[10] Suppose we were to be completely misrepresenting the reality that surrounds us. Then it would be like walking around Berlin with a Paris city map! However, does this adaptiveness of truth also apply to the perception of our emotional and inner world? Here, we may undoubtedly refer to what poet and Nobel laureate T.S. Eliot says in one of his *Four Quartets*: 'Humankind cannot bear very much reality.'[11] What do we like to see, and what do we like less? We wish truth to be beautiful, like Botticelli's Venus emerging from the water with one and all grace. However, isn't truth more often a shame or a horror?[12] This is why, by the way, the liar is always at an advantage. The speaker of truth is bound hand and foot to facts, however incoherent or arbitrary they may be. On the other hand, the liar has every freedom to make their story as pretty as they like.

In any case, Freud's essential lesson is that the mind seems more of an *enemy* of truth.[13] It is, as it were, a censor that forces the disease to speak a secret language. For both Freud and Lacan, the reality of the unconscious is an unbearable, traumatic and primarily sexual truth.[14] Freud approvingly quotes La Rochefoucauld: '*tous les hommes dissimulent la vérité en matière de sexualité*.[15] Pre-eminently in these matters, our most fundamental passion is *'la passion de l'ignorance'*:[16] the passion of not wanting to know. Our erogenous regions are located in Fantasyland. It is a land where unpleasure is banished, and the pleasure principle rules. Psychoanalysis naturally takes the opposite path. It seeks lucidity,[17] breaking through the realm of illusions and the Imaginary.

From the very beginning of this book, we talked about the symptom. It is an abrasive hinge between the surface and what lies beneath, and it contains a hidden core of truth: the subject's being (*'l'être du sujet'*).[18] By speaking freely, the patient collides with the contradictions underlying the symptom. Through the symptom, the door to truth is left ajar, as it were.[19] Lacan repeats it in every tone: psychoanalysis is a method of truth,[20] the psychoanalyst is the master of truth,[21] and acts under the motto: the truth will set you free.[22] Truth most often comes from the mouth of a child, of an idiot, of a madman or from the mouth of a fool. It appears when we do not know it or do not want to know anything about it and not where we *think* we know it or pronounce it.

Referring to Kant, philosophy is concerned with three big questions in their generality: What can I know, what should I do, and what can I hope for? The last two can be taken together as how should I behave, so we can add the political dimension: by whom or what should I let myself be governed? As illustrated in Raphael's fresco, *The School of Athens*, according to Plato, the good life is directed towards a transcendent world of forms and ideas. As the son of a physician, Aristotle seeks it more in the reality surrounding him and, for him, the good life should aim at the golden mean. Happiness (*'eudaimonia'*) will be found there above all. This happiness should not be understood as a simple focus on pleasure. Instead, Aristotle is concerned with a flourishing life in which his virtues of courage, moderation, justice and practical wisdom are cultivated. Alongside an ascetic ideal that starts with them and runs through Stoicism and Christianity, there is traditionally a more materialistic or atomistic thread of hedonism and epicureanism that often becomes somewhat repressed. It can certainly be found partly with British sentimentalists such as John Locke or David Hume and utilitarianists such as Jeremy Bentham and John Stuart Mill. For the former, there is a natural virtue that feels pleasurable and makes one happy. The consequentialism of the latter steers, to a greater or lesser extent, towards the greatest possible pleasure gain for everyone, which, to be precise (at least for the last), is not limited to overly earthly pleasures. Kant's categorical imperative involves an entirely different ethical logic. Instead, it is a doctrine of duty or deontology. With him, ethics obeys an absolute rationale that is most succinctly summarised in his second formulation: never consider your fellow man as a means and only as an end in itself.

Is (more spiritually speaking) a good life a contemplative life as with Socrates, Plato or Aristotle? Is it an active life where you engage in all human activities as much as possible? Is it a fatalistic life characterised by detachment and resignation, as with the Buddha or the stoa? Is it a hedonistic life aimed at avoiding pain and at more or less refined pleasure? Is it, à la Nietzsche, a stylish life in which we must embrace our fate with a certain *grandeur* and sufficient *amor fati*? Is it a life where one can lose oneself in a great cause as it happens (always in moments) to heroes or saints?[23] Perhaps the good life can have something of all this, though. For psychoanalysis, it is mainly about living one's *own* life as consciously and with as much 'inside' knowledge as possible. This pursuit is inevitably painful to a greater or lesser extent. After all, it goes much further than the Kantian 'dare to think' ('*sapere aude*') by which we should free ourselves from our 'heteronomy' (as opposed to autonomy) and insouciance. It is thinking *out loud* and in the presence of someone genuinely listening. Someone with an ear for what we are saying (or not saying), and the often vast difference between the two. In the words of Wilfred Bion, it can be hard labour (especially in domestic affairs) 'to suffer the process of thinking'.[24]

Which brings me back to the clinical situation. In 2013, psychoanalyst Stephen Gross wrote a widely read and acclaimed book of literarily worded psychoanalytic case studies. *The Examined Life* refers to a statement by Socrates that a life not examined is not worth living. The New York psychoanalyst Robert Langs once made a somewhat controversial distinction between two forms of therapy: *truth therapy* and *lie therapy*.[25] However effective, much psychiatric treatment, in his view, belongs to lie therapy. Look, for instance, at pharmaco- (or other biological) therapy. By dampening our feelings, influencing our mood or changing our way of thinking, they can significantly improve or alleviate the course of (especially major) psychiatric disorders as well as their symptoms or complaints. However, everyone will understand that these biological medicines by themselves do not change psychological problems. After all, pharmacotherapy can be applied without any concern for the truth. Even psychotherapy, by the way, does not always have to care about this truth. For instance, a psychotherapist can help by replacing wrong/sick thoughts and feelings with the right/healthy ones in various ways, thus bringing about emotional change. This largely ignores whether feelings have a right and a reason to exist. The main concern is redirecting them in the desired direction as long as the patient or those around them *feel* better.

I refer to an imaginative example of such a therapeutic approach from the famous psychotherapist Milton Erickson.[26] He had a patient in treatment who imagined he was Jesus; he led a passive and withdrawn existence and came to nothing. Erickson said, 'Your father Joseph is a carpenter, so why not take up woodworking?' He got his patient started in that quasi-miraculous way. He used – as in *aikido* – a (psychopathological) movement of the patient to 'floor' him. The delusion is not fought but turned in a more productive or constructive direction. Another example is the so-called paradoxical technique. A person with a fear of blushing ('erythrophobia') is instructed to make his face turn as red as possible several times a day for about five minutes. The same phenomenon changes from undesirable to desirable social behaviour thanks to the therapist's intervention, thus losing function and meaning. This kind of help has its value. If it allows you to avoid someone becoming depressed or acting out destructively, the treatment is considered 'successful' by many.

What is typical of psychoanalytic forms of treatment, however, is that they aim to make things better by truth.[27] Betterment is not pursued magically or chemically. The patient must acquire more knowledge of (their internal) affairs and better understand the actual cause of the origin and persistence of their problems. In the relationship with the psychotherapist, these problems come onto the scene. They can be fathomed and worked through there. The Good that the psychoanalytic approach has in mind is not so much life as survival. It is mainly about what the patient makes of their life, how much sense they make of it and what meaning they give to it. For such reasons, psychoanalysis is both akin to philosophy and science. It is not *philosophy* but *follysophy*. Is it not typical of the true philosopher to prefer truth to happiness and to feel genuine sorrow rather than false joy? According to Spinoza, there is a fundamental difference between the joy of the drunkard and that of the sage!'[28]

Paraphrasing Wilfred Bion, our psyche needs truth as much as oxygen.[29] Only we cannot breathe it in its pure form. After all, it is precisely essential for man to live in falsehood. I recall Belgian writer Hugo Claus: 'He who does not lie lives like a beast'.[30] Whether our bodies can lie is questionable, but our tongues regularly refuse the truth. In a sense 'fortunately', there is also another side. Truth hurts, but what hurts is, nevertheless, not always truth. Psychoanalysis has perhaps suffered too long from a deceptive *a priori*. It is not because it is bad that it is true, nor does the principle apply mordantly: the more gloomy, the more true. Eventually, life may break our hearts, but Freud and '*Freude*' can go together.[31]

Notes

1 Philosophers of distrust see Olivier Dekens (2015).
2 Psychoanalysis is probably most based on an ethic of renunciation: to accept lack, limitation and loss (Lemma, 2022 p 104).
3 The fourth, '*sophia*', only plays a role in philosophy.
4 Michel Thys (2006) rightly argues that in psychoanalysis, we have moved from a gnostic to an experiential meaning of truth. See also Leon Grinberg (1980), Charles Hanly (2009), Wendy Katz (2016) and Thomas Ogden (2016).
5 The Lacanian sinthome is a kind of 'invention' and involves original and idiosyncratic handling of the real, opaque and, in a structural sense, traumatic drive root of the symptom.
6 Slavoj Žižek's book (1992).
7 See Jacques Lacan (1986) or also Kinet (2013).

8 Sigmund Freud (1930b p 139): the magnified minor differences between 'neighbouring and in other respects related communities'.

9 Of Thing, drive and trauma but also of the constitutional component in psychiatric disorders such as the bipolar, the schizophrenic or the autistiform.

10 Maarten Boudry (2015 p 28).

11 From *Burnt Norton* by T.S. Eliot (1944).

12 Embarrassing or an abomination?

13 'The psychic apparatus is intolerant of unpleasure and strives to ward it off at all costs and, if the perception of reality involves unpleasure, that perception-i.e., the truth be sacrificed' (Freud, 1937b p 292).

14 Jacques Lacan (1973 p 138).

15 Sigmund Freud (1896) Freely translated: We all feign/fake the truth in sexual matters.

16 Jacques Lacan (1975a p 110).

17 If not: ludicity.

18 Jacques Lacan (1966a).

19 Clément Fromentin (2021).

20 Jacques Lacan (1953 p 257).

21 Jacques Lacan (1953 p 313).

22 John (8:32) American essayist Gloria Steinem amends: 'The truth will set you free, but first it will piss you off' (2019). See also Jacques Lacan (Lacan 1986 p 32).

23 In his existential psychotherapy, Irvin Yalom talks about four givens of the human condition: isolation, meaninglessness, mortality and freedom. For him, the capstone of such psychotherapy is self-transcendence: '...one comprehends oneself in order not to be preoccupied with oneself'. (1980 p 439).

24 See Wilfred Bion (1970 p 15). I am reminded in this context of an amusing quote by essayist Joseph Epstein: 'A neurotic, when asked why he left psychotherapy after a few sessions, claimed the guy asked too many goddamn personal questions'. Psychoanalytic psychotherapy is not called 'anxiety-provoking' for nothing (Sifneos, 1979). We are led to leave the bastion of our Ego/self and free ourselves from our Ego/self.

25 Robert Langs (1982).

26 Milton Erickson (1992).

27 Michel Thys (2006).

28 Spinoza (1677 in 1979 p 179).

29 See the words of his widow Francesca Bion (1995 p 106): 'First and foremost, he placed respect for the truth, without which effective analysis becomes impossible. It is the central aim and as essential for emotional growth as food is for the body; without it the mind dies of starvation'.

30 Hugo Claus (2011).

31 *Freude* as (life's) joy. I like a quote from Belgian poet-writer Stefan Hertmans (1999), according to whom the poet is characterised by what he calls a 'vital (= vibrant) melancholy'.

List of Abbreviations

AJP American Journal of Psychiatry
BJP British Journal of Psychiatry

Freud
SFNE Sigmund Freud Nederlandse Editie. Amsterdam/Meppel:Boom
FW Freud Werken, 2006. Amsterdam: Boom
FSE Freud Standard Edition
IJPA International Journal of Psychoanalysis
JAPA Journal of the American Psychoanalytical Association

Kinet
AAG Antwerpen/Apeldoorn: Garant
AHGS Antwerpen/'s Hertogenbosch: Gompel&Svacina

Klein
WMK The Writings of Melanie Klein. London: Hogarth Press, 1975

Lacan
E Ecrits
TMPS Texte établi par Jacques-Alain Miller. Paris: Seuil
PQ The Psychoanalytic Quarterly
PSC Psychoanalytic Study of the Child
TVP Tijdschrift voor Psychotherapie
TVPA Tijdschrift voor Psychoanalyse
TVPS Tijdschrift voor Psychiatrie
UP University Press

Winnicott
TPP Through Paediatrics to Psychoanalysis. London: Karnac Books, 1992
MPFE The Maturational Process and the Facilitating Environment, London: Karnac Books, 1990
PR Playing and reality. London: Tavistock, 1971

References

Abbass, A.A., Hancock, J.T., Henderson, J. & Kisley, S. (2006). Short-term psycho-dynamic psychotherapies for common mental health disorders. *Cochrane Database of Systematic Reviews*, Issue 7 Article nr CD004687

Ackrill, J.L. (1994) *Aristoteles*. Groningen: Historische Uitgeverij.

Adler, G. (1979). Aloneness and borderline psychopathology. *IJPA*, 60, 83–96.

Ainsworth, M.D.S., Blehar, M.C., Waters, E., Wall, S. (1978). *Patterns of attachment: a psychological study of the strange situation*. Hillsdale NJ: Erlbaum.

Ainsworth, M.S. & Bowlby, J. (1991). An ethological approach to personality development. *American Psychologist*, 46(4), 333–341.

Alexander, F. & French, T.M. (1946). *Psychoanalytic Therapy*. New York: Ronald.

Allen, J.G. (2013). Treating attachment trauma with plain old therapy. *Journal of Trauma & Dissociation*, 14(4), 367–374.

Allen, J.G. & Fonagy, P. (Eds.). (2006). *Handbook of mentalization-based treatment*. West Sussex, UK: Wiley.

Allison, E. & Fonagy, P. (2016). When is truth relevant? *PQ*, 85(2), 275–303.

Alvarez, A. (1996). The clinician's debt to Winnicott. *Journal of Child Psychotherapy*, 22(3), 377–383.

Almond, R. (1974). *The healing community. Dynamics of the therapeutic milieu*. New York: Jason Aronson.

Andlin-Sobocki, P., Jönsson, B., Wittchen, H.-U., Olesen, J. (2005). Costs of disorders of the brain in Europe. *Eur. J. Neurol.* 12(1), 1–27.

Andreasen, N.C., O'Leary, D.S., Cizadlo, T., Arndt, S., Rezai, K., Watkins, G.L., Ponto, L.L. & Hichwa, R.D. (1995). Remembering the past: two facets of episodic memory explored with positron emission tomography. *AJP* 152(11), 1576–1585.

André, S. (1986). *Que veut une femme?* Paris: Navarin.

André, S. (2003). *Devenir psychanalyste… et le rester*. Paris: Que.

Andreus, H. (1975). *Gedichten 1948–1974*. Amsterdam: Bezige Bij.

Anzieu, D. (1975). *L'autoanalyse de Freud et la découverte de la psychanalyse*. Paris: PUF.

Anzieu, D. (1975). *Le groupe et l'inconscient. L'imaginaire groupal*. Paris: Dunod, 1988.

Anzieu, D. (1994). *Le moi-peau*. Paris: Dunod.

Arendt, H. (1963) *Eichmann in Jerusalem. A report on the banality of evil*. New York: Viking, 2006.

Arlow, J.A. (1982). Psychoanalytic education. A psychoanalytic perspective. *Annual of Psychoanalysis*, 10, 5–20.

Aron, L. (1996) *Meeting of minds: mutuality and psychoanalysis.* Hillsdale NJ: Analytic Press.

Badinter, E. (1998). *L'amour en plus. Histoire de l'amour maternel.* Paris: Flammarion.

Badiou, A. (1988) *L'Être et l'événément.* Paris: Seuil.

Bailly, L. (2012). *Lacan: A beginner's guide.* New York: Simon and Schuster.

Baker, H.S. & Baker, M.N. (1987) Heinz Kohut's self-psychology: an overview. *AJP*, 44, 1–9.

Balint, M. (1952). *Primary love and psychoanalytic technique.* London: Tavistock, 1992.

Balint, M. (1968). *The basic fault. Therapeutic aspects of depression.* London: Tavistock, 1992.

Barthelme, D. (1981) *Sixty Stories.* New York: Putman.

Bateman, A. & Fonagy, P. (1999). Effectiveness of partial hospitalisation in the treatment of borderline personality disorders: a randomised controlled trial. *AJP*, 156(10), 1563–1569.

Bateman, A. & Fonagy, P. (2000). Effectiveness of psychotherapeutic treatment of personality disorders. *BJP*, 177, 138–143.

Bateman, A. & Fonagy, P. (2001). Treatment of borderline personality disorder with psychoanalytically oriented partial hospitalisation: an 18-month follow-up. *AJP*, 158(1), 36–42.

Bateman, A. & Fonagy, P. (2004). *Psychotherapy for borderline personality disorder. Mentalization based treatment.* London: Oxford UP.

Bateman, A. & Fonagy, P. (2008) 8-year follow-up of patients treated for borderline personality disorder. Mentalization-based treatment versus treatment as usual. *AJP*, 165, 631–638.

Baudelaire, C. (1857) *Les Fleurs du Mal.* Paris: Pocket Books, 2018.

Bazan, A. (2011). Phantoms in the voice. A neuropsychoanalytic hypothesis on the structure of the unconscious. *Neuro-Psychoanalysis*, 13(2), 161–176.

Bazan, A. (2016). Trauma en de Dopaminerge Inschrijving van het Evenement. Aan Gene Zijde van het Lustprincipe ligt de Demonische Herhalingsdwang. In M. Kinet (Ed.) *Trauma binnenstebuiten* (pp. 95–116). AAG.

Bazan, A. & Detandt, S. (2013). On the physiology of jouissance: interpreting the mesolimbic dopaminergic reward functions from a psychoanalytic perspective. *Frontiers in Human Neuroscience*, doi:10.3389/fnhum.2013.00709..

Beebe, B. (2005). Mother–infant research informs mother–infant treatment. *PSC*, 60, 7–46.

Beebe, B. & Lachmann, F.M. (2002). *Infant research and adult treatment: co-constructing interactions.* New York: Analytic Press.

Beebe, B., Jaffe, J., Markese, S., Buck, K., Chen, H., Cohen, P., ... & Feldstein, S. (2010). The origins of 12-month attachment: A microanalysis of 4-month mother–infant interaction. *Attachment & Human Development*, 12 (1–2), 3–141.

Beebe, B. & Lachmann, F.M. (2013). *Infant research and adult treatment: co-constructing interactions.* Routledge.

Benjamin, J. (1990). An outline of inter-subjectivity: the development of recognition. *Psychoanalytic Psychology*, 7, 33–46.

Benjamin, L.T. & Baler, D.B. (Eds.). (2000). History of psychology. The Boulder Conference. *American Psychologist*, 55, 233–254.

Bennett, M.R. & Hacker, P.M.S. (2003). *Philosophical Foundations of Neuroscience*. Oxford: Blackwell.

Bercherie, P. (1988). *Géographie du champ psychanalytique*. Paris: Navarin.

Bergin, A.E. & Garfield, S.L. (Eds.). (1994). *Handbook of psychotherapy and behaviour change* (4th ed.). New York: Wiley.

Berk, T. (1980). *Groepsanalytische psychotherapie*. Deventer: Van Loghum Slaterus.

Berk, T. (2001). *Handboek korte psychodynamische psychotherapie: context, theorie en praktijk*. Amsterdam: Boom.

Berk, T. (2005). *Leerboek groepspsychotherapie*. Utrecht: de Tijdstroom.

Bernfeld, S. (1949). Freud's scientific beginnings. *American Imago*, 6(3), 163–196.

Bettelheim, B. (1983). *Freud and Man's soul*. London: Hogarth.

Bettelheim, B. (1990). *Niet volmaakt maar goed genoeg*. Amsterdam: Contact.

Bibring, E. (1954). Psychoanalysis and the dynamic psychotherapies. *JAPA*, 2, 754–770.

Bion, F. (1995). The days of our years. *The Journal of Melanie Klein & Object Relations Journal*, 13(1), 1995.

Bion, W.R. (1959). Attacks on linking. In *Second thoughts* (1967, pp 93–119). London: Maresfield, 1967.

Bion, W.R. (1961). *Experiences in groups and other papers*. London: Tavistock.

Bion, W.R. (1962a). A theory of thinking. In *Second Thoughts* (1967, pp. 110–119). London: Maresfield, 1967.

Bion, W.R. (1962b). *Learning from experience*. London: Karnac, 1984.

Bion, W.R. (1963). *Elements of psychoanalysis*. London: Heinemann.

Bion, W.R. (1965). *Transformations*. London: Heinemann.

Bion, W.R. (1967). *Second thoughts*. London: Maresfield.

Bion, W.R. (1970). *Attention and interpretation*. London: Karnac, 1986.

Bion, W.R. (1974). *Bion's Brazilian lectures*. London: Karnac, 1990.

Bion, W.R. (1975a). *A memoir of the future*. London: Karnac, 1991.

Bion, W.R. (1975b). Brasilia clinical seminars. In W.R. Bion & F. Bion (Eds.), *Clinical seminars and four papers*. Abingdon: Fleetwood Press.

Bion, W.R. (1982). *The long weekend*. Abingdon: Fleetwood Press.

Bion, W.R. (1987). *Clinical seminars and four papers*. Abingdon: Fleetwood Press.

Bion, W.R. (1997). *Taming wild thoughts*. F. Bion (Ed.). London: Karnac.

Bion, W.R. (2013) *Los Angeles seminars and supervision*. J. Aguayo & B. Malin (Eds.). London: Karnac.

Blackburn, S. (2008) *Goed leven. Een tegendraadse beschouwing over ethiek*. Amsterdam: Lemniscaat.

Blass, R.B. (2011). On the immediacy of unconscious truth: Understanding Betty Joseph's 'here and now' through comparison with alternative views of it outside of and within Kleinian thinking. *IJPA* 92(5), 1137–1157.

Blass, R.B. (2016) The quest for truth as the foundation of psychoanalytic practice: a traditional Freudian-Kleinian perspective, *PQ*, 85(2), 305–337.

Blatt, S.J. (1992) The differential effect of psychotherapy and psychoanalysis with anaclitic and introjective patients: The Menninger Psychotherapy Research Project revisited. *JAPA*, 40, 691–724.

Blatt, S.J. (2004). *Experiences of depression: theoretical, clinical and research perspectives*. Washington DC: American Psychological Association.

Blatt, S.J. (2008) *Polarities of experience: Relatedness and self-definition in personality development, psychopathology and the therapeutic process.* Washington, DC: American Psychological Association.

Blatt, S.J. & Levy, K.N. (2003) Attachment theory, psychoanalysis, personality development and psychopathology. *Psychoanalytic Inquiry*, 23, 102–150.

Blatt, S.J. & Luyten, P. (2010) Reactivating the psychodynamic approach to the classification of psychopathology. In T. Millon, R.F. Krueger & E. Simonsen (Eds.) *Contemporary directions in psychopathology: scientific foundations of the DSM-and ICD-11* (pp. 483–514) New York: Guilford.

Bloch, S. & Crouch, E. (1985). *Therapeutic factors in group psychotherapy.* Oxford: Oxford UP.

Boerwinkel, A.R., Gomperts, W.J. (2001). *Alleen en met z'n tweeën: one- en two-person psychologie in de psychoanalyse.* Assen: Van Gorcum.

Bloom, H. (1994) *The western canon: the books and school of the ages.* New York: Riverhead.

Bloom, H. (1998) *The invention of the human.* New York: Riverhead.

Bögels, G.F. (2001). Verbindingslijnen tussen babyobservatie en psychoanalytische behandeling. In A. De Bruyne & W. Heuves (Eds.), *Bij nader inzien. Over kijken en psychoanalyse* (pp. 21–43). Amsterdam: Boom.

Bollas, C. (1987). *The shadow of the object: psychoanalysis of the unthought known.* New York: Columbia UP.

Bollas, C. (1993) *Being a character: psychoanalysis and self-experience.* London/New York: Routledge.

Bolten, M.P., Hesselink, A.J. & Vreeswijk, L. (1988). Heilzame factoren in klinische psychotherapie. *TVP*, 14(2), 16–36.

Bornstein, R.F. (2001). The impending death of psychoanalysis. *Psychoanalytic Psychology*, 18, 3–20.

Boudry, M. (2015) *Illusies voor gevorderden.* Antwerp: Polis.

Bourdieu, P. (1989). *Opstellen over smaak, habitus en het veldbegrip.* Amsterdam: Van Gennep.

Bowlby, J. (1940). The influence of early environment in the development of neurosis and neurotic character. *IJPA*, XXI, 1–25.

Bowlby, J. (1951). Maternal care and mental health. *World Health Organization Monograph* (Serial No. 2).

Bowlby, J. (1958), The nature of the child's tie to his mother. *IJPA*, XXXIX, 1–23.

Bowlby, J. (1959). Separation anxiety. *IJPA*, XLI, 1–25.

Bowlby, J. (1960). Grief and mourning in infancy and early childhood. *PSC*, VX, 3–39.

Bowlby, J. (1969). *Attachment and loss, Vol. 1: Attachment.* New York: Basic Books, 1989 (2nd ed.).

Bowlby, J. (1973). *Attachment and loss, Vol. 2: Separation.* New York: Basic Books.

Bowlby, J. (1980). *Attachment and loss, Vol. 3: Loss, sadness and depression.* New York: Basic Books.

Bowlby, J. (1988). *A secure base: clinical applications of attachment theory.* London: Routledge.

Bowlby, J. (1990). *Charles Darwin: a new life.* New York/London: Norton.

Bradshaw, G., Schore, A., Brown, J.*et al.* (2005) Elephant breakdown. *Nature*, 433, 807.

Braeckman, J. (2001). *Darwins moordbekentenis: de ontwikkeling van het denken van Charles Darwin.* Utrecht: Nieuwezijds.

Bremner, J.D. (1999). Does stress damage the brain? *Biological Psychiatry*, 45: 797–805.

Brenner, C. (1983). *The mind in conflict*. New York: International UP.

Bretherton, I. (1992). The origins of attachment theory: John Bowlby and Mary Ainsworth. *Developmental Psychology*, 28(5), 759–775.

Brown, L.J. (2011). *Intersubjective processes and the unconscious: an integration of Freudian, Kleinian and Bionian perspectives*. Hove: Routledge.

Brown, D., Scheflin, A.W. *et al.* (1998). *Memory, trauma treatment and the law: an essential reference on memory for clinicians, researchers, attorneys and judges*. New York: Norton.

Bruffaerts, R., Bonnewyn, A., Demarest, S., Van Oyen, H., Demyttenaere, K. (2004). Prevalentie van mentale stoornissen in de Belgische bevolking. Resultaten van de European Study of the Epidemiology of Mental Disorders (ESEMeD). *Tijdschrift voor Geneeskunde*, 60, 75–85.

Bucci, W. (1997). *Psychoanalysis and cognitive science: a multiple code theory*. New York: Guilford.

Caldwell, L., & Joyce, A. (Eds.) (2011). *Reading Winnicott* (Vol. 4). New York/London: Routledge.

Cambien, J. (1981). De (on)wetenschappelijkheid van de psychoanalyse. *TVPS*, 23, 203–215.

Cambien, J. (1987). De (on)wetenschappelijkheid van de psychotherapie. *TVPA*, 29, 528–539.

Cambien, J. (1988). Fantasie in het werk van Melanie Klein. *TVP*, 14, 258–268.

Cambien, J. (1999). De geschiedenis van O. *Psychoanalyse*, 9 (pp. 169–177). Leuven: Peeters.

Cambien, J. (2002). Als het denken de passie preekt. In A.R. Boerwinkel & A. De Bruyne (Eds.), *Psychoanalyse en passie* (pp. 83–97). Amsterdam: Boom.

Cambien, J. (2005). Vier personages. In M. Kinet & L. Moyson (Eds.), *Grootse patiënten, kleine therapeuten. Narcisme en psychotherapie*. AAG.

Camon, F. (1981). *De ziekte die mens heet*. Amsterdam: Arbeiderspers, 1992.

Carver, R. (1981). *What we talk about when we talk about love*. New York: Picador.

Carveth, D.L. (2023) *Guilt: a contemporary introduction*. London/New York: Routledge.

Cassidy, J. & Shaver, P.R. (Eds.) (2008) *Handbook of attachment: theory, research, and clinical applications* (2nd ed.) New York: Guilford.

Ceysens, E. (2005). Hyperindividualisme: narcisme aan het begin van de 21ste eeuw. In M. Kinet & L. Moyson (Eds.), *Grootse patiënten, kleine therapeuten. Narcisme en Psychotherapie*. AAG.

Chalmers, D. (1995). *The conscious mind: in search of a fundamental theory*. New York: Oxford UP.

Chiesa, M., Fonagy, P. & Holmes, J. (2003). When less is more: an exploration of psychoanalytically oriented hospital-based treatment for severe personality disorder. *IJPA*, 84, 637–650.

Cicchetti, D. & Rogosch, F.A. (1996) Equifinality and multifinality in developmental psychopathology. *Development and Psychopathology*, 8, 597–600.

Cioran, E.M. (1986) *Aveux et Anathèmes*. Paris: Gallimard.

Civitarese, G. (2014). Bion and the sublime: The origins of an aesthetic paradigm. *IJPA*, 95(6), 1059–1086.

Clarkin, J.F., Yeomans, F.E. & Kernberg, O.F. (1999). *Psychotherapy for borderline personality*. New York: Wiley.

Clarkin, J.F., Levy, K.N., Lenzenweger, M.F. & Kernberg, O.F. (2007) Evaluating three treatments for borderline personality disorder: a three-wave study. *AJP*, 164, 922–928.

Claus, H. (2011) *De Wolken*. Amsterdam: Bezige Bij.

Cloitre, M (2015) The 'one size fits all' approach to trauma treatment: should we be satisfied? *European Journal of Psychotraumatology*, 6, Article 27344.

Cluckers, G. & Meurs, P. (2005). Bruggen tussen denk-wijzen. In M. Kinet & R. Vermote (Eds.), *Mentalisatie*. AAG.

Cluckers, G., Vliegen, N. & Leroy, C. (Eds.) (2012). *Het raadsel autism: psychoanalytische therapie?* AAG.

Cocteau, J. (1934). *La machine infernale*. Paris: Bernard Grasset.

Conrad, P. (1999). *De ovementose van de wereld: de cultuurgeschiedenis van de twintigste eeuw*. Amsterdam: Anthos/Manteau.

Corveleyn, J., Luyten, P. & Blatt, S. (2005). *The theory and treatment of depression: towards a dynamic interactionism model*. Leuven: Peeters UP.

Courteaux, W. (1987). *William Shakespeare: verzameld werk*. Kapellen: DNB/Pelckmans.

Crits-Cristoph, P. & Barber, J.P. (1991). *Handbook of short-term dynamic psychotherapy*. New York: Basic Books.

Daenen, E.W.P.M., van Reekum, A.C., Knapen, P.M.F.J.J., Verheul, R. (2005). Langerdurende psychotherapie is effectief. Een kritisch literatuuroverzicht per stoornis. *TVPS*, 47(9), 603–611.

Damasio, A.R. (1994). *Descartes' error: emotion, reason, and the human brain*. New York: Putnam.

Davanloo, H. (1990). *Unlocking the unconscious*. New York: Wiley.

Dawkins, R. (1986). *The blind watchmaker*. New York: Norton.

De Block, A. (2003). *Psychoanalyse en de menselijke natuur*. Amsterdam: Boom.

De Block, A. & Moyaert, P. (Eds.) (2004). *Oneigenlijk gebruik. De psychoanalyse voorbij haar grenzen*. Kapellen: Pelckmans.

De Jonghe, F, Rynierse, P. & Janssen, R. (1987). Uitzicht op inzicht: een psycho-analytisch beschreven spectrum van behandelingsmethoden. *TVP*, 13(4), 180–190.

De Jonghe, F, Rynierse, P. & Janssen, R. (1988a). Uitzicht op inzicht II: een psycho-analytisch beschreven spectrum van persoonlijkheidsstructuren. *TVP*, 14, 12–15.

De Jonghe, F, Rynierse, P. & Janssen, R. (1988b). Uitzicht op inzicht III: over het mogelijke en het nodige. *TVP*, 14(2), 91–99.

De Kesel, M. (2002). *Eros en Ethiek*. Leuven/Leusden: Acco.

De Kesel, M. (2019). *Het Münchhausenparadigma. Waarom Freud & Lacan ertoe doen*. Nijmegen: Vantilt.

De Klyen, M. & Greenberg, M.T. (2008). Attachment and psychopathology in childhood. In J. Cassidy & P.R. Shaver (Eds.) *Handbook of attachment: theory, research, and clinical applications* (2nd ed., pp. 637–665). New York: Guilford.

De Saussure, F. (1916). *Course in General Linguistics*. Columbia UP, 2011.

De Waal, F. (2005). *De aap in ons*. Amsterdam: Olympus, 2020.

De Wolf, H.M.H. (2002). *Inleiding in de psychoanalytische psychotherapie*. Bussum: Boutinho.

Declercq, F. (2000). *Het Reële bij Lacan*. Gent: Idesça.

Dehing, J. (Ed.) (1998). *Een bundel intense duisternis: psychoanalytische opstellen rond W.R. Bion*. Leuven/Apeldoorn: Garant.

Dehing, J. (Ed.) (2007). *Hysterie en psychoanalyse: springlevend ondanks onrustwekkende verdwijning.* AAG.

Dekens, O. (2015). *Le structuralisme.* Paris: Collin.

Deleuze, G. (1992). Postscript on the societies of Control. https://libcom.org/library/postscript-on-the-societies-of-control-gilles-deleuze.

Dennett, D. (1995). *Darwin's dangerous idea: evolution and the meanings of life.* New York: Allen.

Derksen, J. & Markx, O. (Eds.) (2003). *Steungevende psychotherapie op psychoanalytische basis.* Utrecht: De Tijdstroom.

Descartes, R. (1641). *Meditaties.* Amsterdam: Boom, 1989.

Desmet, M. (2018). *The pursuit of objectivity in psychology.* Antwerp: Owl.

Didier-Weill, A. (2001). *Quartier Lacan.* Paris: Denoël.

Dilthey, W. (1988). *Introduction to the human sciences: an attempt to lay a foundation for the study of society and history.* Detroit: Wayne State UP.

Doering, S., Horz, S., Rentrop, M., Fischer-Kern, M., Schuster, P., Benecke, C.*et al.* (2010). Transference-focused psychotherapy vs treatment by community psychotherapists for borderline personality disorder: Randomised controlled trial. *BJP,* 196, 389–395.

Doidge, N., Simon, B., Gilles, L.A. & Ruskin, R. (1994). Characteristics of psychoanalytic patients under a nationalized health plan: DSM-IIIR diagnoses, previous treatment and childhood trauma. *AJP,* 151, 586–590.

Doidge, N. (1997). Empirical evidence for the efficacy of psychoanalytic psychotherapies and psychoanalysis: an overview. *Psychoanalytic Inquiry,* 17 (suppl), 102–150.

Dor, J. (1988). *L'Ascientificité de la psychanalyse.* Paris: Denoël.

Dor, J. (1997). *The clinical Lacan.* Northvale NJ: Jason Aronson.

Doran, R. (2015). *The theory of the sublime from Longinus to Kant.* London: Cambridge UP.

Dresden, S. (1952). *Montaigne: de spelende wijsgeer.* Leiden: Leiden UP.

Dufrenne, M. (1967). *Phénoménologie de l'experience esthétique.* Paris: PUF.

Dunn, J. (1995). Intersubjectivity in psychoanalysis: a critical review. *IJPA,* 76, 723–738.

Duras, M. (1984). *L'amant.* Paris: Minuit.

Eco, U. (1962). *The Open Work.* Tr. A. Cancogni. Cambridge MA: Harvard UP, 1989.

Durkin, H.E. (1964). *The group in depth.* New York: International UP.

Edelman, G.M. (1993). *Bright air, brilliant fire: on the matter of the mind.* New York: Basic Books.

Eigen, M. (1998). *The psychoanalytic mystic.* London/New York: Free Association Press.

Eigen, M. (2004). *The sensitive self.* Middletown CT: Wesleyan UP.

Eissler, K. (1965). *Medical orthodoxy and the future of psychoanalysis.* New York: International UP.

Eliot, T.S. (1941). *A choice of Kipling's verse made by T.S. Eliot.* London: Faber and Faber, 1963.

Eliot, T.S. (1944). *Four quartets.* London: Faber and Faber, 2019.

Ellenberger, H. (1970). *The discovery of the unconscious: the history and evolution of dynamic psychiatry.* New York: Basic Books.

Emde, R.N. (1988). Development terminable and interminable. Innate and motivational factors from infancy. *IJPA,* 69: 23–42.

Engel, G. (1962). *Psychological development in health and disease.* Philadelphia: Saunders.

Erickson, M. (1992). *Onbewust leren.* Drempt: Uitgeverij Karnak.

Erikson, E. (1950). *Childhood and society.* New York: Vintage, 2010.

Etchegoyen, R.H. & Miller, J.-A. (1996). *Silence brisé: entretien sur le mouvement psychanalytique.* Paris: Seuil.

Etchegoyen, R.H. (1999). *The fundamentals of psychoanalytic technique* (2nd ed.). London/New York: Karnac.

Evans, D. (2006). *An introductory dictionary of Lacanian psychoanalysis.* London/New York: Routledge.

Eysenck, H.J. (1985). *Decline and fall of the Freudian empire.* London: Viking.

Farberman, H. A. (1985). The foundations of symbolic interaction: James, Cooley, and Mead. *Studies in Symbolic Interaction,* Suppl 1, 13–27.

Ferbos, C. (1986). La notion de structure dans la théorie psychanalytique. In C. Ferbos & A. Magoudi, *Approche psychanalytique des toxicomanes* (pp. 45–80). Paris: PUF.

Ferro, A. (1996). *In the analyst's consulting room.* Hove: Brunner-Routledge, 2002.

Ferro, A. (2015). *Torments of the soul: psychoanalytic transformations in dreaming and narration.* London/New York: Routledge.

Ferry, L. (2009). *Après Heidegger: l'oeuvre philosophique expliquée.* Paris: Gallimard.

Ferry, L. (2010). *La bohème, le bourgeois et l'amour: l'éthique de la mondialisation.* Paris: Gallimard.

Fink, B. (1997). *A clinical introduction to Lacanian psychoanalysis.* London: Harvard UP.

Fisher, H. (2004). *Why we love: the nature and chemistry of romantic love.* London: Macmillan.

Fisher, S. & Greenberg, R.P. (1996). *Freud scientifically reappraised: testing the theories and therapy.* New York: Wiley.

Florence, J. (1985). *Ouvertures psychanalytiques.* Bruxelles: Publications des Facultés Univ. St-Louis.

Flückiger, C., Del Re, A.C., Wampold, B.E., Symonds, D., & Horvath, A.O. (2012). How central is the alliance in psychotherapy? A multilevel longitudinal meta-analysis. *Journal of Counseling Psychology,* 59(1), 10.

Fonagy, P. (1999). The process of remembering: recovery and discovery. *IJPA,* 80, 961–978.

Fonagy, P. (2001). *Attachment theory and psychoanalysis.* London: Karnac.

Fonagy, P. (2003a). Genetics, developmental psychopathology and psychoanalytic theory: the case for ending our (not so) splendid isolation. *Psychoanalytic Inquiry,* 23, 218–247.

Fonagy, P. (2003b). Some complexities in the relationship of psychoanalytic theory to technique. *PQ,* 72(1), 13–47.

Fonagy, P. (2008). A genuinely developmental theory of sexual enjoyment and its implications for psychoanalytic technique. *JAPA,* 56 (II), 11–36.

Fonagy, P. & Target, M. (1997). Attachment and reflective functioning: their role in self-organization. *Development & Psychopathology,* 9, 679–700.

Fonagy, P., Kächele, H., Krausen, R., Jones, E., Perron, R., Lopez, L. (1999). *An open-door review of outcome studies in psychoanalysis.* London: IPA.

Fonagy, P. & Target, M. (2003). *Psychoanalytic theories: perspectives from developmental psychopathology.* England: Whurr.

Fonagy, P., Gergely, G., Jurist, E. & Target, M. (2002). *Affect regulation, mentalization and the development of the self.* New York: Other Press.

Fonagy, P., Target, M., Gergely, G. (2006). Psychoanalytic perspectives on developmental psychopathology. In D. Cicchetti & D.J. Cohen (Eds.), *Developmental psychopathology, Vol 1: Theory and method* (2nd ed. pp 701–749) Hoboken, NJ: Wiley.

Ford, J.D. & Courtois, C.A. (Eds.) (2009). *Treating complex traumatic stress disorders: an evidence-based guide.* New York: Guilford.

Ford, J.D., Fallot, R.D. & Harris, M. (2009). Group therapy. In C.A. Courtois & J.D. Ford (Eds.), *Treating complex traumatic stress disorders: an evidence-based guide* (pp. 415–440). New York: Guilford.

Foucault, M. (1961). *Histoire de la folie à l'âge classique.* Paris: Gallimard.

Foulkes S.H. (1964). *Therapeutic Group Analysis.* New York: International UP, 1977.

Foulkes, S.H. & Anthony, E.J. (1967). *Group psychotherapy: the psychoanalytic approach.* Harmondsworth: Penguin.

Frances, A. (2013). *Terug naar normaal.* Amsterdam: Nieuwezijds.

Franckx, C. & Hebbrecht, M. (2023). *Het kinderlijk trauma: verloren tussen tederheid en passie.* AHGS.

Freud, A. (1927). Four lectures on child analysis. In *The writings of Anna Freud* (Vol I). New York: International UP, 1974.

Freud, A. (1936). The Ego and the mechanisms of defence. In *The writings of Anna Freud* (Vol II). New York: International UP, 1974.

Freud, S. (1895a). *Het Ontwerp.* Tr. G. Van de Vijver & F. Geerardyn. Gent: Idesça, 1992.

Freud, S. (1895b). *Studies over hysterie.* K.B.**5**. SFNE: 39–354. FW1: 441–702. SE2.

Freud, S. (1896). *Over de etiologie van de hysterie.* K.B.**1**. SFNE: 13–45. FW1: 787–813. SE31: 91–222.

Freud, S. (1900). *De droomduiding.* P.D.**2/3**. SFNE: 1–713. FW2: 22–582. SE4: 1–338. SE5: 339–627.

Freud, S. (1901a). *Psychopathologie van het dagelijks leven.* PD1. SFNE: 23–319. FW3: 64–310. SE6: 1–279.

Freud, S. (1901b). *On Dreams.* SE5: 633–686.

Freud, S. (1905a). *Drie verhandelingen over de theorie van de seksualiteit.* KB1 SFNE: 55–177. FW4: 9–105. SE7: 123–243.

Freud, S. (1905b). *Fragment van de analyse van een geval van hysterie.* Z.G.**2**. SFNE: 17–145. FW4: 124–225.

Freud, S. (1905c). *De grap en haar relatie tot het onbewuste.* P.D.**5**. SFNE: 17–263. FW3: 346–557. SE8: 1–236.

Freud, S., (1908). *Infantiele theorieën over seksualiteit.* K.B.**2**. SFNE: 83–99. FW4: 374–387. SE9: 205–226.

Freud, S. (1909). *Analyse van de fobie van een vijfjarige jongen ('kleine Hans').* Z.G.**1**. SFNE: 17–159. FW4: 431–543. SE10: 1–147.

Freud, S. (1910). *De toekomstkansen van de psychoanalytische therapie.* P.B.**1**. SFNE. p 11–24. FW5 p 278–287. SE11: 139–151.

Freud, S. (1912a). *Bijdragen tot de psychologie van het liefdeleven II: over de meest verbreide vernedering in het liefdeleven.* K.B.**2**. SFNE: 183–198. FW5: 480–491. SE11: 177–190.

Freud, S. (1912b). *Adviezen voor de arts bij de psychoanalytische behandeling.* K.B.**4**. SFNE: 87–99. FW5: 494–502. SE11: 109–122.

Freud, S. (1912–1913). *Totem en taboe*. C.R.**4**. SFNE: 21–211. FW6: 15–167. SE13 VII–XIV:1–161.

Freud, S. (1913). *De dispositie tot dwangneurose (Een bijdrage aan het probleem van de neurosekeuze)*. KB2 SFNE: 153–163. FW6: 246–254. SE12: 311–326.

Freud, S. (1914a). *Verdere adviezen over de psychoanalytische techniek (II) Her- inneren*, herhalen en doorwerken. K.B.**4**: 133–143.SFNE. FW6: 425–433. SE12: 145–156.

Freud, S. (1914b). *Over de geschiedenis van de psychoanalytische beweging*. P.B. **1**. SFNE: 59–132. FW6: 359–416. SE14: 7–66.

Freud, S. (1914c). *Ter introductie van het narcisme*. P.T. **1**. SFNE: 27–64. FW6: 329– 355. SE14: 67–102.

Freud, S. (1915a). *Driften en hun lotgevallen*. PT2 SFNE: 39–65. FW7: 23–44. SE14: 109–140.

Freud, S. (1915b). *Verslag van een met de psychoanalytische theorie strijdig geval van paranoia*. ZG2 SFNE: 163–174. FW7: 169–180. SE14: 261–272.

Freud, S. (1916–1917a). *Colleges inleiding tot de psychoanalyse I.P.* **1/2**. SFNE: 19– 498. FW7: 217–606. SE15–16:1–463.

Freud, S. (1916–1917b). *Rouw en melancholie*. PT1 SFNE: 73–91. FW7: 129–148. SE14: 237–258.

Freud, S. (1917). *A metapsychological supplement to the theory of dreams*. SE14: 217– 235.

Freud, S. (1918). *Uit de geschiedenis van een kinderneurose ('de Wolvenman')*. Z.G.**3**. SFNE: 21–159; FW6: 474–482. SE17: 1–122.

Freud, S. (1919). *Wegen der psychoanalytische therapie*. K.B.**4**. SFNE: 179–189. FW8: 50–58. SE17: 157–168.

Freud, S. (1920). *Aan gene zijde van het lustprincipe*. P.T.**1**. SFNE. p 95–163; FW162– 218. SE18: 1–64.

Freud, S. (1921). *Massapsychologie en Ik-analyse*. C.R.**5**. SFNE. p 11–93; FW8 p. 225–292. SE18 p 65–143.

Freud, S. (1923a). *Het Ik en het Es*. PT3 SFNE: 22–82. FW8 371–427. SE19 1–59.

Freud, S. (1923b). *De genitale organisatie bij het kind*. K.B. **3**. SFNE: 75–80. FW8: 482–486. SE19: 139–145.

Freud, S. (1924a). *Het masochisme als economisch probleem*. PT1 SFNE: 171–185. FW9: 18–31. SE19: 155–170.

Freud, S. (1924b). *De ondergang van het Oedipus-complex*. K.B. **3**. SFNE. p 85–92. FW9 34–40. SE19 p 171–179.

Freud, S. (1925a). *De weerstanden tegen de psychoanalyse*. P.B.**2**. SFNE: 93–103. FW9: 140–148. SE19: 213–222.

Freud, S. (1925b). *Zelfportret*. PB2 SFNE: 15–83. FW9: 75–137. SE20: 7–70.

Freud, S. (1925c). *Notitie over het 'Toverblok'*. PT3 SFNE: 103–112. FW9: 68–74. SE19: 225–232.

Freud, S. (1926a). *Remming, symptoom en angst*. P.T.**3**. SFNE: 125–228; FW9: 186– 271. SE20: 75–172.

Freud, S. (1926b). *Het vraagstuk van de lekenanalyse*. P.B. **2**. SFNE: 111–186. FW9: 276–338. SE20: 177–250.

Freud, S. (1928). *Dostojevski en de vadermoord*. CR2 SFNE: 203–223. FW9: 430–449. SE21: 173–194.

Freud, S. (1930a). *Goetheprijs. Brief aan Dr Alfons Paquet*. FW10: 11–19. SE21: 205–207.

Freud, S. (1930b). *Het onbehagen in de cultuur.* C.R. **3**. SFNE: 79–173; FW9: 456–532. SE21: 57–145.

Freud, S. (1931). *Over de vrouwelijke seksualiteit.* K.B.**3**. SFNE: 123–145. FW: 41–58. SE21: 221–243.

Freud, S. (1933). *Colleges inleiding tot de psychoanalyse.* Nieuwe Reeks. I.P.3. SFNE: 13–202. FW10: 79–232. SE22: 1–182.

Freud, S. (1937a). *De eindige en de oneindige analyse.* K.B.**4**. SFNE: 225–265. FW10: 270–305. SE23: 209–253.

Freud, S. (1937b). *Constructies in de analyse.* K.B.**4**. SNFE: 271–283. FW10: 308–319. SE23: 255–269.

Freud, S. (1940). *Hoofdlijnen van de psychoanalyse.* I.P. **1/ 2**. SFNE: 73–150. FW10: 446–503. SE 23: 144–207.

Fromentin C. (2021) La vérité de la clinique psychanalytique. *L'Évolution Psychiatrique,* 86(2), 229–244.

Gabbard, G.O. (1997). A reconsideration of objectivity in the analyst. *IJPA*, 78(1), 15.

Gabbard, G.O. (2000a). Empirical evidence and psychotherapy: a growing scientific base. *AJP*, 158(1), 1–3.

Gabbard, G.O. (2000b). Psychotherapy of personality disorders. *Journal of Psychotherapy: Practice and Research*, 9(1), 1–6. Review.

Gabbard, G.O. (2001). Psychodynamic psychotherapy of borderline personality disorder: a contemporary approach. *Bulletin of the Menninger Clinic*, 65(1), 41–57. Review.

Gabbard, G.O. (2014) *Psychodynamic psychiatry in clinical practice* (5th ed.). Arlington: American Psychiatric Publishing.

Galatzer-Levy, R., Bachrach, H., Skolnikoff, A. & Waldron, S. (2000). *Does psychoanalysis work?* New Haven: Yale UP.

Gay, P. (1989). *Sigmund Freud: zijn leven en werk.* Baarn: Tirion.

Geldhof, A. (2014). *Alleen met kunst: drie gevalstudies over het sinthoom.* Leuven-Den Haag: Acco.

Geyskens, T. & Van Haute, P. (2003). *Van doodsdrift tot hechtingstheorie: het primaat van het kind bij Freud, Klein en Hermann.* Amsterdam: Boom.

Gilliéron, E. (1983). *Aux confins de la psychanalyse.* Paris: Payot.

Gilliéron, E. (1997). *Manuel de psychothérapies brèves.* Paris: Dunod.

Godfrind, J. (1993). *Les deux courants du transfert.* Paris: PUF.

Goldner, E.M. & Bilsker, D. (1995). Evidence-based psychiatry. *Canadian Journal of Psychiatry*, 4, 97–101.

Goethe, J.W. (1790). *Faust.* Amsterdam: Arbeiderspers, 2012.

Gould, S.J. (1981). *The mismeasure of man.* New York: Norton.

Grant, S., Norton, S., Weiland, R.F., Scheeren, A.M., Begeer, S. & Hoekstra, R.A. (2022). Autism and chronic ill health: an observational study of symptoms and diagnoses of central sensitivity syndromes in autistic adults. *Molecular Autism*, 13 (1), 7.

Green, A. (1972). Note sur les processus tertiaires: a propos des critères psychanalytique de la normalité. *Revue française de psychanalyse*, 36(3), 407–410.

Green, A. (1983). *Narcissisme de vie, narcissisme de mort.* Paris: Minuit.

Green, A. (1988). Pourquoi le mal? In J.B. Pontalis (Ed.), *Le Mal* (pp. 399–438). Paris: Gallimard.

Green, A. (1995a). *La causalité psychique: entre nature et culture*. Paris: Odile Jacob.

Green, A. (1995b). Has sexuality anything to do with psychoanalysis? *IJPA*, 76, 871–883.

Green, A. (2007). *Pourquoi les pulsions de destruction ou de mort?* Paris: Éditions du Panama.

Green, A.*et al.* (1986). La pulsion de mort. *Premier symposium de la Fédération Européenne de Psychanalyse* (Marseille, 1984). Paris: PUF.

Greenson, R. (1967). *The technique and practice of psycho-analysis*. London: Hogarth.

Grinberg, L. (1980). The closing phase of the psychoanalytic treatment of adults and the goals of psychoanalysis: 'The search for truth about one's self'. *IJPA*, 61(1), 25–37.

Grinberg, L., Sor, D. & Tabak de Bianchedi, E. (1971). *New introduction to the work of Bion*. Northvale NJ: Jason Aronson, 1996 revised edition.

Groen, J.A. (1986). *Afgunst regeert de wereld*. Meppel: Boom.

Grosskurth, P. (1987). *Melanie Klein: her world and her work*. Cambridge MA: Harvard UP.

Grosz, S. (2013). *The examined life: how we lose and find ourselves*. London/New York: Norton.

Grotjahn, M. (1963). *Sigmund Freud–Oskar Pfister: Briefe [Letters]. 1909–1939*. E.L. Freud & H. Meng (Eds.). Frankfurt-am-Main: Fischer.

Grotstein, J. (1981). *Who is the dreamer who dreams the dream and who is the dreamer who understands it? Do I dare disturb the universe?* London: Karnac.

Gunderson, J.G., Frank, A.F., Katz, H.M.*et al.* (1984). Effects of psychotherapy in schizophrenia. II. Comparative outcome of two forms of treatment. *Schizophrenia Bulletin*, 10, 564–596.

Gunderson, J.G. & Gabbard, G.O. (1999). Making the case for psychoanalytic therapies in the current psychiatric environment. *JAPA*, 47, 679–704.

Hanly, C. (2006). Tradition and truth in psychoanalysis. *American Imago*, 63(3), 261–282.

Hanly, C. (2009). On truth and clinical psychoanalysis, *IJPA*, 90(2), 363–373.

Harari, Y.N. (2011). *Sapiens: een kleine geschiedenis van de mensheid*. Amsterdam: Thomas Rap.

Hardy, T. (1874). *Far from the madding crowd*. London: Penguin, 2003.

Harlow, H.F. (1958). The nature of love. *American Psychologist*, 13, 673–685.

Harlow, H.F., Gluck, J.P. & Suomi, S.J. (1972). Generalization of behavioural data between nonhuman and human animals. *American Psychologist*, 27(8), 709–716.

Harlow, H.F., Plubell, P.E. & Baysinger, C.M. (1973). Induction of psychological death in rhesus monkeys. *Journal of Autism and Childhood Schizophrenia*, 3(4), 299–307.

Hartman, J. (1982). PSM. Ideologie en praktijk. In J. van de Lande (Ed.), *Opgenomen in de groep: psychotherapeutische gemeenschappen in Nederland*. Amsterdam: Van Loghum Slaterus.

Hebbrecht, M. (1997). Behandelen met liefde. *TVPS*, 39, 912–922.

Hebbrecht, M. (1998). Spelen met grenzen. *TVPA*, 4, 192–204.

Hebbrecht, M. (2001). Beschouwingen over regressie op afdelingsniveau. *TVPA*, 7, 221–232.

Hebbrecht, M. (2004). De psychiater als steunfiguur. *TVPS*, 4, 211–222.

Hebbrecht, M. (2005). Zoals een liefdevol sprekende spiegel. De narcistische patiënt in psychoanalytische psychotherapie. In M. Kinet & L. Moyson (Eds.), *Grootse patiënten, kleine therapeuten: psychotherapie en narcisme*. AAG.

Heim, E. (1985). *Praxis der Milieutherapie*. Berlin: Springer.

Herman, J.L. (1992). *Trauma and recovery*. New York: Basic Books.

Herman, J.L. (1993). Sequelae of prolonged and repeated trauma: Evidence for a complex posttraumatic syndrome. In J.R.T. Davidson & E.B. Foa (Eds.), *Posttraumatic stress disorder: DSM-IV and beyond* (pp. 213–228). Washington DC: American Psychiatric Press.

Herman, J.L., Perry, J.C., Kolk, B.A. van der. (1989). Childhood trauma in borderline personality disorder. *AJP*, 147, 490–495.

Hertmans, S. (1999). *Waarover men niet spreken kan*. Brussels: VUB press.

Heyde, L. (2000). *De maat van de mens: over autonomie, transcendentie en sterfelijkheid*. Amsterdam: Boom.

Heyes, C.M. (1998). Theory of mind in Nonhuman Primates. *Behavioural and Brain Sciences*, 21, 101–134.

Hill, C. E., Sim, W., Spangler, P., Stahl, J., Sullivan, C. & Teyber, E. (2008). Therapist immediacy in brief psychotherapy: Case study II. *Psychotherapy: Theory, Research, Practice, Training*, 45(3), 298–315.

Hillenaar, H. (1982). *Roland Barthes: existentialisme, semiotiek, psychoanalyse*. Assen: Van Gorcum.

Hinshelwood, R.D. (1987). *What happens in groups, psychoanalysis, the individual and the community*. London: Free Association Books.

Hinshelwood, R.D. (2005). Group psychotherapy as psychic containing. *International Journal of Group Psychotherapy*, 58, 283–302.

Hoff, P. & Hippius, H. (2001). Wilhelm Griesinger (1817–1868): sein Psychiatrieverständnis aus historischer und aktueller Perspektive. *Der Nervenarzt*, 72, 885–892.

Hoffer, W. (1952). The mutual influences in the development of Ego and Id: earliest stages. *The Psychoanalytic Study of the Child*, 7(1), 31–41.

Høglend, P., Amlo, S., Marble, A., Bøgwald, K.P., Sørbye, Ø., Sjaastad, M.C. & Heyerdahl, O. (2006). Analysis of the patient-therapist relationship in dynamic psychotherapy: An experimental study of transference interpretations. *AJP*, 163 (10), 1739–1746.

Høglend, P., Bøgwald, K.P., Amlo, S., Marble, A., Ulberg, R., Sjaastad, M.C., ... & Johansson, P. (2008). Transference interpretations in dynamic psychotherapy: do they really yield sustained effects? *AJP*, 165(6), 763–771.

Høglend, P., Hersoug, A.G., Bøgwald, K.P., Amlo, S., Marble, A., Sørbye, Ø., ... & Crits-Christoph, P. (2011). Effects of transference work in the context of therapeutic alliance and quality of object relations. *Journal of Consulting and Clinical Psychology*, 79(5), 697–706.

Holmes, J. (2014). *John Bowlby and attachment theory*. London/New York: Routledge.

Houellebecq, M. (1988). *Elementaire deeltjes*. Amsterdam: Arbeiderspers, 2009.

Hubble, M.A., Duncan, B.L. & Miller, S.D. (Ed.) (1999). *The heart and soul of change: what works in therapy*. Washington DC: APA.

Hull *et al.* (2017). "Putting on my best normal": social camouflaging in adults with autism spectrum conditions, https://discovery.ucl.ac.uk/id/eprint/1558346/1/Hull%20Putting%20On%20My%20Best%20Normal%20JADD.pdf.

Hunter, G.K. (Ed.) (1968). *Macbeth*. New Penguin Shakespeare.

Ingenhoven, T.J.M., Abraham, R.E. & Hartman, J. (2000). Persoonlijkheidsstoornissen. In C. Janzing, A. van den Berg & F. Kruisdijk (Eds.), *Handboek voor milieutherapie* (pp. 30–55), Assen: Van Gorcum.

Janis, I.L. (1972). *Victims of groupthink: a psychological study of foreign-policy decisions and fiascoes.* Boston: Houghton, Mifflin.

Janzing, C. & Lansen, J. (1985). *Milieutherapie.* Maastricht: Van Gorcum.

Jaspers, K. (1913). *Algemeine Psychopathologie.* Berlin: Springer.

Johansson, P., Høglend, P., Ulberg, R., Amlo, S., Marble, A., Bøgwald, K.P., ... & Heyerdahl, O. (2010). The mediating role of insight for long-term improvements in psychodynamic therapy. *Journal of consulting and clinical psychology,* 78(3), 438–448.

Jones, E. (1953). *The life and works of Sigmund Freud.* 3 Vols. London: Hogarth/New York: Basic Books.

Jones, M. (1968). *Social psychiatry in practice: the idea of the therapeutic community.* Harmondsworth: Penguin.

Jongerius, P.J. (1981). De psychiater als milieukundig ingenieur. *TVPS,* 23, 317–325.

Jongerius, P.J. & Rylant, R.F. (1989). *Milieu als methode: theorie en praktijk van de methodische milieuhantering in de GGZ.* Amsterdam: Boom.

Jongerius, P.J. & Eyckman, J.C.B. (1993). *Praktijkboek groepstherapie.* Assen: Van Gorcum.

Jonkers, P. (2020). Philosophy and wisdom. *Algemeen Nederlands T voor Wijsbegeerte,* 12(3), 261–277.

Jordan, J.F. (2012). Projective identification and the weight of intersubjectivity. In E. Spillius & E. O'Shaughnessy (Eds.), *Projective identification* (pp. 354–364). London/New York: Routledge.

Joseph, B. (1985). Transference: the total situation. *IJPA,* 66, 447–454.

Joseph, B. (1987). *Projective identification: some clinical aspects.* In J. Sandler (Ed.), *Projection, identification, projective identification* (pp. 65–76). London: Karnac.

Joyce, J. (1922). *Ulysses.* Paris: Shakespeare and Company.

Jung, C.G. (1961). *Memories, dreams, reflections.* New York: Random House.

Kächele, H. (2001). The spectrum of psychoanalysis: does psychoanalysis work? *JAPA,* 34, 1041–1047.

Kaës, R. (1994). *La parole et le lien: processus associatifs dans les groupes.* Paris: Dunod.

Kaës, R. (2000). *L'appareil psychique groupal.* Paris: Dunod.

Kaës, R. (2004). *Le groupe et le sujet du groupe.* Paris: Dunod.

Kandel, E.R. (1998). A new intellectual framework for psychiatry. *AJP,* 155, 457–469.

Kandel, E.R. (1999). Biology and the future of psychoanalysis. *AJP,* 156, 505–524.

Kant, I. (1790). *Over schoonheid.* J.-P. Rondas & J. De Visscher (Eds.) Amsterdam: Boom, 1987.

Kaplan, M.J. (1997). Psychoanalysis, psychiatry and psychobiology: how do we help patients as we search for a new equilibrium? *Journal of Clinical Psychoanalysis,* 6 (3), 417–438.

Kaplan-Solms, K. & Solms, M. (2000). *Clinical studies in neuropsychoanalysis: introduction to a depth neuropsychology.* London: Karnac.

Katz, W.W. (2016). The experience of truth in psychoanalysis today, *PQ,* 85(2), 503–530.

Kazdin, A.E. (1986). Comparative outcome studies of psychotherapy: methodological issues and strategies. *Journal of Consulting and Clinical Psychology,* 54, 95–105.

Kemp, R. & Lorentzatou, D. (2013). The place of truth in psychoanalysis: a Heideggerian contribution, *European Journal of Psychotherapy & Counselling,* 15(1), 5–17.

Kennedy, R. (1993). *Freedom to relate: psychoanalytic explorations.* London: Free Association Books.

Kernberg, O.F. (1976). *Object relations theory and clinical psychoanalysis.* New York: Jason Aronson.

Kernberg, O.F. (1984a). Psychoanalytic studies of group and organizational leadership. *International Journal of Group Psychotherapy,* 34, 5–24.

Kernberg, O.F. (1984b). *Severe personality disorders.* New Haven: Yale UP.

Kernberg, O.F. (1988). Psychic structure and structural change: an ego psychology-object relations theory viewpoint. *JAPA,* 36, 315–337.

Kernberg, O.F. (1993). Convergences and divergences in psychoanalytic technique. *IJPA,* 74, 659–673.

Kernberg, O.F. (1996). The analyst's authority in the psychoanalytical situation. *PQ,* LXV, 137–157.

Kernberg, O.F. (1999). Psychoanalysis, psychoanalytic psychotherapy and supportive psychotherapy: contemporary controversies. *IJPA,* 80, 1075–1091.

Kernberg, O.F., Clarkin, J.F., Yeomans, F.E. (2002). *A primer of transference-focused psychotherapy for the borderline patient.* New York: Jason Aronson.

Kernberg, O.F. & Caligor, E. (2005). A psychoanalytic theory of personality disorders. In M.F. Lenzenweger & J.F. Clarkin (Eds.), *Major theories of personality disorder* (2nd ed., pp. 114–156). New York: Guilford Press.

Kets de Vries, M.F.R. (2021). *Leadership unhinged: essays on the ugly, the bad, and the weird.* London: Palgrave.

Khan, M.M.R. (1963). The concept of cumulative trauma. *The Psychoanalytic Study of the Child,* 18(1), 286–306.

Kienstra, N. (2020). Reconnecting Wisdom and Philosophy. *Algemeen Nederlands Tijdschrift voor Wijsbegeerte,* 112(3), 253–259.

Kinet, M. (1996). Weerzien met…Melanie Klein. *TVP,* 22, 197–211.

Kinet, M. (2002a). Adolescentie en passieprincipe. In A.R. Boerwinkel & A. De Bruyne (Eds.), *Psychoanalyse en passie: over hartstocht en loutering* (pp 25–40). Amsterdam: Boom.

Kinet, M. (2002b). Het passieprincipe: noThing but the Real Thing. In M. Thys & M. Kinet (Eds.) *Liefdesverklaringen* (pp. 155–173). Leuven/Leusden: Acco.

Kinet, M. (2003). Klinische psychotherapie bij angst-, stemming- en persoonlijkheidsstoornissen. Een poging tot integratie tussen psychiatrie en psychoanalyse. In C. Janzing, A. van den Berg, F. Kruisdijk (Eds.), *Handboek milieutherapie deel II.* Assen: Van Gorcum.

Kinet, M. & Moyson, L. (Eds.) (2005a). *Grootse patiënten, kleine therapeuten: over psychotherapie en narcisme.* AAG.

Kinet, M. & Vermote, R. (Eds.) (2005b). *Mentalisatie.* AAG.

Kinet, M. (2005c). Poëzie en psychoanalyse, Muze en mentalisatie. In M. Kinet & R. Vermote (Eds.), *Mentalisatie* (pp. 111–128). AAG.

Kinet, M. (2005d). Reflections in a golden I. In M. Kinet & L. Moyson (Eds.), *Grootse patiënten, kleine therapeuten: over psychotherapie en narcisme* (pp 7–19). AAG.

Kinet, M. (2006). *Freud & Co in de psychiatrie: klinisch-psychotherapeutisch perspectief.* AAG.

Kinet, M. (2006b). Een langgerekte kortsluiting. In M. Kinet (Ed.), *Zuchtigheid en afhankelijkheid in hun relatie met middelenmisbruik.* AAG.

Kinet, M. (2007). Psychoanalytische renaissance. Van interpretatie tot mentalisatie. In M. Kinet & W. Vanmechelen (Eds.), *Tussen ruis en storingen: de golflengte vinden in psychoanalytische therapie* (pp. 11–20). AAG.

Kinet, M. (2007). De groep bestaat niet. In M. Hebbrecht & M. Willemsen (Eds.), *De borderlinepatiënt in dagbehandeling*. AAG.

Kinet, M. (2008). Empathie en empathologie. Als het register van het imaginaire. In M. Hebbrecht & I. Demuynck (Eds.), *Empathie: hoeksteen of struikelblok in psychoanalytische psychotherapie*. AAG.

Kinet, M. (2009). Een Berk met andere takken. De psychoanalytische grondregel vs de groep. In M. Kinet (Ed.), *De groep in psychoanalyse* (pp. 309–338). AAG.

Kinet, M. (2010). A cry in the dark. Appel en antwoord in psychoanalytisch perspectief. In W. Roelofsen*et al.* (Ed.), *Psychoanalytische psychotherapie over grenzen* (pp. 41–50). Assen: Van Gorcum.

Kinet, M. (2011). De groep is/als geschiedenis: in reactie op Berk en Verhagen. *Groepen. Tijdschrift voor Groepsdynamica & Groepspsychotherapie*, 1, 63–73.

Kinet, M. (2013). De vierkantswortel van super. Supervisie vanuit klinisch psychotherapeutisch perspectief. In M. Hebbrecht & N. Vliegen (Eds.), *Supervisie: van psychoanalyse en psychoanalytische therapie* (pp. 123–140). AAG.

Kinet, M. (2014). Op het scherp van de gulden snede. *TVPA*, 3, 219–220.

Kinet, M. (2015a). Tussen diepte- en metaseksuologie: psychoanalyse met het Es van seks. In M. Kinet & K. Baeten (Eds.), *Psychoanalyse als seksuologie? Libido van gesel tot gezel* (pp. 61–86). AAG.

Kinet, M. (2015b). Van Queen Victoria tot Victoria's secret. Een sexy geschiedenis. In M. Kinet & K. Baeten (Eds.), *Psychoanalyse als seksuologie? Libido van gesel tot gezel* (pp. 269–290). AAG.

Kinet, M. (2015). Het sinthoom als kunstgreep. *TVPA*, 1, 70–72.

Kinet, M. (Ed.) (2016). *Trauma binnenstebuiten: verbanden bij psychische wonden*. AAG.

Kinet, M. (2018). *Een psychotherapeutische praktijk: in 7 premissen en 77 portretten*. AHGS.

Kinet, M. (2019). Enkele oedipale variaties: van Darwin tot Lacan. In M. Kinet & W. Heuves (Eds.), *Driehoeksverhoudingen Actuele oedipale variaties* (pp. 51–70). AHGS.

Kinet, M. (2021). *Beter en wijzer door psychotherapie: 31 patiënten vertellen het zelf*. AHGS.

Kinet, M. (2022a). De groep: het onbewuste live on stage. Groepen . *Tijdschrift Nederlandse Vereniging voor Groepsdynamica en Groepspsychotherapie*, 2, 24–41.

Kinet, M. (2022b). *De geest van de drift: over neuropsychoanalyse*. AHGS.

Kinet, M. (2023a). *The spirit of the drive in neuropsychoanalysis*. London/New York: Routledge.

Kinet, M. (2023b). Tien nawoorden. Tussen ça voir en faire ainsi. In C. Franckx & M. Hebbrecht (Eds.), *Het kinderlijk trauma. Verloren tussen tederheid en passie* (pp. 293–305). AHGS.

Kinet, M. (2023c). Psychoanalytische seksualiteit. Tien nawoorden. In W. Heuves & N. Silvester (Eds.), *Seks in de praktijk* (pp. 125–142). AHGS.

Kinet, M. (2023d). Saving Private Ryan. In C. Schmidt-Hellerau, M. Erlich-Ginor (Eds.), *Mind in the line of fire/Mente en la linea de fuego* (pp. 502–506). IPA in the Community & The World Committees.

Kinet, M. (Ed.) (2006). *Zuchtigheid en afhankelijkheid in hun relatie met middelenmisbruik*. AAG.

Kinet, M. & Baeten, K. (Eds.) (2015). *Psychoanalyse als seksuologie? Libido van gesel tot gezel*. AAG.

Kinet, M. & Thys, M. (Eds.) (2016). *Psychoanalytische praktijk tussen onbewuste en wetenschap*. AAG.

Kinet, M. & Heuves, W. (Eds.) (2019). *Driehoeksverhoudingen: actuele oedipale variaties*. AHGS.

King, P. & Steiner, R. (Eds.) (1991). *The Freud-Klein controversies 1941–1945*. London: Tavistock.

King, P. (2003). *No ordinary psychoanalyst: the exceptional contributions of John Rickman*. London: Karnac.

Klein, M. (1926). The psychological principles of early analysis. In *WMK (Vol I)*. London: Hogarth Press (1975).

Klein, M. (1927). Criminal tendencies in normal children. In *Love, guilt and reparation & other works 1921–1945* (pp. 170–185). London: Virago, 1988.

Klein, M. (1928). Early stages of the Oedipus complex. In *WMK (Vol I)*. London: Hogarth, 1975.

Klein, M. (1932). *The psycho-analysis of children*. London: Virago, 1989.

Klein, M. (1935). A contribution to the psychogenesis of manic-depressive states. In *WMK (Vol I)*. London: Hogarth, 1975.

Klein, M. (1940). Mourning and its relation to manic-depressive states. In *WMK (Vol I)*. London: Hogarth, 1975.

Klein, M. (1945). The Oedipus complex in the light of early anxieties. In *WMK (Vol I)*. London: Hogarth, 1975.

Klein, M. (1946). Notes on some schizoid mechanisms. In *Envy and Gratitude & other works 1946–1963* (pp. 1–24). London: Virago, 1988.

Klein, M. (1952). The origins of transference. In *WMK (Vol IV)*. London: Hogarth.

Klein, M. (1955). The psycho-analytic play technique: its history and significance. In *WMK (Vol IV)*. London: Hogarth.

Klein, M (1957). Envy and gratitude. In *WMK (Vol IV)*. London: Hogarth.

Klein, M. (1959). Our adult world and its roots in infancy. In *WMK (Vol IV)*. London: Hogarth.

Klein, M. (1961). *Narrative of a child analysis*. London: Hogarth Press.

Klein, M. (1975). *The Writings of Melanie Klein. (Vols I–IV)*. London: Hogarth.

Klein, R.-H. & Brown, S.-L. (1987) Large group processes and the patient-staff community meeting. *International Journal of Group Psychotherapy*, 2, 219–237.

Klein, Y. (1959). Sorbonne Lecture. In C. Harrison & P. Wood (Eds.), *Art in Theory 1900–1990: an anthology of changing ideas* (pp. 803–805). Oxford UK/Cambridge MA: Blackwell, 1992.

Kluft, R.P. (2000). The psychoanalytic psychotherapy of dissociative identity disorder in the context of trauma therapy. *Psychoanalytic inquiry*, 20(2), 259–286.

Kohut, H. (1968). The evaluation of applicants for psychoanalytic training (A letter written by Anna Freud – p 533). *IJPA*, 49, 548–554.

Kohut, H. (1971). *The analysis of the self*. New York: International UP.

Kohut, H. (1977). *The restoration of the self*. New York: International UP.

Kohut, H. (1984). *How does analysis cure?* Chicago: University of Chicago Press.

Kristeva, J. (1984). *Revolution in poetic language*. New York: Columbia University Press.

Kudler, H.S., Krupnick, J.L., Blank, A.S., Jr., Herman, J.L. & Horowitz, M.J. (2009). Psychodynamic therapy for adults. In E.B. Foa, T.M. Keane, M.J. Friedman & J.A. Cohen (Eds.), *Effective treatments for PTSD: practice guidelines from the*

International Society for Traumatic Stress Studies (2nd ed, pp. 346–369). New York: Guilford.

Kuhn, T.S. (1970). *The structure of scientific revolutions.* Chicago: Chicago UP.

Kulish, N. (2019). Reckoning with sexuality, *IJPA*, 100(6), 1216–1236.

Kunneman, H. (2003). *Kritisch humanisme.* Utrecht: Utrecht UP.

Lacan, J. (1938). *Les complexes familiaux dans la formation de l'individu.* Paris: Navarin, 1984.

Lacan, J. (1947). La psychiatrie anglaise et la guerre. In *Travaux et interventions.* Paris: AREP Editeurs, 1977.

Lacan, J. (1949). Le stade du miroir comme formateur de la fonction du Je. In *E*, 93–100.

Lacan, J. (1950). Propos sur la causalité psychique. In *E*, 151–196.

Lacan, J. (1952). Intervention sur le transfert. In *E*, 215–228.

Lacan, J. (1953). Fonction et champ de la parole et du langage en psychanalyse. In *E*, 237–322.

Lacan, J. (1955a). Variantes de la cure-type. In *E*, 323–362.

Lacan, J. (1955b). La chose freudienne ou Sens du retour à Freud en psychanalyse. In *E*, 401–436.

Lacan, J. (1956). Le Séminaire sur 'la lettre volée'. In *E*, 11–61.

Lacan, J. (1957). L'instance de la lettre dans l'inconscient ou la raison depuis Freud. In *E*, 521.

Lacan, J. (1958a). La direction de la cure et les principes de son pouvoir. In *E*, 585–645.

Lacan, J. (1958b). La signification de phallus. In *E*, 685–696.

Lacan, J. (1958c). La jeunesse de Gide ou la lettre et le désir. In *E*, 739–764.

Lacan, J. (1958d). La psychanalyse vraie, et la fausse. In *Autres ecrits* (pp. 165–174). Paris: Seuil, 2001.

Lacan, J. (1958e) Le rendez-vous chez le psychanalyste. In *La psychanalyse: les psychoses (Vol. 4).* Paris: PUF.

Lacan, J. (1959). Sur la théorie du symbolisme d'Ernest Jones. In *E*, 697–717.

Lacan, J. (1960a). Remarque sur le rapport de Daniel Lagache: psychanalyse et structure de personnalité. In *E*, 647–684.

Lacan, J. (1960b). Propos directifs pour un Congrès sur la sexualité féminine. In *E*, 725–738.

Lacan, J. (1962). Kant avec Sade. In *E*, 765–790.

Lacan, J. (1966a). *Ecrits.* Paris: Seuil.

Lacan, J. (1966b). De nos antécédents. In *E*, 65–72.

Lacan, J. (1966c). La science et la vérité. In *E*, 855–877.

Lacan, J. (1966d). Problèmes cruciaux de la psychoanalyse. In *Autres ecrits* (pp. 199–202). Paris: Seuil, 2001.

Lacan, J. (1971). *Le séminaire. Livre XIX. …Ou pire.* 1971–1972/ Unpublished.

Lacan, J. (1973). *Le séminaire. Livre XI: les quatre concepts fondamentaux de la psychanalyse. 1964.* TMPS.

Lacan, J. (1975a). *Le séminaire. Livre I: les écrits techniques de Freud. 1953–1954.* TMPS.

Lacan, J. (1975b). *Le séminaire. Livre XX: encore. 1972–1973.* TMPS.

Lacan, J. (1975c). *Télévision.* Paris: Du Seuil.

Lacan, J. (1977) *Ecrits: a selection.* Tr. A. Sheridan. New York: Norton.

Lacan, J. (1978). *Le séminaire. Livre II: le moi dans la théorie de Freud et dans la technique de la psychanalyse. 1954–1955.* TMPS.

Lacan, J. (1981a). *Le séminaire de Caracas. 1981.* L'âne no 1.

Lacan, J. (1981b). *Le séminaire. Livre III: les psychoses. 1955–1956.* TMPS.

Lacan, J. (1986). *Le séminaire. Livre VII: l'éthique de la psychanalyse. 1959–1960.* TMPS.

Lacan, J. (1991a). *Le séminaire. Livre VIII: le transfert. 1960–1961.* TMPS.

Lacan, J. (1991b). *Le séminaire. Livre XVII: l'envers de la psychanalyse. 1969–1970.* TMPS.

Lacan, J. (1994). *Le séminaire. Livre IV: la relation d'objet. 1956–1957.* TMPS.

Lacan, J. (1998). *Le séminaire. Livre V: les formations de l'inconscient. 1957–1958.* TMPS.

Lacan, J. (2001). *Autres ecrits.* Paris: Du Seuil.

Lacan, J. (2005a). *Des noms-du-père. 1953/1963.* Paris: Du Seuil.

Lacan, J. (2005b). *Le séminaire. Livre XXIII: le sinthome. 1975–1976.* Texte établi par J.A. Miller. Paris: Du Seuil.

Ladan, A. (2007). De analyticus als 'desillusionist'. *TVPA*, 4, 280–291.

Laermans, R. (1997). *Schimmenspel: essays over de hedendaagse onwerkelijkheid.* Leuven: Van Halewijck.

Langs, R. (1982). *Psychotherapy: a basic text.* New York/London: Jason Aronson.

Laplanche, J. (1976). *Life and death in psychoanalysis.* Baltimore/London: Johns Hopkins UP.

Laplanche, J. (1987). *Nouveaux fondements pour la psychanalyse: la séduction originaire.* Paris: PUF.

Laplanche, J. (1999). *Essays on otherness.* London/New York: Routledge.

Laplanche, J. (2002). Sexuality and attachment in metapsychology. In D. Widlöcher (Ed.), *Infantile sexuality and attachment* (pp. 37–45). New York: Other Press.

Laplanche, J. (2011). *Freud and the sexual: essays, 2000–2006.* Tr. J. Fletcher, J. House & N. Ray. New York: International Psychoanalytic Books.

Laplanche, J. & Pontalis, J.B. (1967). *Vocabulaire de la psychanalyse.* Paris: PUF.

Lasch, C. (1979). *The culture of narcissism.* New York: Warner Books.

Latané, B. & Darley, J. M. (1970). *The unresponsive bystander: why doesn't he help?* New York: Appleton-Century-Croft.

Laufer, M. (1976). The central masturbation fantasy, the final sexual organisation, and adolescence. *PSC*, 31, 297–316.

Le Boulengé, C. (2004). La séance courte: editorial. *Nouvelle Revue de Psychanalyse*, 56, 10–11.

Le Guen, C. (1974). *L'oedipe originaire.* Paris: Payot.

Ledoux, M. (2004). *Waar zijn we toch mee bezig. Institutionele psychotherapie in weerstand en dialoog met de kwaliteitspsychiatrie.* Kessel-Lo: Literarte.

Leichsenring, F. & Leibing, E. (2003). The effectiveness of psychodynamic therapy and cognitive behaviour therapy in the treatment of personality disorders: a meta-analysis. *AJP*, 160, 1223–1232.

Leichsenring, F., Rabung, S. & Leibing, E. (2004). The efficacy of short-term psychodynamic psychotherapy in specific psychiatric disorders: a meta-analysis. *Archives of General Psychiatry*, 61(12), 1208–1216.

Leichsenring, F. (2005). Are psychodynamic and psychoanalytic therapies effective? A review of empirical data. *IJPA*, 86, 841–868.

Leichsenring, F. & Rabung, S. (2011). Effectiveness of long-term psychodynamic psychotherapy in complex mental disorders: update of a meta-analysis. *BJP*, 199, 15–22.

Leichsenring, F., Steinert, C. & Ioannidis, J.P.A. (2019). Toward a paradigm shift in treatment and research of mental disorders. *Psychological Medicine*, 49, 2111–2117.

Leichsenring, F., Steinert, C., Rabung, S. & Ioannidis, J.P.A. (2022). The efficacy of psychotherapies and pharmacotherapies for mental disorders in adults: an umbrella review and meta-analytic evaluation of recent meta-analyses. *World Psychiatry*, 21, 133–145.

Leichsenring, F., Fonagy, P., Heim, N., Kernberg, O.F., Leweke, F., Luyten, P., Salzer, S., Spitzer, C., Steinert, C. (2024). Borderline personality disorder: a comprehensive review of diagnosis and clinical presentation, etiology, treatment, and current controversies. *World Psychiatry*, 23, 4–25.

Lemma, A. (2022). *Transgender identities: a contemporary introduction*. London/New York: Routledge.

Leuzinger-Bohleber, M. (1996). Erinnern in der Ubertragung. Zum interdisziplinären Dialog zwischen Psychoanalyse und biologischer Gedachtnisforschung, *Psychotherapie, Psychosomatik, Medizinische Pscychologie*, 46, 217–227.

Leuzinger-Bohleber, M. (2002). DPV: a representative multicentre study of long-term psychoanalytic therapies. In M. Leuzinger-Bohlever & M. Target (Eds), *Outcomes of Psychoanalytic Treatment*. London: Whurr.

Levine, H.B. (2016). Psychoanalysis and The Problem of Truth, *PQ*, 85(2), 391–409.

Levine, H.B. (2020). The compulsion to repeat: An introduction. *IJPA*, 101(6), 1162–1171.

Levi-Strauss, C. (1949). *Les structures élémentaires de la parenté*. Paris: Ehess, 2017.

Levi-Strauss, C. (1962). *Het wilde denken*. Amsterdam: Meulenhoff, 2009.

Lilliengren, P. (2023). A comprehensive overview of randomized controlled trials of psychodynamic psychotherapies. *Psychoanalytic Psychotherapy*, 37(2), 117–140.

Linden, P.T.H.M. van der (1984). Wat herhaald wordt moet herinnerd worden. Over reconstructieve psychotherapie met gebruikmaking van de klinische setting. *TVPS*, 26, 621–634.

Livesley, W.J., Jang, K.L., Jackson, D.N. & Vernon, P.A. (1993). Genetic and environmental contributions to dimensions of personality disorder. *AJP*, 150(12), 1826–1831.

Lohser, B. & Newton, P.M. (1996). *Unorthodox Freud*. New York: Guilford.

Lombardi, R. (2015). *Formless infinity: clinical explorations of Matte Blanco and Bion*. London/New York: Routledge.

Luborsky, L. (1984). *Principles of psychoanalytic psychotherapy: a manual for supportive-expressive treatment*. New York: Basic Books.

Luborsky, L., Rosenthal, R., Diguer, L., Andrusyna, T.P., Berman, J.S., Levitt, J.T., *et al.* (2002). The dodo bird verdict is alive and well—mostly. *Clinical Psychology: Science and Practice*, 9, 2–12.

Lucebert (1974), *Verzamelde Gedichten*. Amsterdam: Bezige Bij.

Luyten, P. (2001). Psychoanalyse: de berichten over mijn dood zijn (opnieuw) sterk overdreven. *TVPA*, 1, 5–23.

Luyten, P. (2015). Unholy questions about five central tenets of psychoanalysis that need to be empirically verified. *PQ*, 35(1), 5–23.

Luyten, P. & Vliegen, N. (2005). Lost in translation. De invloed van de ziektemetafoor op de classificatie en behandeling van psychopathologie: assumpties en bevindingen. *Tijdschrift Klinische Psychologie*, 4, 243–252.

Luyten, P., Vliegen, N., Van Houdenhove, B. & Blatt, S.J. (2008). Equifinality, multifinality, and the rediscovery of the importance of early experiences. *PSC*, 63, 27–60.

Luyten, P., Blatt, S.J. & Corveleyn, J. (2006). Minding the gap between positivism and hermeneutics in psychoanalytic research. *JAPA*, 54(2), 571–610.

Luyten, P., Mayes, L.C., Fonagy, P., Target, M. & Blatt, S.J. (2015). *Handbook of psychodynamic approaches to psychopathology*. New York: Guilford Press.

Luyten, P. & Lowyck, B. (2016). De effectiviteit van psychodynamische psychotherapie. *Tijdschrift Klinische Psychologie*, 46(4), 271–288.

Luyten, P., Campbell, C., Allison, E. & Fonagy, P. (2020). The mentalizing approach to psychopathology: State of the art and future directions. *Annual review of clinical psychology*, 16, 297–325.

Lyotard, J.F. (1983). *Le différend*. Paris: Minuit.

Mahler, M. (1975). *The psychological birth of the human infant*. New York: Basic Books.

Main, M. & Goldwyn, S. (1995). Interview-based adult attachment classification: related to infant-mother and infant-father attachment. *Developmental Psychology*, 19, 237–239.

Main, M. (1996). Introduction to the special section on attachment and psychopathology: 2. Overview of the field of attachment. *Journal of Consulting and Clinical Psychology*, 64(2), 237–243.

Malan, D. (1979) *Individual Psychotherapy and The Science of Psychodynamics*. Kent: Butterworth.

Malin, A. & Grotstein, J.S. (1966). Projective identification in the therapeutic process. *IJPA*, 47, 26–31.

Malloch, S. & Trevarthen, C. (2018). The human nature of music. *Frontiers in psychology*, 9, 1680.

Masson, J. M. (Ed.) (1985). *The complete letters of Sigmund Freud to Wilhelm Fliess, 1887–1904*. Cambridge/London: Harvard UP.

Matet, J.-D. & Wachsberger, H. (Ed.) (1994). *Comment finissent les analyses. Textes réunis par l'Association Mondiale de Psychanalyse*. Paris: Seuil.

Matte-Blanco, I. (1975), *The unconscious as infinite sets*. London: Duckworth.

McDougall, J. (1982). *Théâtres du Je*. Parix: Gallimard.

McDougall, J. (1996). *Eros aux mille et un visages*. Paris: Gallimard.

McDougall, J. (1978). *Plaidoyer pour une certaine anormalité*. Paris: Gallimard.

McDougall, J. (2003). *Donald Winnicott the man: reflections and recollections*. London: Karnac.

McKay, K.M., Imel, Z.E. & Wampold, B.E. (2006). Psychiatrist effects in the psychopharmacological treatment of depression. *Journal of Affective Disorders*, 92, 287–290.

McWilliams, N. (2011). *Psychoanalytic diagnosis: Understanding personality structure in the clinical process* (2nd ed.) New York: Guilford.

Mendelson, M. (1993). *Psychoanalytic concepts of depression* (2nd ed.). New York/London: Jason Aronson.

Meltzer, D. (1986). *Studies in extended metapsychology*. Perthshire: Clunie.

Midgley, N. (2007). Anna Freud: The Hampstead War Nurseries and the role of the direct observation of children for psychoanalysis. *IJPA*, 88, 939–959.

Migone, P. & Liotti, G. (1998). Psychoanalysis and cognitive-evolutionary psychology: an attempt at integration. *IJPA*, 79, 1071–1095.

Milgram, S. (1974). *Obedience to authority: an experimental view*. London: Tavistock.

Miller, S.D., Duncan, B.L., & Hubble, M.A. (1997). *Escape from Babel: toward a unifying language for psychotherapy practice*. New York/London: Norton.

Miller, J.A. (2002). La théorie du partenaire. *Quarto*, 77/Juillet, 6–33.

Monjauze, M. (1999). *La part alcoolique du soi: la prise en charge clinique des patients alcooliques*. Paris: Dunod.

Mooij, A. (1988). *De psychische realiteit: over psychiatrie als wetenschap*. Amsterdam: Boom.

Mooij, A. (2002). *Psychoanalytisch gedachtegoed*. Amsterdam: Boom.

Mooij, A. (2005). Het vreemde van de psychoanalyse. *TVPA*, 11(1), 24–36.

Moyaert, P. (1991). Fenomenologie van de eros. In H. Bleijendaal, J. Goud & E. Van Hove (Eds.), *Emanuel Levinas over psyche, kunst en moral* (pp. 33–45). Baarn: Ambo.

Moyaert, P. (1994). *Ethiek en sublimatie: over de ethiek van de psychoanalyse van Jacques Lacan*. Nijmegen: SUN.

Moyaert, P. (1998). *De mateloosheid van het Christendom*. Nijmegen: SUN.

Moyaert, P. (2004). Psychoanalyse en seksuologie. In A. De Block & P. Moyaert (Eds.), *Oneigenlijk gebruik: de psychoanalyse voorbij haar grenzen*. Kapellen: Pelckmans.

Mülisch, H. (1984). *Het Ene*. In *De zuilen van Hercules*. Amsterdam: Bezige Bij (1990).

Mülisch, H. (1990). *Oedipus als Freud*. In *De Zuilen van Hercules*. Amsterdam: Bezige Bij.

Murakami, H. (2008). *Na de aardbeving*. Amsterdam: Atlas.

Muran, J.C., Safran, J.D., Gorman, B.S., Samstag, L.W., Eubanks-Carter, C. & Winston, A. (2009). The relationship of early alliance ruptures and their resolution to process and outcome in three time-limited psychotherapies for personality disorders. *Psychotherapy: Theory, Research, Practice, Training*, 46(2), 233–248.

Nader, K. & Hardt, O. (2009). A single standard for memory: the case for reconsolidation. *Nature Reviews Neuroscience*, 10, 224–234.

Nagel, T. (1986). *A view from nowhere*. London: Oxford UP.

Nai, A. & Toros, E. (2020). The peculiar personality of strongmen: comparing the Big Five and Dark Triad traits of autocrats and non-autocrats. *Political Research Exchange*, 2(1), 1701697.

Nasio, J.-D. (1988). *Enseignement de 7 concepts cruciaux de la psychanalyse*. Paris: Rivages.

Nasio, J.-D. (1992). *Cinq leçons sur la théorie de Jacques Lacan*. Paris: Rivages.

Neri, C. (2007). La notion élargie de champ. *Psychothérapies*, 27, 1.

Neri C. (2009). La capacité négative du psychothérapeute de groupe. In R. Kaës & P. Laurent (Eds.), *Le processus thérapeutique dans le groupe* (pp. 53–66). Toulouse: Érès.

Nietzsche, F. (1882). *De vrolijke wetenschap*. Amsterdam: Arbeiderspers, 2003.

Nieweg, E.H. (2005a). De psychiater in spagaat: over de kloof tussen natuur- en geesteswetenschappen. *TVPS*, 47, 239–248.

Nieweg, E.H. (2005b). Wat wij van Jip en Janneke kunnen leren: over reïficatie (verdinglijking) in de psychiatrie. *TVPS*, 47, 687–696.

Nobus, D. (1997). *Key concepts of Lacanian psychoanalysis*. London: Karnac.

Nobus, D. & Quinn, M. (2005). *Knowing nothing, staying stupid: elements for a psychoanalytic epistemology*. London/New York: Routledge, 2013.

Obholzer, K. & Pankejeff, S. (1982). *The Wolf-Man: conversations with Freud's patient – sixty years later*. New York: Continuum/London: Routledge.

Ogata, S.N., Silk, K.R., Goodrich, S. (1990). Childhood sexual and physical abuse in adult patients with borderline personality disorder. *AJP*, 147, 1008–1013.

Ogden, T. (1979). On projective identification. *IJPA*, 60, 357–373.

Ogden, T. (1983). The concept of internal object relations. *IJPA*, 64, 227–241.

Ogden, T. (1994). The analytic third: working with intersubjective clinical facts. *IJPA*, 75, 3–20.

Ogden, T. (1997). *Reverie and interpretation: sensing something human*. Northvale NJ: Jason Aronson.

Ogden, T. (1999). The music of what happens in poetry and psychoanalysis. *IJPA*, 80, 979–994.

Ogden, T.H. (2001). Reading Winnicott. *PQ*, 70(2), 299–323.

Ogden, T. (2002). *Conversations at the frontier of dreaming*. London: Karnac.

Ogden, T.H. (2004). On holding and containing, being and dreaming. *IJPA* 85(6), 1349–1364.

Ogden, T. (2016). On Language and Truth in Psychoanalysis. *PQ*, 85(2), 411–426.

Ogrodniczuk, J.S. & Piper, W.E. (2001). Day treatment for personality disorders: a review of research findings. *Harvard Review of Psychiatry*, 9, 105–117.

Ormel, J., Hollon, S.D., Kessler, R.C., Cuijpers, P., Monroe, S.M. (2022). More treatment but no less depression: the treatment-prevalence paradox. *Clinical Psychology Review*, 91, 102–111.

Ormel, J. (2023). Meer behandeling, maar niet minder depressie: een ongemakkelijke paradox. *Tijdschr Psychiatr*, 65(8), 484–490.

Osswald-Rinner, I. (2011). *Oversexed and underfucked: uber die gesellschaftliche Konstruktion der Lust*. Wiesbaden: Springer.

Paglia, C. (1992). *Het seksuele masker*. Amsterdam: Prometheus.

Panksepp, J. (1998). *Affective Neuroscience: The Foundations of Human and Animal Emotions*. New York: Oxford UP.

Paris, J. (1999). *Nature and nurture in psychiatry: a predisposition-stress model of mental disorder*. Washington DC/London: The American Press.

Pascal, B. (1669). *Pensées*. Paris: Gallimard Folio, 1977.

PDM Task Force (2006). *Psychodynamic diagnostic manual*. Silver Spring, MD: Alliance of Psychoanalytic Organizations.

Peelen, G.J. (Ed.) (2001). *Dichter bij de waarheid: gedachten over poëzie en wetenschap*. Zoetemeer: Meinema.

Perry, J.C., Banon, E. & Ianni, F. (1999). Effectiveness of psychotherapy for personality disorders. *AJP*, 156(9), 1312–1321.

Person, D.S. (1989). *Dreams of love and fateful encounters*. New York: Penguin.

Phillips, A. (1988). *Winnicott*. Cambridge MA: Harvard UP.

Philonenko, M. (2004). Le notre père. *Nouvelle Revue de Psychanalyse*, 56, 15–24.

Pico della Mirandolla, G. (1486). *Rede over de menselijke waardigheid*. Amsterdam: Boom klassiek, 2008.

Pierloot, R.A. & Thiel, J.H. (1986). *Psychoanalytische therapieën*. Deventer: Van Loghum Slaterus.

Pieters, G. (1998). Science wars. *TVPS*, 40, 65–67.

Pieters, G. (2000). Psychoanalyse en evidence based psychiatrie. *TVPA*, 6(3), 124–134.

Pine, F. (1990). *Drive, Ego, Object, and Self: a synthesis for clinical work*. New York: Basic Books.

Pine, F. (1998). *Diversity and direction in psychoanalytic technique.* New Haven CT: Yale UP.

Pines, M. (1984). Reflections on mirroring. *International Review of Psychoanalysis,* 11, 27–37.

Popper, K.R. (1963). *Conjectures and refutations.* London: Routledge.

Porge, E. (1989). *Se compter trois: le temps logique de Lacan.* Paris: Erès.

Postel, J. (1981). *Genèse de la psychiatrie.* Paris: Sycamore.

Proust, M. (1920–1921). *De kant van Guermantes.* Amsterdam: Bezige Bij, 1981.

Quinodoz, D. (2003). Words that touch. *IJPA,* 84, 1469–1485.

Quinodoz, J.M. (2013). *Reading Freud: a chronological exploration of Freud's writings.* London/New York: Routledge.

Racker, H. (1957). The meaning and uses of countertransference. *PQ,* 26, 303–357.

Rangell, L. (2006). An analysis of the course of psychoanalysis: The case for a unitary theory. *Psychoanalytic Psychology,* 23(2), 217.

Rimbaud, A. (1871). Lettre à Georges Izambard 13/05/1871. In *Œuvres* (pp. 305–306). Paris: Mercure, 1958.

Roazen, P. (1971). *Freud and his followers.* Middlesex: Penguin, 1979.

Robinson, G.E. (2004). Genome mix: beyond nature and nurture. *Science,* 304, 397–399.

Rockland, L.H. (1989). *Supportive therapy: a psychodynamic approach.* New York: Basic Books.

Rodman, F.R. (Ed.) (1987). *The spontaneous gesture: Selected letters of D.W. Winnicott.* Cambridge MA: Harvard UP.

Romains, J. (1924). *Le docteur Knock ou le triomphe de la médecine.* Paris: Gallimard.

Rorty, R. (1967). *The linguistic turn.* Chicago: Chicago UP, 1989.

Rose, H., & Rose, S. (Eds.) (2000). *Alas, poor Darwin: arguments against evolutionary psychology.* New York: Vintage.

Rosolato, G. (1999). *Les cinq axes de la psychanalyse.* Paris: PUF.

Roth, A. & Fonagy, P. (2004). *What works for whom? A critical review of psychotherapy research* (2nd ed.). New York: Guilford.

Roudinesco, E. (1993). *Jacques Lacan. Esquisse d'une vie, histoire d'un système de pensée.* Paris: Fayard.

Rousseau, J.J. (1754). *Vertoog over de ongelijkheid.* Amsterdam: Boom klassiek, 2003.

Rude, S.S. & Burnham, B.L. (1995). Connectedness and neediness: factors of the DEQ and SAS dependency scales. *Cognitive Therapy and Research,* 19, 323–340.

Rustin, M. & Rustin, M. (2016). *Reading Klein.* London/New York: Routledge.

Rylant, R.F.A. (1992). Klinische psychotherapie: de stand van zaken in de jaren negentig. *TVP,* 18(4), 202–206.

Sacks, O. (1984). *A leg to stand on.* London: Duckworth.

Safouan, M. (2005). *Lacaniana: les séminaires de Jacques Lacan. 1964–1979.* Paris: Fayard.

Sandell, R., Blomber, J., Lazar, A., Carlsson, J., Broberg, J. & Schubert, J. (2000). Varieties of long-term outcome among patients in psychoanalysis and long-term psychotherapy. *IJPA,* 81(5), 921–942.

Sandler, J. (1987). The concept of projective identification. *Bulletin of the Anna Freud Centre,* 10, 33–49.

Sandler, J., Holder, A., Dare, C. & Dreher, U. (1998). *Freud's models of the mind: an introduction.* Madison: International UP.

Sartre, J.P. (1943). *L'être et le néant: essai d'ontologie phénoménologique.* Paris: Gallimard, 1976.

Sartre, J.P. (1970). *L'existentialisme est un humanisme.* Paris: Gallimard Folio, 1996.

Say, J. (2011). Projective identification simplified: recruiting your shadow. *International Journal of Group Psychotherapy*, 61(2), 239–261.

Schaeffer, J. (1989). Les cartes et le territoire. *Revue Française de Psychanalyse*, LIII, 781–794.

Schiller, F. (1796). *Brieven over de esthetische opvoeding van de mens.* Amsterdam: Octavo, 2009.

Schokker, J. & Schokker, T. (2000). *Extimiteit: Jacques Lacans terugkeer naar Freud.* Amsterdam: Boom.

Schönau, W. (2002). De moeder-taal van de poëzie. In H. Hillenaar & K. Nuyten (Eds.), *Psychoanalyse en poëzie* (pp. 17–44). Amsterdam: Dutch UP.

Schopenhauer, A. (1818). *De wereld als wil en voorstelling.* Amsterdam: Wereldbibliotheek, 2012.

Schore, A. (1994). *Affect regulation and the origin of the self: the neurobiology of emotional development.* Hove: Laurence Erlbaum.

Schotte, J. (1990). *Szondi avec Freud: sur la voie d'une psychiatrie pulsionnelle.* Brussels: De Boeck.

Schotte, J. (1994). Sporen: voor een anthropopsychiatrie. In A. Nijs (Ed.), *De mens... in samenspraak, in tegenspraak...* (pp. 14–48). Leuven: Peeters.

Scott, A. (1996). *Real events revisited: fantasy, memory and psychoanalysis.* London: Virago.

Segal, H. (1957). Notes on symbol formation. In *The work of Hanna Segal: a Kleinian approach to clinical practice* (Chapter 4). New York: Jason Aronson, 1981.

Segal, H. (1964). *Introduction to the work of Melanie Klein.* London: Karnac, 1988.

Segal, H. (1979). *Melanie Klein.* New York: Viking.

Shahar, G. (2010). Poetics, pragmatics, schematics and the psychoanalysis-research dialogue. *Psychoanalytic Psychotherapy*, 24, 315–328.

Shapiro, T & Emde, R.N. (Ed.). (1995). *Research in psychoanalysis: process, development, outcome.* Madison CT: International UP.

Shedler, J. & Westen, D. (2007). Refining personality disorder diagnoses: integrating science and practice. *AJP*, 161, 1–16.

Shea, M.T., McDevitt-Murphy, M., Ready, D.J. & Schnurr, P.P. (2009). Group Therapy. In E.B. Foa, T.M. Keane, M.J. Friedman & J.A. Cohen (Eds.), *Effective treatments for PTSD: practice guidelines from the International Society for Traumatic Stress Studies* (2nd ed., pp. 306–326). New York: Guilford Press.

Sifneos, P.E. (1979). *Short-term dynamic psychotherapy: evaluation and technique.* New York: Plenum.

Sigrell, B. (1992). The long-term effects of group psychotherapy: a thirteen-year follow-up study. *Group Analysis*, 25, 333–352.

Skodol, A.E. (2012). Personality disorders in DSM-5. *Annual Review of Clinical Psychology*, 8, 317–344.

Smet, J., Van Bouwel, L. & Vandenborre, R. (2003). *Spreken en gesproken worden: psychoanalyse en psychose.* AAG.

Sokal, A. & Bricmont, J. (1997). *Impostures intellectuelles.* Paris: Odile Jacob.

Soler, C. (1987). *Quelle place pour l'analyste? Actes de l'ECF*, Vol XIII.

Soler, C. (2019). *Lacan: the unconscious reinvented.* London/New York: Routledge.

Solms, M. (2018a). The scientific standing of psychoanalysis. *BJP International*, 15, 5–8.

Solms M. (2018b). The neurobiological underpinnings of psychoanalytic theory and therapy. *Frontiers in Behavioral Neuroscience*, 12, 1–12.

Solms, M. (2021a). Revision of drive theory. *JAPA*, 69(6), 1033–1091.

Solms, M. (2021b). A revision of Freud's theory of the biological origin of the Oedipus complex. *PQ*, 90(4), 555–581.

Spiegel, D. (1991) Dissociation and trauma. In A. Tasman & S.M. Goldfinger (Eds.), *American Psychiatric Press Review of Psychiatry* (pp. 261–275). Washington: American Psychiatric Press.

Spinoza, B. (1979). *Ethica*. Tr. N. Van Suchtelen. Amsterdam: Wereldbibliotheek.

Spitz, R.A. (1945). Hospitalism: an inquiry into the genesis of psychiatric conditions in early childhood. *PSC*, 1, 53–74.

Spitz, R.A. (1946). Anaclitic depression: an inquiry into the genesis of psychiatric conditions in early childhood, II. *PSC*, 2, 313–342.

Spitz, R.A. (1965). *The first year of life: a psychoanalytic study of normal and deviant development of object relations*. New York: International UP.

Steinem, G. (2019). *The truth will set you free but first it will piss you off*. London: Murdoch.

Stern, D. N. (1985), *The interpersonal world of the infant*. New York: Basic Books.

Stern, D.N. (1995). *The motherhood constellation*. New York: Basic Books.

Stern, D.N. (2004). *The present moment in psychotherapy and everyday life*. New York: Norton.

Stern, D.N.*et al.* (1998). Non-interpretative mechanisms in psychoanalytic therapy: the something more than interpretation. *IJPA*, 79, 903–921.

Stolorow, R.D., Brandchaft, B. & Atwood, G.E. (1987). *Psychoanalytic treatment: an intersubjective approach*. Hillsdale NJ: Analytic Press.

Stone, M.H. (1990). *The fate of borderline patients: successful outcome and psychiatric practice*. New York: Guilford.

Stroeken, H. (1987). *En analyse avec Freud*. Paris: Payot.

Sulloway, F.J. (1979). *Freud, biologist of the mind: beyond the psychoanalytic legend*. New York: Basic Books.

Symington, N. (1986). *The analytic experience*. London: Free Association Books.

Symington, N. (2004). *The blind man sees: Freud's awakening and other essays*. London: Karnac.

Target, M. (2005). Psychoanalyse, (re-) constructie, mentalisatie. In: M. Kinet & R. Vermote (Eds.), *Mentalisatie* (pp. 35–54). AAG.

Target, M. (2007). Is our sexuality our own? A developmental model of sexuality based on early affect mirroring. *British Journal of Psychotherapy*, 23, 530.

Tessier, H. (2014). The sexual unconscious and sexuality in psychoanalysis: Laplanche's theory of generalized seduction, *PQ*, 83(1), 169–183.

Thase, M.E. & Jindal, R.D. (2004). Combining psychotherapy and psychopharmacology for treatment of mental disorders. In M. Lambert, A.E. Bergin & S.L. Garfield, *Handbook of psychotherapy and behavior change* (pp. 743–766). New York: Wiley.

Thys, M. (1998). Tussen psychose en mystiek: Bion en de filosofie. In J. Dehing (Ed.), *Een bundel intense duisternis* (pp. 85–100). Leuven/Apeldoorn: Garant.

Thys, M. (2006). Beter worden van waarheid. *TVPA*, 2, 136–142.

Thys, M. (2009). The group-as-a-hole: siblingoverdracht en fantasieën over de groep. In M. Kinet (Ed.), *De groep in psychoanalyse* (pp. 149–164). AAG.

Thys, M. (2015). Projectieve identificatie tussen doodsdrift en intersubjectiviteit. *TVPA*, 2, 82–96.

Thys, M. & Vermote, R. (Eds.) (1995). *Trauma en taboe*. Leuven/Apeldoorn: Garant.

Thys, M. & Kinet, M. (Eds.) (2002). *Liefdesverklaringen: over perversie, liefde en passie*. Leuven/Leusden: Acco.

Tomkins, S.S. & Demos, E.V. (1995). *Exploring affect: selected writings of Silvan S. Tomkins*. Cambridge: Cambridge UP.

Toulmin, S. (2001). *Terug naar de rede*. Kampen/Kapellen: Agora/Pelckmans.

Trevarthen, C. (Ed.) (1990). *Brain circuits and functions of the mind*. Cambridge: Cambridge University Press.

Tronick, E.Z. (1998). Implicit relational knowing: its role in development and psychoanalytic treatment. *Infant Mental Health Journal: Official Publication of The World Association for Infant Mental Health*, 19(3), 282–289.

Tucker, L.*et al.* (1987). Long-term hospital treatment of borderline patients: a descriptive outcome study. *AJP*, 144, 1443–1448.

Tulving, E. (1972). Episodic and semantic memory. In E. Tulving & W. Donaldson (Eds.), *Organization of memory* (pp. 381–403). New York: Academic Press.

Tuymans, L. (1996). *Luc Tuymans*. London: Phaidon.

Tzara, T. (1924). *Sept manifestes Dada: lampisteries*. Paris: Fayard, 1978.

Ubbels, J. (2000). Psychiatrie en psychoanalyse in beweging: relevante kwesties. *TVPA*, 3, 13–145.

Vaillant, G.E. (1992). *Ego mechanisms of defense: a guide for clinicans and researchers*. Arlington: American Psychiatric Publishing.

Van Belzen, J.A. (1988). *Fenomenologie en psychiatrie: essays van H.C. Rümke*. Kampen: Kok Agora.

Van Bouwel, L. (1998). De oneindigheid van het heelal: Bion en de psychose. In J. Dehing Ed.), *Een bundel intense duisternis* (pp. 27–51). Leuven/Apeldoorn: Garant.

Van Coillie, F. (2000). Psychoanalyse en psychiatrie: interview met professor Jacques Schotte. *TVPA*, 4, 214–231.

Van Coillie, F. (2004). *De ongenode gast: zes psychoanalytische essays over het verlangen en de dood*. Amsterdam: Boom.

Van den Berg, J.H. (1960). *Metabletica of de leer der veranderingen*. Nijkerk: Callenbach.

Van den Hoofdakker, R.H. (1976). *Een pil voor Doornroosje*. Amsterdam: Van Gennep.

Van der Horst, F.C.P. & Van der Veer, R. (2008). Loneliness in infancy: Harry Harlow, John Bowlby and issues of separation. *Integrative Psychological and Behavioral Science*, 42(4), 325–335.

Van der Kolk, B.A. (2005). Developmental trauma disorder. *Psychiatric Annals*, 35, 401–408.

Vandenberg, P. (2006). *L'important, c'est le kamikaze. Œuvre 2000–2006*. Ghent: On-Line.

Vandenberghe, J. (2007). De psychiater: clinicus en manager? Het spanningsveld tussen klinisch denken en management denken. *TVPS*, 10, 689–691.

Van Haute, P. (1990). *Het imaginaire en het symbolische in het werk van Jacques Lacan*. Leuven: Peeters.

Van Haute, P. (2000). *Tegen de aanpassing*. Nijmegen: SUN.

Van Haute, P. (2005). Lacan leest Klein: over symbolisatie en de ontwikkeling van het Ik. In M. Kinet & R. Vermote (Eds.), *Mentalisatie* (pp. 55–67). AAG.

Van Haute, P. & Geyskens, T. (2002). *Spraakverwarring: het primaat van de seksualiteit bij Freud, Ferenczi en Laplanche.* Nijmegen: SUN.

Vanheule, S. (2015). *Psychodiagnostiek anders bekeken: kritieken op de DSM. Een pleidooi voor functiegerichte diagnostiek.* Leuven: LannooCampus.

Van Hoorde, H. (1992). *Psychiatrie en psychoanalyse: scheiding van tafel en bank?* Gent: Idesça.

Van Hoorde H. (2000). Psychiatrie en psychoanalyse: toetsing van een egelstelling. *TVPA*, 3, 168–177.

Van Os, J., Guloksuz, S., Vijn, T.W., Hafkenscheid, A. and Delespaul, P. (2019). The evidence-based group-level symptom-reduction model as the organizing principle for mental health care: time for change? *World Psychiatry*, 18, 88–96.

Van Rosmalen, L., van der Horst, F.C.P. & van der Veer, R. (2012). Of monkeys and men: Spitz and Harlow on the consequences of maternal deprivation. *Attachment & Human Development*, 14(4), 425–437.

Van Tilburg, W. (2000). Psychoanalyse en psychiatrie. *TVPA*, 3, 113–123.

Verbruggen, G. (1999). Van doodsdrift naar violence fondamentale. *TVPA*, 2, 89–101.

Vergote, A. (1978). *Bekentenis en begeerte in religie: psychoanalytische verkenning.* Amsterdam: DNB/Pelckmans.

Verhaeghe, P. (1989). Spreken en de waarheid. *Cahier*, 3.

Verhaeghe, P. (1994a). *Klinische psychodiagnostiek vanuit Lacans discourstheorie.* Gent: Idesça.

Verhaeghe, P. (1994b). Psychotherapy, Psychoanalysis and Hysteria. *The Letter*, Autumn, 47–68.

Verhaeghe, P. (1995). Neurosis and perversion: il n'y a pas de rapport sexuel. *Journal of the Centre for Freudian Analysis and Research*, 6, 39–63.

Verhaeghe, P. (1996). *Tussen vrouw en hysterie.* Leuven/Amersfoort: Acco.

Verhaeghe, P. (1997). Trauma en hysterie bij Freud en Lacan. *TVPA*, 3, 86–99.

Verhaeghe, P. (1998). *Liefde in tijden van eenzaamheid.* Leuven: Acco.

Verhaeghe, P. (2002a). *Over normaliteit en andere afwijkingen.* Leuven: Acco.

Verhaeghe, P. (2002b). Causality in science and psychoanalysis. In J. Glynos & Y. Stavrakakis (Eds.), *Lacan & Science* (pp. 119–145). London/New York: Karnac.

Verhaeghe, P. (2003). *Beyond gender: from subject to drive.* New York: Other Press.

Verhaeghe, P. (2005a). Pleidooi tegen gelijkheid. *Tijdschrift Cliëntgerichte Psychotherapie* 43(2), 101–110.

Verhaeghe, P. (2005b). De essentie van de psychotherapie vanuit een psychoanalytisch perspectief. *Tijdschrift Klinische Psychologie*, 35(2), 109–118.

Verhaeghe, P. (2007). Aktuaalpathologie: hoe luisteren als het spreken niet dragend is. In M. Kinet & W. Vanmechelen (Eds.), *Tussen ruis en storingen: de golflengte vinden in psychoanalytische therapie.* AAG.

Verhaeghe, P. (2011). *Identiteit.* Amsterdam: Bezige Bij.

Verhaeghe, P. (2013). Psychoanalytische opleiding-een contradictio in terminis. Welke kennis voor wie? In M. Hebbrecht & N. Vliegen (Eds.), *Supervisie in psychoanalyse en psychoanalytische therapie* (pp. 87–106). AAG.

Verhaeghe, P. (2015). *Autoriteit.* Antwerpen/Amsterdam: Bezige Bij.

Verhaeghe, P. (2022). *Intieme vreemden.* Rotterdam: MVDF.

Verhaest, S. (1986). Psychoanalytische groepstherapie. In R.A. Pierloot & J.H. Thiel (Eds.), *Psychoanalytische therapieën* (pp. 135–157). Deventer: Van Loghum Slaterus.

Verheugt-Pleiter, A & Deben-Mager, M. (2005). Transference Focused Psychotherapy en Mentalization Based Treatment: broer en zus? *TVPA*, 3, 169–183.

Verheul R., Brink, W. van den. (1999). Persoonlijkheidsstoornissen. In A. de Jong, W. van den Brink, J. Orme & D. Wiersma (Eds.), *Handboek psychiatrische epidemiologie*. Amsterdam: Boom.

Vermote, R. (1994). Le mythe d'Oedipe à la lumière du Sphinx. *Revue Belge de Psychanalyse*, 24, 29–42.

Vermote, R. (1997). Psychose en lijden. In M. De Hert*et al.* (Eds.), *Zin in waanzin*. Berchem: EPO.

Vermote, R. (1998a). De grid en de caesura in het werk van Bion. In J. Dehing (Ed.) *Een bundel intense duisternis*. Leuven/Apeldoorn: Garant.

Vermote, R. (1998b). A psychoanalytic hospital unit for people with severe personality disorders. In J. Pestalozzi, S. Frisch, R.D. Hinshelwood*et al.* (Eds.), *Psychoanalytic psychotherapy in institutional settings* (pp. 75–93). London: Karnac.

Vermote, R. (2000). Psychoanalytische en psychiatrische diagnostiek bij persoonlijkheidsstoornissen. *TVPS*, 9, 7–674.

Vermote, R. (2005a). Mentaliseren en psychopathologie. In M. Kinet & R. Vermote (Eds.), *Mentalisatie* (pp. 69–89). AAG.

Vermote, R. (2005b). *Touching inner change. Psychoanalytically informed Hospitalization based treatment of personality disorders. A process-outcome study*. Doctoraal proefschrift ter behaling van doctoraat in de psychologische wetenschappen KUL 27.06.05.

Vermote, R. (2011). Seksualiteit. In J. Dirkx, M. Hebbrecht, A.W.M. Mooij, R. Vermote (Eds.), *Handboek psychodynamiek* (pp. 65–72). Utrecht: Tijdstroom.

Vermote, R. (2018). *Reading Bion*. London/New York: Routledge.

Vermote, R., Goldberg, A. & Rousillon, R. (2003). Two sessions with Catherine: the analyst at work. *IJPA*, 84, 1415–1429.

Verschaffel, B. (1989). *De glans der dingen*. Mechelen: Vlees en Beton.

Vestdijk, S. (1960). *De glanzende Kiemcel*. Amsterdam: Nijgh & Van Ditmar.

Vliegen, N. (2003). Psychotherapie: erkennen en ver-drijven? *Tijdschrift voor Klinische Psychologie*, 33(2), 86–90.

Vliegen, N. & Meurs, P. (1998). *Het voorjaarsontwaken: de adolescentie in psychodynamische theorie en therapie*. Leuven/Apeldoorn: Garant.

Vliegen, N. & Cluckers, G. (2001a). Babyobservatie en therapeutisch proces. In N. Vliegen & C. Leroy (Eds.), *Het Moederland? De vroegste relatie tussen moeder en kind in de psychoanalytische therapie* (pp. 21–43). Leuven: Acco.

Vliegen, N. & Leroy, C. (Eds.) (2001b). *Het Moederland? De vroegste relatie tussen moeder en kind in de psychoanalytische therapie*. Leuven: Acco.

Wallerstein, R. (1986). *Forty-two lives in treatment: a study of psychoanalysis and psychotherapy*. New York: Guilford.

Wallerstein, R.S. (1988a). One psychoanalysis or many? *IJPA*, 69, 5–22.

Wallerstein, R.S. (1988b). Psychoanalysis and psychotherapy: relative roles reconsidered. *Annual of Psychoanalysis*, 16, 129–151.

Wallerstein, R.S. (Ed.) (1992). *The common ground of psychoanalysis*. Northvale/London: Jason Aronson.

Wallerstein, R.S. (2002). The trajectory of psychoanalysis: a prognostication. *IJPA*, 83, 1247–1267.

Wampold, B.E. (2001). *The great psychotherapy debate: models, methods and findings*. Mahwah NJ: Erlbaum.

Wampold, B.E., Mondin, G.W., Moody, M.*et al.* (1997). A meta-analysis of outcome studies comparing bona fide psychotherapies: empirically 'all must have prizes'. *Psychological Bulletin*, Nov. 122, 203–215.

Wampold, B.E. & Imel, Z.E. (2015). *The great psychotherapy debate: the evidence for what makes psychotherapy work.* New York: Routledge.

Wasch, K. (1998). *Dylan Thomas.* Zeist: Indigo.

Watson, P. (2001). *Wrede schoonheid.* Utrecht: Spectrum/Manteau.

Westen, D. & Morrison, K. (2001). A multi-dimensional meta-analysis of treatments for depression, panic, and generalized anxiety disorder: an empirical examination of the status of empirically supported therapies. *Journal of Consulting and Clinical Psychology*, 69, 841–845.

Westen, D., Novotny, C.M. & Thompson-Brenner, H. (2004). The empirical status of empirically supported psychotherapies. Assumptions, findings and reporting in controlled clinical trials. *Psychological Bulletin*, 130, 631–663.

Whorf, B. (1940). *Language, thought and reality.* Cambridge: MIT Press.

Willi, J. (1983). *De partnerrelatie.* Rotterdam: Ad Donker.

Williams, G. (1997). *Internal landscapes and foreign bodies: eating disorders and other pathologies.* London/New York: Routledge.

Wilson, G (2018). *Het pornobrein.* Amsterdam: Boom.

Winner, J.-A & Ornstein, E. (1994). Relational themes in the inpatient community meeting. *International Journal of Group Psychotherapy*, 44, 313–332.

Winnicott, D.W. (1939). Aggression and its roots. In C. Winnicott*et al.* (Eds.), *Deprivation and delinquency.* London: Tavistock, 1984.

Winnicott, D.W. (1945). *Primitive emotional development.* In TPP.

Winnicott, D.W. (1950). Some thoughts on the meaning of the word 'democracy'. In C. Winnicott*et al.* (Eds.), *Home is where we start from.* London: Penguin, 1986.

Winnicott, D.W. (1951). *Transitional objects and transitional phenomena.* In TPP.

Winnicott, D.W. (1952). *Anxiety associated with insecurity.* In TPP.

Winnicott, D.W. (1954). *Metapsychological and clinical aspects of regression.* In TPP.

Winnicott, D.W. (1956). *Primary maternal preoccupation.* In TPP.

Winnicott, D.W. (1958). *The capacity to be alone.* In MPFE.

Winnicott, D.W. (1960). *Theory of the parent-infant relationship.* In MPFE.

Winnicott, D.W. (1962). *Ego integration in child development.* In TPP.

Winnicott, D.W. (1963a). *Communicating and not communicating leading to a study of certain opposites.* In MPFE.

Winnicott, D.W. (1963b). *The development of the capacity for concern.* In MPFE.

Winnicott, D.W. (1967). *The location of cultural experience.* In PR.

Winnicott, D.W. (1968a). *The use of an object and relating through identifications.* In PR.

Winnicott, D.W. (1968b). Communication between infant and mother, and mother and infant, compared and contrasted. In C. Winnicott*et al.* (Eds.), *Babies and their mothers.* London: Free Association Books, 1987.

Winnicott, D.W. (1969a). *Symposium on envy and jealousy.* In C. Winnicott*et al.* (Eds.), *Psycho-analytic explorations.* London: Karnac, 1989.

Winnicott, D.W. (1969b). *The mother-infant experience of mutuality.* In C. Winnicott*et al.* (Eds.), *Psycho-analytic explorations.* London: Karnac, 1989.

Winnicott, D.W. (1971a). *Creativity and its origins.* In PR.

Winnicott, D.W. (1971b). *Playing: a theoretical statement.* In PR.

Winnicott, D.W. (1986). *Holding and interpretation: fragment of an analysis*. London: Karnac, 1989.

Winnicott, D.W. (1987). *The spontaneous gesture: selected letters*. Cambridge MA: Harvard University Press.

Winnicott, D.W. (1988). *Human nature*. London/New York: Routledge, 2015.

Wolf, A. & Schwartz, E.K. (1962). *Psychoanalysis in groups*. New York: Grune & Stratton.

Wolf, A., Kutash, I. & Nattland, C. (1993). *The primacy of the individual in psychoanalysis in groups*. New York: Jason Aronson.

Yalom, I.O. (1970). *The theory and practice of group psychotherapy*. New York: Basic Books.

Yalom, I.O. (1980). *Existential psychotherapy*. New York: Basic Books.

Zanarini, M.C., Frankenbrug, F.R., Dubo, E.D.*et al.* (1998). Axis I comorbidity of borderline personality disorder. *AJP*, 155, 1733–1739.

Zegerius, L., Waldinger, M.D. (2000). De neurobiologische basis van de psychoanalyse. *TVPA*, 3, 156–167.

Zeuthen, K. & Gammelgaard, J. (2010). Infantile sexuality: the concept, its history and place in contemporary psychoanalysis, *The Scandinavian Psychoanalytic Review*, 33(1), 3–12.

Zimbardo, P. (2007). *The Lucifer effect: understanding how good people turn evil*. New York: Random.

Žižek, S. (1992). *Enjoy your symptom!* London/New York: Routledge.

Žižek, S. (1996). *Schuins beziend*. Amsterdam: Boom.

Žižek, S. (1997a). *Het subject en zijn onbehagen*. Amsterdam: Boom.

Žižek, S. (1997b). *The plague of fantasies*. London/New York: Verso.

Žižek, S. (2009a). *In defense of lost causes*. New York: Verso.

Žižek, S. (2009b). *The Parallax view*. Cambridge MA: MIT Press.

Žižek, S. (2014). *Event: philosophy in transit*. London: Penguin.

Žižek, S. (2019). *The sublime object of ideology*. New York: Verso.

Zupančič, A. (2017). *What is sex?* Cambridge MA: MIT Press.

Index

Page numbers in **bold** indicate Tables.